Radiographic Positioning and Related Anatomy

ISADORE MESCHAN, M.A., M.D.

Professor and Director of the Department of Radiology,
The Bowman Gray School of Medicine of Wake Forest University
Winston-Salem, North Carolina; Consultant in Radiology,
Department of Radiology, Walter Reed Army Hospital,
Washington, D.C.

with the assistance of

R.M.F. FARRER-MESCHAN, M.B., B.S. (Australia)**, M.D.**

Research Associate, Department of Radiology,
The Bowman Gray School of Medicine of Wake Forest University
Winston-Salem, North Carolina

W. B. SAUNDERS COMPANY
Philadelphia — London — Toronto

W. B. Saunders Company: West Washington Square
Philadelphia, Pa. 19105

12 Dyott Street
London, WC1A 1DB

833 Oxford Street
Toronto, Ontario M8Z 5T9, Canada

Radiographic Positioning and Related Anatomy   ISBN 0-7216-6275-7

Print No.:   9

TO
OUR PARENTS

PREFACE

The companion volume to this text—*An Atlas of Normal Radiographic Anatomy*—has furnished the basic material and approach for this book. Since the *Atlas* was published in its first edition in 1951, and thereafter, in its second edition in 1959, numerous requests have been received to present this material specifically as a practical manual of radiographic positioning and related anatomy, eliminating much of the text, which was oriented to the physician and medical student.

In the present volume, this objective has been followed, utilizing the basic format of the *Atlas* illustrations. For each position commonly used in our radiologic practice, we have presented the radiograph so obtained, and either an adjoining labeled radiograph, or its appropriately labeled line tracing.

No effort has been made to dilute the presentation with other facets of x-ray technology, such as the specific utilization of certain physical factors, the Bucky diaphragm, or types of cassettes or film. Frequently, comments relating to these matters are provided with the illustrations, but not in every instance.

It has been our desire that this book fill a need for a succinct, practical, well-illustrated text of radiographic positioning and the anatomy of the films so obtained — that it be a book not completely encyclopedic, as are some of the large, multivolume texts referred to in the bibliography, yet one that can be utilized widely for reference in daily activities of x-ray technicians and in their training. Also, the present text includes a number of positions and techniques omitted in the *Atlas*.

A chapter on special procedures has been included for introductory indoctrination of the student. From the technical standpoint, these procedures must be learned in the laboratory of experience; this section is designed to assist in this practical approach.

The publishers have collaborated to provide instructors with good teaching slides that duplicate the illustrations in the book. We have found this adjunct useful for demonstrations and lectures.

We are extremely grateful to those who have helped us in this endeavor:

Mrs. Edna Snow, our Executive Secretary, who has taken the brunt of the secretarial work involved.

Mrs. Rolene Ward, Chief Technician and Senior Instructor in the School of X-Ray Technology of the North Carolina Baptist Hospital, who has checked the position drawings for accuracy, and whose suggestions and encouragement have been very helpful.

Mrs. Polly Story, Assistant Chief Technician, who has provided us with the appropriate films needed for illustrative material.

Mr. George Lynch, Professor of Medical Illustration at the Bowman Gray School of Medicine, and Director of the Department of Audio-visual Aids, whose artwork has formed the basis of this text.

Mrs. Erika Love, Head Librarian of the Bowman Gray School of Medicine, who has checked all references in the bibliography for accuracy.

Our Publishers, without whose constant help and encouragement this text would not have been written.

ISADORE MESCHAN, M.D.

RACHEL FARRER MESCHAN, M.D.

CONTENTS

Chapter 1 — The Production of X-rays, Principles of Radiography and Radiation Protection

GENERAL PRINCIPLES

X-rays are produced when fast-moving electrons with sufficient energy strike a target. Most of the electron energy is converted to heat, but a very minute amount — less than 1 per cent — is converted to x-ray.

The device which produces the fast-moving electrons is the x-ray tube (Fig. 1-1). The electrons are produced when a filament within the tube is heated. A large electrical force drives these electrons onto a target or focal spot. Upon impact with this focal spot, the electrons give rise to a stream of x-rays which are emitted over a 180-degree hemispherical angle surrounding the focal spot.

A lead-shielded window, along with a lead tube casing, is provided as part of the housing of the x-ray tube, so that only a small fraction of these x-rays pass through the portal of the tube.

The intricate details of the tube and the circuitry responsible for producing the electrons are outside the scope of this text. For a more comprehensive review of this subject the student is referred to the bibliography for other text material.

There are two properties of x-rays which become particularly useful in diagnostic radiology. These are the fluorescent and photosensitization effects of x-rays.

The radiographer, however, must also be familiar with other fundamental properties of x-rays, particularly from the standpoint of radiation protection. When x-rays strike matter, particles are ionized, and this ionization produces various phenomena in biological material. In practically all instances this is a destructive effect, at least to some degree. Some reparative processes do occur, but in any case the utilization of x-rays must be carried forward extremely judiciously and with every care taken to ensure protection. These protective measures are briefly summarized on page 20.

NECESSARY ACCESSORIES FOR RECORDING THE X-RAY IMAGE

Introduction

The radiographer must first familiarize himself with the operation of the x-ray machine. Once having mastered the technique for production of x-rays, and the importance of radiation protection, the student must next familiarize himself with those accessories which make radiography possible: the x-ray film; the x-ray cassette with the enclosed intensifying screen (Fig. 1-2); the x-ray film that does not require an intensifying screen and conventional cassette, but is contained within a plastic or cardboard film holder; the stationary and moving grids, such as the Potter-Bucky diaphragm (Fig. 1-3); various cones, apertures and adjustable diaphragms for delimiting the x-ray beam to the body part in question (Fig. 1-4); and such additional accessories as equipment for body-section radiography (Fig. 1-5), stereoradiography (Fig. 1-6) and x-ray ky-

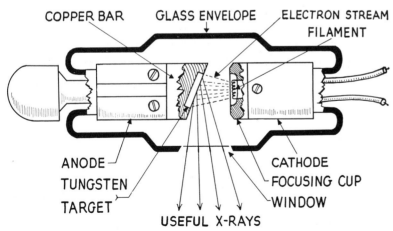

COPPER BAR   GLASS ENVELOPE   ELECTRON STREAM
FILAMENT

ANODE
TUNGSTEN
TARGET

USEFUL X-RAYS

CATHODE
FOCUSING CUP
WINDOW

FIGURE 1-1.   Diagram of standard stationary anode x-ray tube.

mography (Fig. 1-7), and the various contrast media which must be employed in the several examinations.

The fluoroscopic screen (Fig. 1-8, A, B, C) also is frequently employed by the radiologist. This, in essence, is a specially constructed intensifying screen that converts most of the x-rays to visible light rather than to ultraviolet light, as does the radiographic screen. It offers the immediate advantage of visualization of an x-ray image, but this image is not nearly so clearly delineated as is the photographic image on the x-ray film. The screen is ordinarily covered with lead glass so that the penetrating x-rays that are not absorbed by the intensifying screen are in turn absorbed by the lead and do not strike the observer (Fig. 1-8C).

The fluoroscope contains a shutter mechanism to delimit the x-ray beam and adequate filtration for protection—usually 2 to 4 mm. of aluminum added to the inherent filtration of the x-ray tube—and very often is equipped to take spot-film radiographs instantaneously during the fluoroscopic procedure. Thus, the fluoroscope permits the physician to position the patient accurately prior to obtaining the radiograph so that he may obtain the x-ray depiction instantaneously after viewing a particular anatomic part.

In recent years "image amplifiers" have been used in conjunction with radiography and fluoroscopy. These are complex systems employing either mirrors or electronic amplification or a combination of both (Figs. 1-9 and 1-10). Such amplification has the decided advantages of both greater accuracy and less x-ray exposure for patient and physician alike. The amplified image may be photographed by an appropriate camera, or it may be televised so that the physician or even large groups may view the image simultaneously. Movie cameras have also been employed in conjunction with this device to obtain "cine radiographs." In general, a detailed discussion of these many accessories is outside the scope of this text, since we shall be concentrating primarily on x-ray positioning and the related anatomy.

The miniature (indirect) radiograph or "photoroentgenogram" has been used for many years (Fig. 1-11). Fundamentally, this is a photograph of the fluoroscopic image. It may be an intensified image obtained with variously designed image intensifiers (Fig. 1-9) or mirror and lens systems. This technique is becoming more frequently employed in making "spot films"—especially when image amplifiers are used in fluoroscopy.

The Radiographic Cassette (Figure 1-2)

The x-ray cassette is a permanent lightproof container for two intensifying screens which permits the easy introduction of the x-ray film between them. A diagrammatic section of the x-ray cassette is illustrated in Figure 1-2. A layer of felt is usually interposed between the outer screen and the cassette back.

Cardboard Film Holder

This is a lightproof cardboard or plastic holder into which the film can be placed. Ordinarily the back cardboard, which is away from the x-ray tube, contains lead foil to absorb the x-rays which penetrate the upper cardboard and film to prevent the scattering effect from the table top. Adequately light-protected and individually wrapped nonscreen films are also available commercially (with or without the lead backing). Their use avoids the necessity for darkroom loading and prevents confusion from storage of both nonscreen and screen films in the darkroom.

Ordinarily, the x-ray image is not produced nearly as efficiently with this method of radiography as it is with intensifying screens. There is, however, no loss of detail from fluorescent diffusion of light and, in the thinner parts of the body, it is advantageous. Also, when it is necessary to look for extremely minute foreign bodies, as in the case of the eye, this method offers greater accuracy, since no artifacts are interposed between the film and the intensifying screen.

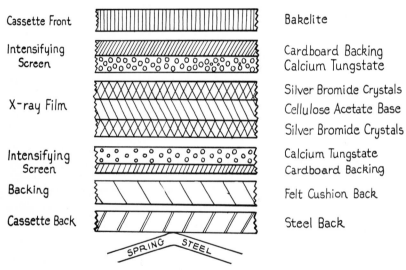

Cassette Front	Bakelite
Intensifying Screen	Cardboard Backing Calcium Tungstate
X-ray Film	Silver Bromide Crystals Cellulose Acetate Base Silver Bromide Crystals
Intensifying Screen	Calcium Tungstate Cardboard Backing
Backing	Felt Cushion Back
Cassette Back	Steel Back

SPRING STEEL

FIGURE 1-2A. Diagrammatic cross section of the x-ray cassette.

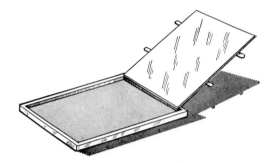

1. AVOID INJURY OR DROPPING.
2. AVOID CHEMICAL CONTACT WITH SCREENS.
3. HANDLE ON DRY BENCH.
4. AVOID STORAGE OF ITEMS ABOVE LOADING BENCH.
5. DO NOT LEAVE CASSETTE OPEN.
6. INSPECT FREQUENTLY TO DETECT WEARING OF FELT OR BENDING OF HINGES.
7. TEST SCREEN FILM CONTACT WITH FLAT WIRE MESH.

FIGURE 1-2B. The cassette and its care.

Stationary and Moving Grids *(Figure 1-3)*

When an x-ray beam strikes any matter, some of the x-rays are absorbed, some are deflected and partially absorbed, and others pass directly through. There is a considerable percentage of x-rays scattered in all directions by the atoms of the target struck. This is known as "secondary radiation," and although the wave lengths of such radiation are longer than that of the primary beam, nevertheless, they are photographically effective and overcast the x-ray image with a consequent loss of image detail. It is desirable in radiography to reduce the secondary radiation to a minimum.

The grid, a device for eliminating much of the scattered radiation, is composed of a series of very thin strips of lead held in position by intervening strips of wood, Bakelite or plastic. It is interposed between the part to be radiographed and the film. The lead strips are placed so that the plane of each is parallel to the ray projections from the x-ray focal spot. Thus, a special grid must be employed for each major change in grid-to-tube target distance; this is called the "grid radius." The wood-filled slots between the lead strips are usually about 6 to 32 times as deep as they are wide; this ratio of the height to the width of the wood slot is the "grid ratio." The strips of lead have the function of absorbing the scattered rays as they come from the body part before they can strike the beam, so that the image is formed by the primary parallel radiation that has penetrated the body part. The greater the grid ratio, the more efficient is the grid in absorbing scattered radiation—but the greater is the amount of radiation necessary to obtain a given suitable exposure.

If the grid is stationary, the lead lines are reproduced on the radiograph and are objectionable unless the lead strips are extremely fine; but if the grid is placed in motion by a spring or motor device while the exposure is being made, the grid lines are not seen and the efficiency of the grid is improved. This moving grid is called the "Potter-Bucky diaphragm." In the Camp grid cassette, a stationary grid of special design has been incorporated into the cover

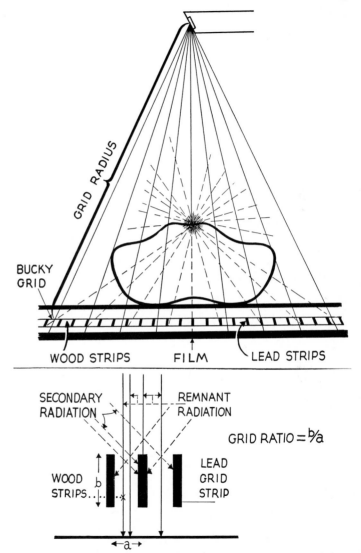

FIGURE 1-3. Diagram of a Potter-Bucky diaphragm and how it is used.

of the cassette. Although such cassettes are expensive, they delimit scattered radiation very efficiently, and the grid lines are visible only on closest inspection. Great care must be exercised in the handling of these wafer-thin grids, since the slightest bending of the grid will distort the relationship of the lead strips to the primary beam and diminish the efficiency of the grid.

It is also important to recognize that a focused grid has a "tube side" and a "film side." These must not be reversed or a virtually blank radiograph will result. If the lead strips are all perpendicular to the grid surface (an unfocused grid) either side may be used as the tube side, but a sufficient target-to-grid distance (usually in excess of 40 inches) must be employed.

A focused grid must be carefully centered with respect to the x-ray tube. Otherwise more radiation will be absorbed on one side of the grid than on the other, and an uneven radiograph will result.

The grid method of eliminating the major portion of secondary radiation requires considerably more exposure; therefore, intensifying screens are usually employed along with the grid. These devices increase the distance of the part to be radiographed from the film and thereby increase the distortion of the image unless a long tube target-to-skin distance is employed with a small focal spot.

Cones and Aperture Diaphragms (Figure 1-4)

Cones and aperture diaphragms are applied to the tube window to delimit the x-ray beam and thus reduce the secondary radiation. There are various designs of these coning devices, but it is generally desirable to choose the cone best suited to the anatomical part and to the size of the film being exposed. Adjustable cones are also available for this purpose. In these devices a reflected visible light source contained within it will give the radiographer the cone's exact field of visualization. Cones have the additional advantage of reducing the stray radiation toward the operator, and thus they furnish a very important protective mechanism as well.

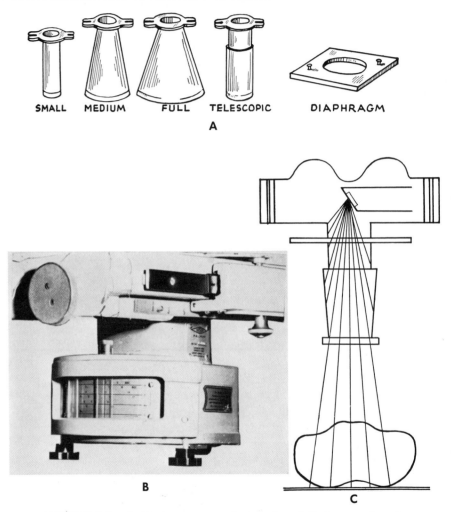

FIGURE 1-4. A, Various accessories used to delimit secondary irradiation. **B,** An adjustable cone for various field sizes with a light localizer and centering device. **C,** Diagram illustrating effect of cone in delimiting scattered radiation.

SPECIAL TYPES OF X-RAY IMAGES

Body-Section Radiography *(Figure 1-5)*

The body-section radiograph is known by various names, depending on slightly different operating principles (i.e., laminograph, stratograph, tomograph). The main factor in each of these is the rotation of the x-ray tube and the x-ray film about a fixed axis or center of rotation, so that all images are blurred except that at the chosen axis or center. By this means a certain section of the body is brought into clear focus while other interfering parts are diffused and a clear image at the chosen level is obtained. This is a useful adjunct, particularly in the visualization of certain partially concealed structures such as those within the skull, the lung, the brain, the larynx or the nasopharynx.

Stereoscopic Radiography *(Figure 1-6)*

A single radiographic image is a two-dimensional representation and does not possess perspective. To some extent our mind's eye can be trained to overcome this deficiency when we project our knowledge of gross anatomy into the x-ray image and visualize the structure in three dimensions. This projection process is not a true visualization in space, but is most helpful in roentgenographic interpretation. To obtain radiographs that can give a true stereoscopic effect, two slightly different views are obtained—first as though one eye were looking at the part, and then as though the other eye were seeing it. This is done by making two radiographs from two separate tube positions, the amount of tube shift being in a definite ratio to the normal interpupillary distance. These two radiographs are then placed in a stereoscope or viewed with special prismatic lenses so that each eye will see the separate image. The brain fuses the two images into one in which the various parts stand out in striking relief in their true perspective and correct spatial relationship.

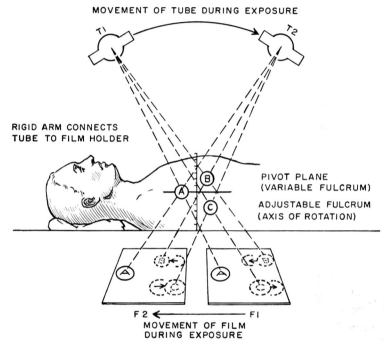

FIGURE 1-5. The principles of body-section radiography. The image of an object, such as *A,* located on the pivot plane remains in focus during movement of tube and film. An object above the pivot plane, *B,* or below, *C,* blurs due to its realignment between tube and film as they move during exposure.

Contrast Media

The differential radiopacity and radiolucency of many of the organs of the body are very similar, and it would be difficult to diagnose many structural aberrations and abnormalities, were it not possible to introduce substances within these organs to afford contrast. It is desirable that the substance so introduced should be physiologically inert or harmless. The many substances that have been devised for this purpose fall into two main categories: those that are radiopaque, and those that are radiolucent. The commonly used radiopaque compounds are as follows.

Barium sulfate is particularly useful in studies of the gastrointestinal tract. It is inert and is not absorbed, nor does it alter the normal physiologic function of the gastrointestinal tract. At times it is used in colloidal suspension to obtain a particular type of coating of the gastrointestinal tract more effective for demonstration of small filling defects.

Gallbladder contrast agents such as Telepaque, Priodax, Teridax or Monophen may be given orally, or Cholografin (Biligrafin) intravenously, to visualize the biliary ducts and gallbladder.

Organic iodides are *selectively concentrated by the normal kidney*. There are many of these water-soluble compounds available but the most frequently used in this country at the present writing are Hypaque (sodium diatrizoate), Renografin (meglumine diatrizoate), and for cardiac visualization iothalamate compounds. Hypaque or Renografin in low concentration may also be used for visualization of hepatic and biliary radicals by T-tube or operative cholangiography.

Iodized oils such as Pantopaque or Dionosil (oily). Pantopaque is used for myelography in the spinal column and Dionosil for bronchography for visualization of the bronchial tree.

Other absorbable organic iodides such as Skiodan Acacia and Salpix are used in hysterosalpingography.

The common radiolucent substances used are mostly gases: air, oxygen, nitrogen, helium and carbon dioxide. These are most commonly employed for visualization of the brain (pneumoenceph-

(Text continues on page 12.)

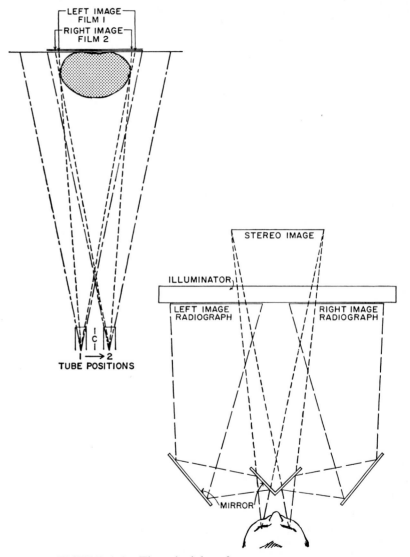

FIGURE 1-6. The principles of roentgen stereoscopy.

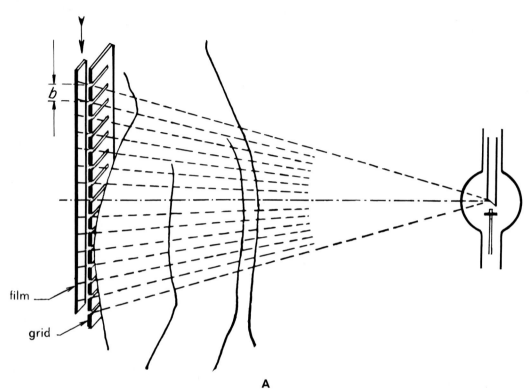

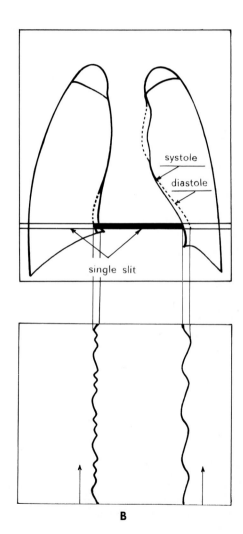

A

FIGURE 1-7A. Diagram of parallel-slit kymograph. The slit-bearing grid is placed between the patient and the film. Either the grid or the film can be moved downwards; in the first case a *plane* kymogram is obtained; in the second a *linear* kymogram. The distance traveled by the grid or film is the same as that between one slit and the next (*b,* slit space). (From Juliani, G., and Quaglia, C.: *Atlas of Cardiovascular Kymography,* translated by J. L. Maurice. Charles C Thomas.)

FIGURE 1-7B. The linear kymogram (with moving film) obtained with a single-slit kymograph (modified by Bordet and Fischgold). The movements of the two points on the cardiac contour intercepted by the slit are recorded graphically on the film as it moves downwards; the resulting waves are traced on the kymogram from the bottom upwards and must therefore be read in this order. (From Juliani, G., and Quaglia, C.: *Atlas of Cardiovascular Kymography,* translated by J. L. Maurice. Charles C Thomas.)

B

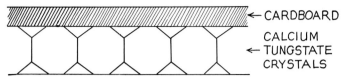

FIGURE 1-8B. Diagrammatic presentation of intensifying screen in cross section.

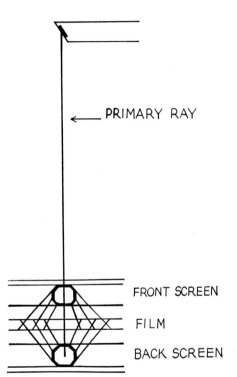

FIGURE 1-8A. Diagram illustrating fluorescence from intensifying screen.

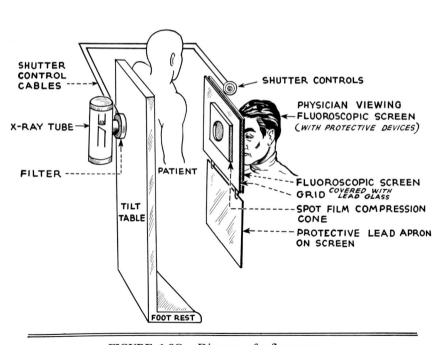

FIGURE 1-8C. Diagram of a fluoroscope.

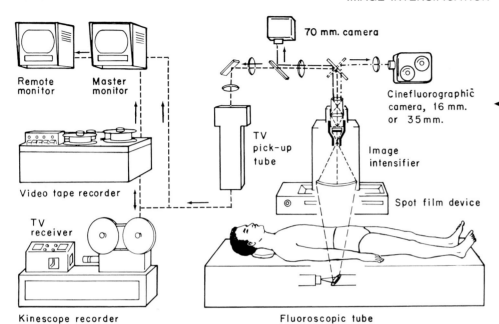

Remote monitor

Master monitor

Video tape recorder

TV receiver

Kinescope recorder

70 mm. camera

TV pick-up tube

Cinefluorographic camera, 16 mm. or 35mm.

Image intensifier

Spot film device

Fluoroscopic tube

◄ **FIGURE 1-9.** Diagram of presently available fluoroscopic equipment, containing image amplification, cinefluoroscopy, cineradiography, and kineradiography. The amplified image from the output phosphor may be conducted through a lens and mirror system directly to the human eye, directly to a stationary or movie camera device, through a television camera to a television receiver, or through a television camera to a television tape recorder. The image on the television screen may be viewed by the human eye or by an additional camera.

FIGURE 1-10. Diagram of image intensifier tube. ► X-rays which pass through an object form an image on the input phosphor screen emitting visible light proportional to the impinging radiation. The photocathode in contact with this screen is an alkali metal layer that emits electrons proportional to the brightness of the fluorescing screen. This electron image is focused by electrostatic lenses on the output phosphor screen. The electrons are also accelerated by a potential difference of 25,000 volts, and a further increase in brightness results. The proper optical system permits the eye to view the brilliant image. To obtain cineradiography or television fluoroscopy one needs only to substitute a movie or television camera for the eye, or a mirror system, to obtain simultaneous viewing and filming.

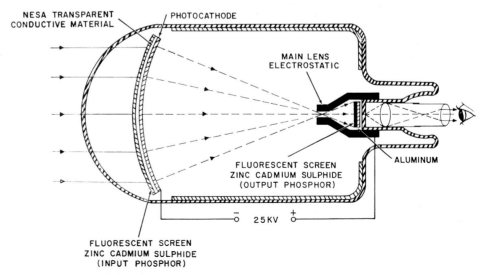

NESA TRANSPARENT CONDUCTIVE MATERIAL

PHOTOCATHODE

MAIN LENS ELECTROSTATIC

FLUORESCENT SCREEN ZINC CADMIUM SULPHIDE (OUTPUT PHOSPHOR)

ALUMINUM

25 KV

FLUORESCENT SCREEN ZINC CADMIUM SULPHIDE (INPUT PHOSPHOR)

alograms and ventriculograms), in the demonstration of some of the joint spaces such as the knee joint, and occasionally in the spinal canal. Air is also used as a contrast medium in the pleural, peritoneal and pericardial spaces as well.

Carbon dioxide is achieving particular importance since it is resorbed extremely rapidly, and it is well tolerated even when injected directly into the bloodstream.

THE FUNDAMENTAL GEOMETRY OF X-RAY IMAGE FORMATION AND INTERPRETATION

X-rays obey the common laws of light. The manner in which any object placed in the path of the x-ray beam is projected depends on five factors: the size of the light source (focal spot), i.e., whether pinpoint or a larger surface; the alignment of the object with respect to the light source and the screen or film; the distance of the object from the light source; the distance of the object from the screen or film; and the plane of the object with respect to the screen or film.

When an image is projected from a pinpoint light source, its borders are sharp, but if the light source is a larger surface, as in the case of the focal spot of an x-ray tube, the image is ill-defined at its periphery owing to penumbra formation (Fig. 1-12). Measures must be taken to reduce the penumbra as much as possible. To accomplish this the focal spot must be as small as possible, and the object-to-film distance as short as possible. The object-to-focal-spot distance should be as long as possible (Fig. 1-13). Also, the film should be perpendicular to the central ray arising from the focal spot.

When the object is not centrally placed with respect to the central ray its image will be distorted, and this distortion may be considerable (Fig. 1-14). Sometimes this distortion is unavoidable if one is to visualize a part, and in some of the radiographic positions, this distortion brings into view a part which otherwise would be

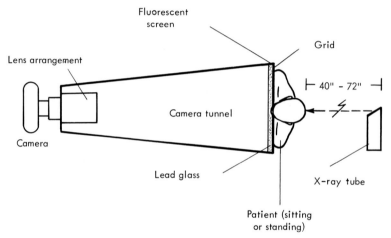

FIGURE 1-11.   Miniature (indirect) radiographs.

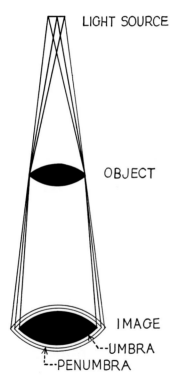

LIGHT SOURCE

OBJECT

IMAGE

---UMBRA

---PENUMBRA

FIGURE 1-12. Diagram of penumbra formation from surface light source.

hidden (Fig. 1-15). Thus, the phenomenon of projection may be utilized to good advantage.

The farther an object is from the light source and the closer it is to the film, the less will be the magnification (Fig. 1-13). The magnification of an object as much as 15 cm. from the film when a relatively usual focal-spot-to-film distance is employed (such as 36 inches) is approximately 20 per cent. Such magnification must be considered in interpreting the size of the heart, the pelvis or any other structure which is to be measured.

These various phenomena of magnification, projection, distortion and penumbra formation must be constantly borne in mind in viewing radiographic images.

THE NECESSITY FOR DIFFERENT VIEWS OR PROJECTIONS OF AN ANATOMIC PART

The obvious method of examining a part is to look at it from several different aspects. This allows a proper perspective of the entire structure. Similarly, in an x-ray examination, it is radiographed from a minimum of two different views, and a three-dimensional concept is thus obtained.

This method of obtaining several views of a given anatomic part has the additional advantage of separating overlying or overlapping structures — of separating the gallbladder, for example, from interfering gas shadows, the stomach from the spine, and so on.

DIRECT ROENTGENOGRAPHIC MAGNIFICATION TECHNIQUES

When effective x-ray tube focal-spot size of 0.2 to 0.3 mm. is employed, the x-ray source is virtually a pinpoint, and very little sharpness is lost in the image even if the anatomic part is at a con-

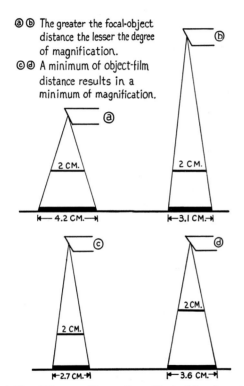

FIGURE 1-13. Diagram illustrating effect of focal-spot-to-object distance and object-to-film distance on magnification.

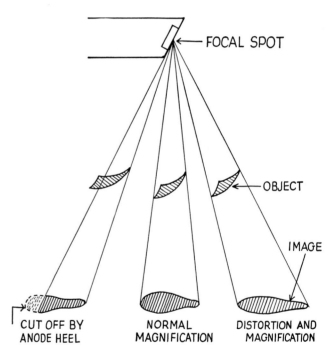

FIGURE 1-14. Diagram illustrating effect of position of object with respect to central ray on distortion, magnification, and anode-heel effect.

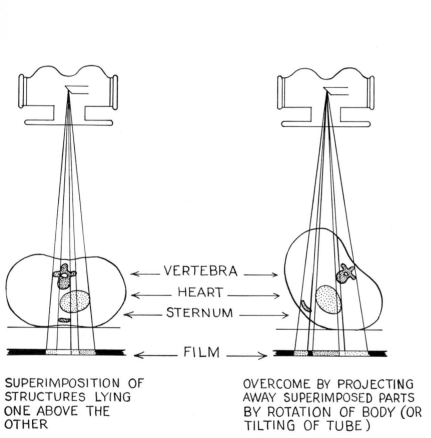

SUPERIMPOSITION OF
STRUCTURES LYING
ONE ABOVE THE
OTHER

OVERCOME BY PROJECTING
AWAY SUPERIMPOSED PARTS
BY ROTATION OF BODY (OR
TILTING OF TUBE)

FIGURE 1-15. Diagram illustrating utilization of projection to overcome superimposition of anatomic parts.

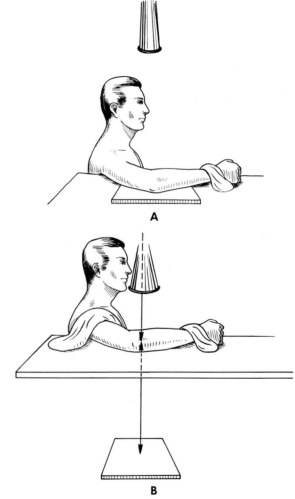

FIGURE 1-16. A, When the film is in close contact with the part being radiographed, and the x-ray tube target is 36 to 40 inches from the film, very little magnification of the part ensues. **B,** When the film is at a considerable distance from the part being radiographed, and the target-to-film distance is 24 to 30 inches, considerable magnification results.

siderable distance from the film (Fig. 1-16). Two- to threefold enlargement may thus be accomplished, depending upon the geometric relationship of the tube target to the body part, and body part to the film. When the two are equal, a 2 × enlargement results; when the target-to-object distance is half the object-to-film distance, a 3 × enlargement is obtained.

Such magnification techniques are especially useful in detailed bone, skull and chest examinations.

FILM IDENTIFICATION

Various methods of film identification include: (1) lead markers;

(2) photographic transfer in the darkroom from a card to a previously unexposed corner of the film; or (3) the insertion of a special data card into the cassette in the lighted room just prior to radiographic exposure. This latter is accomplished by using a special slot identification cassette designed by the author (Fig. 1-17).

The following data are essential: (1) name and address of the radiologist or institution; (2) name and identification number of the patient; (3) the date of the examination; (4) the side of the body being examined, or a clear label of one side; (5) stereoradiography, if employed; (6) time intervals between films, if films are obtained in sequence; (7) distances of laminographic cuts, if body-section studies are done.

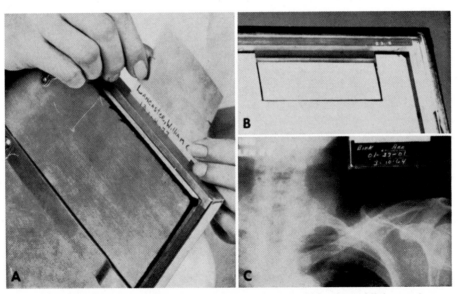

FIGURE 1-17.   Slot identification cassette. **A,** Side view of lightproof slot with the Cronaflex identification card in position. **B,** View of open cassette, showing guides and special depressed area for introduction of identification data card. **C,** The appearance of the data on the final film, obtained at the same time that the routine exposure is made. (Meschan Printab Cassette, Picker X-ray Corp.)

STEPS IN THE PRODUCTION OF A RADIOGRAPH

There are many steps in the production and final interpretation of a radiograph (Fig. 1-18), and it is well to have some concept of all of them. Given the problem of the radiography of an anatomic part, the following steps are pursued:

1. Proper positioning of the patient or his anatomic part with respect to the central ray.

2. Proper choice of grid and cone.

3. Choice of screen (cassette) or nonscreen technique.

4. Choice of optimum exposure factors.

5. Exposure.

6. Removal of film from cassette in darkroom and transfer of the film to a hanger (for wet film developing) or to an automatic processing unit.

7. Passage of film, either automatically or manually, through development, stop-bath, fixation, wash and dry.

8. Sorting and attachment of dried films to consultation request form and old film envelope, ready for interpretation by the radiologist.

9. Submission of consultation report to the referring physician and return of the duplicate report as well as the films to the appropriate files.

There are numerous commercially available rapid film processors which allow one to have the film processed automatically from "dry to dry" in as little as 90 seconds. Such rapid film processing ordinarily requires careful control of temperatures and chemistry of solutions and even special films. It is very likely that in the not too distant future such "dry to dry" automatic processors will be available even in smaller offices and the need for the more complicated wet film processing will disappear. The special technical care and maintenance of such processors is beyond the scope of this text.

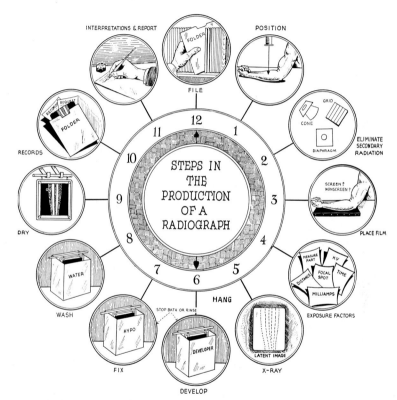

FIGURE 1-18. Diagrammatic presentation of all the steps in the production of a radiograph.

PROTECTIVE MEASURES IN X-RAY DIAGNOSIS

For the Patient (Figure 1-19)

In x-ray diagnosis, exposure of the patient may be considered from the standpoint of protection against the acute effects and the chronic effects of overexposure, each being dealt with in relation to fluoroscopy on the one hand and radiography on the other. The acute effects are epilation and erythema; the chronic effects may be reflected in the blood-forming organs, may cause induction of malignant tumors or cataracts, impaired fertility, reduction of the life span, and genetic changes.

The methods of diminishing x-ray exposure of the patient may be outlined as follows.

Maximum Filtration of the Primary Beam. The inherent filtration of the tube structure is ordinarily equivalent to 0.5 mm. of aluminum. The addition of 2.0 to 4.0 mm. of aluminum is highly desirable. In the usually employed voltage range (40 kvp to 120 kvp), 1 mm. of aluminum will reduce the dose to the skin about 60 per cent; 2 mm. of aluminum about 80 per cent at 50 kvp and 60 per cent at 130 kvp; and 3 mm. of aluminum about 80 to 85 per cent.

It is also interesting that added filtration of this order has very little effect on the resulting roentgenograms. The effective radiation is that which is transmitted through the part being radiographed and hence is the more penetrating, hard type. The addition of a filter increases the transmission by a large factor, at the same time reducing the percentage of soft radiations. The quality of the resulting radiograph is not materially altered by the additional filtration, and the necessary increase in the exposure time is relatively small.

It is concluded that it is advisable to use 2 mm. of aluminum filter for voltages of 50 to 70 kvp and 3 mm. of aluminum for voltages above 70 kvp. If voltages above 100 kvp are employed, use 0.25 mm. of copper added filtration.

Higher Voltages. Whenever possible without significantly altering the quality of the radiograph, higher voltages should be used. This expedient also increases the penetration of the beam, thereby relatively diminishing the total quanta of rays which must strike the skin of the patient to produce a satisfactory radiograph.

This, of course, is of particular importance in pregnancy examinations.

Increased Target-to-skin Distance. As far as this is practicable, on the basis of the inverse square law, it increases the intensity of the remnant radiation (producing the radiographic or fluoroscopic image) for a given entry dose. In fluoroscopy a minimum target-to-skin distance of 18 inches should be used. In radiography, a minimum target-to-film distance of 36 inches is recommended.

Small Field of Radiation. The use of as small a field of radiation as is necessary to achieve the desired diagnostic result may be achieved with cones in radiography and an adjustable diaphragm in fluoroscopy.

Diminished Fluoroscopic Exposure. Using an 18-inch target-to-table-top distance, 80 kvp, and 4 ma., with 3 mm. of aluminum filtration added, fluoroscopy adds 5 to 8 roentgens per minute to the skin of the irradiated area. Five minutes of fluoroscopy to one area must be considered maximum.

Calculation of Dosage to Patients in Diagnostic Examinations. Various tables and nomograms have been provided which permit ready calculation of dose delivered. Table 1-1 is representative.

Needless to say, these are representative values and will vary with the technique employed. It is advised that each radiologist become familiar with the dosages obtained by his techniques.

Although maximum tolerance doses for workers with radiation are established at 0.3 roentgen per week, the maximum permissible dose to patients is not established.

We do not actually know the limitation to impose on diagnostic procedures except to avoid untoward reaction or visible reactions of any kind. Radiation hazards to the embryo and fetus are particularly important to bear in mind. The developing embryos of a

TABLE 1-1. Radiation Dose Received by the Skin and Gonads in
Radiographic Examinations (per film)

Examination	kV.	mAs.	Focus-film distance	Added filtration	Dose per exposure (with back scatter)		
					Skin dose (mr)	Male gonad dose (mr)	Female gonad dose (mr)
Sinuses	80	40	27 in.	3 mm. Al	1040	0.1	0.05
Hand and wrist, postero-anterior	46	50	27 in.	3 mm. Al	100	0.04	0.01
Chest, postero-anterior	90	3	27 in.	3 mm. Al	8	0.01	0.02
Chest, tomogram (apices) antero-posterior	85	12B	100 cm.	3 mm. Al	110	0.01	0.02
Dorsal spine, antero-posterior	75	80B	110 cm.	3 mm. Al	480	1.0	1.3
Lumbar spine, antero-posterior	75	80B	110 cm.	3 mm. Al	480	0.5*	95.0
Lumbar spine, lateral	85	300B	110 cm.	3 mm. Al	2000	2.25	270.0
Lumbar sacral joint, lateral	90	400B	110 cm.	3 mm. Al	3000	2.0	350.0
Pelvis, antero-posterior	75	80B	110 cm.	3 mm. Al	480	20.0*	80.0
Abdomen, antero-posterior	75	60B	110 cm.	3 mm. Al	360	0.5*	75.0
Abdomen, B meal, prone (H.V.)	90	20B	110 cm.	3 mm. Al	130	1.5	20.0
I.V.P. renal, antero-posterior	75	80B	110 cm.	3 mm. Al	480	0.5*	95.0
I.V.P. bladder, antero-posterior	75	80B	110 cm.	3 mm. Al	480	10.0*	80.0
Knee, antero-posterior	82	25B	110 cm.	3 mm. Al	180	1.25	0.4
Ankle, antero-posterior	70	30B	36 cm.	1 mm. Al	200	0.1	0.025
Duodenal cap series, postero-anterior (H.V.)	90	15G	18 in.	5 mm. Al + TT	130	0.05	0.05
Fluoroscopy chest (I.I.)	75	90G (3 min.)	18 in.	5 mm. Al + TT	900	3.0	3.0
Fluoroscopy B meal (I.I.)	75	150G (5 min.)	18 in.	5 mm. Al + TT	1500	5.0	5.0

* Lead rubber protection.
B—Bucky.
G—Stationary grid.
H.V.—High voltage screen–Ilford Red Seal film. Other examinations Par Speed
    screens and Red Seal film extremities.
Ilfex film.
I.I.—Image intensifier, tube current, 0.5 to 1.0 Ma.
From Ardran, G. M., and Crooks, H. E.: Gonad Radiation Dose from Diagnostic
    Procedures. Brit. J. Radiol., *30*:295–297, 1957.

great variety of animals, including several mammals, are highly susceptible to the induction of malformations by radiation. These occur in a well-defined critical period for each genus. There is no reason to doubt that this also applies to human embryos. In man this would correspond to the second to the sixth week of gestation for the majority of characters, when doses of less than 25 roentgens may be detrimental. Beyond this period, the effects are less obvious or possibly delayed with such doses. *Certainly, if pregnancy is known, radiation should, at all costs, be avoided in the first trimester and as much as possible thereafter.*

For the Physician and Technician

Protection Against Radiation Hazard. Most local injuries sustained by the physician or technician are of the hands. Such injuries can be avoided by certain protective measures:

1. Personnel working near an x-ray machine (who are not behind a proper screen) should at all times wear protective lead gloves of at least 0.5 mm. lead equivalent, as well as a lead-lined apron or its equivalent. Roentgenoscopic screens with lead-rubber drapes also diminish radiation exposure.

2. The physician's or technician's unprotected hands, wrists, arms or other parts should never be exposed to the x-ray beam.

3. Eye accommodation preceding fluoroscopy without image amplification should be at least 20 minutes.

4. Suitable kilovoltage and milliamperage settings at fluoroscopy should be adopted, as follows:

Abdomen	80 kvp	3-4 ma.
Chest	70 kvp	3.0 ma.
Thick extremities	60 kvp	3.0 ma.
Thin extremities	50 kvp	3.0 ma.
Children	50-55 kvp	3.0 ma.

5. The following general principles of fluoroscope use should be adhered to.

(a) Shutters must be closed down to no more than 30 to 40 square centimeters.

(b) The fluoroscope should be used intermittently, and should be avoided when the patient is not intercepting the beam.

(c) The examination should be concluded as quickly as possible, usually within five minutes. It is well to have a special timing device in the circuit to turn off the machine automatically when this time is exceeded.

(d) When fractures are being set or foreign bodies located, alternating radiography with intermittent manipulation should be used, if possible, rather than fluoroscopy.

(e) Head fluoroscopy should never be used.

Metabolic changes are perhaps incurred by physicians even though sufficient protection is worn. There is a high incidence of leukemia in radiologists, and even among nonradiologists; it is pos-

TABLE 1-2. Methods to Insure Adequate Protection

For Patient	For Physician
1. Avoid examination in the first trimester of pregnancy.	1. Wear lead impregnated gloves and apron.
2. Work with a minimum of 2 to 3 mm. of aluminum filter over aperture of tube.	2. Never expose unprotected areas to x-ray beam.
3. Use as high a kilovoltage as possible.	3. Always use repeated x-ray film examination rather than fluoroscopic unit in the setting of fractures.
4. Increase target-skin distance as much as possible.	
5. Use narrow shutter for fluoroscopy screen and use unit intermittently with limitation of time.	4. Avoid head fluoroscopy.
	5. Accommodate eyes for 20 minutes prior to fluoroscopy.

sible that when certain susceptible individuals receive even the minimal exposure allowed for in the foregoing methods, they ultimately develop leukemia.

Protection Against Electrical Hazard. In addition to the radiation hazard, an electrical hazard may also be present. The voltages used to energize x-ray tubes are highly dangerous. The best assurance of safety is the enclosure of all high voltage parts in a shockproof container. Most x-ray machines now being made for diagnostic use are of shockproof design, but where the design is such that high voltage conductors are exposed, operators should keep at a liberal distance from them and should guard against spark-gap formation. A space of at least 1 foot should always be allowed between such a conductor and any body part.

X-ray apparatus should not be installed or operated in dangerous locations. When used in a room with anesthetic gases, the machine and all switches should be explosion-proof, or all electrical contacts should be 5 feet or more above floor level. Provision should be made to protect all exposed cables from mechanical damage, and these should be periodically inspected for defects or abrasions. All the exposed non-current-carrying parts of the apparatus should be permanently grounded in acceptable fashion with good ground leads.

It is well to bear in mind first aid practices such as artificial respiration and emergency treatment for burns, in the event the need for these should arise.

Although the high tension does not extend to the darkroom, the hazard of electrical shock there is great. Lighting fixtures are the greatest potential hazard and must be carefully installed with every attention to proper insulation and grounding.

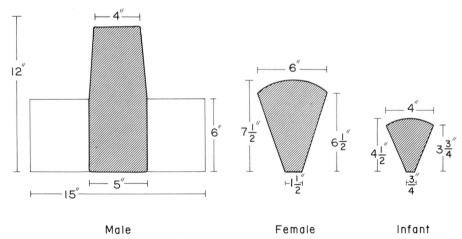

Male   Female   Infant

FIGURE 1-19A. Design of lead gonad shields useful in radiography. These should be 1/8 inch lead (or equivalent) in thickness. They should be placed over the patient's gonads whenever such exposure is not required as part of the diagnostic test.

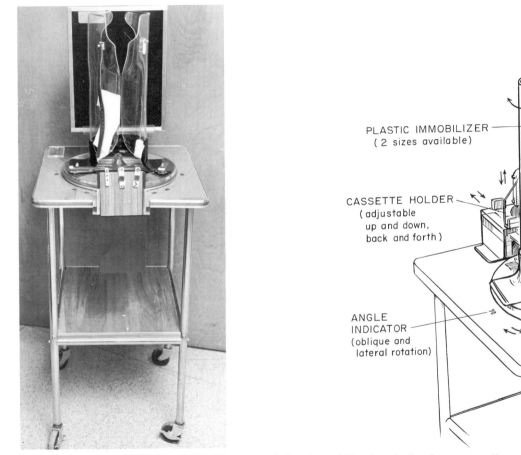

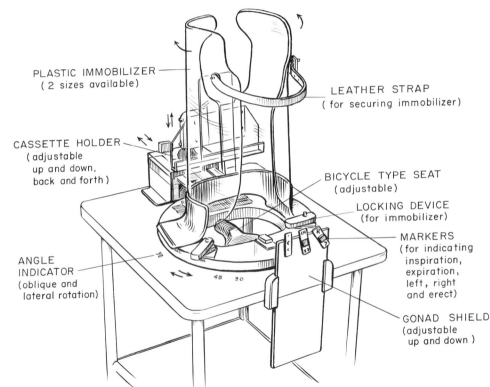

PLASTIC IMMOBILIZER
(2 sizes available)

LEATHER STRAP
(for securing immobilizer)

CASSETTE HOLDER
(adjustable
up and down,
back and forth)

BICYCLE TYPE SEAT
(adjustable)

LOCKING DEVICE
(for immobilizer)

MARKERS
(for indicating
inspiration,
expiration,
left, right
and erect)

ANGLE
INDICATOR
(oblique and
lateral rotation)

GONAD SHIELD
(adjustable
up and down)

FIGURE 1-19B. Pigg-o-stat infant immobilization device for erect radiography (made by Modern Way Immobilizers, Memphis, Tennessee).

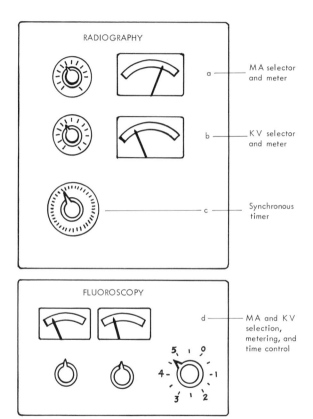

RADIOGRAPHY

a — M A selector and meter

b — K V selector and meter

c — Synchronous timer

FLUOROSCOPY

d — M A and K V selection, metering, and time control

5 0
4 1
3 2

FIGURE 1-19C. Diagram of x-ray control panel to emphasize control of physical factors in radiation protection.

Fundamental Rules of Radiation Protection — the Key to Good Basic Understanding of X-ray Technology (Figure 1-19)

There are a few good fundamental rules that, when followed by the well-trained x-ray technician, produce the best results for the patient and his doctor and the greatest protection against the hazards of radiation for the technician and patient.

(a) The milliamperage setting should be the maximum which the tube target will tolerate without being damaged, for the time necessary to produce the "amount of x-ray photons" necessary for the examination.

(b) The kilovoltage setting should be sufficient to give the x-rays enough penetrating power for the anatomic part in question — not so much, that good differentiation of different tissue structure is not possible, not too much for the characteristics of the tube and circuit, not so little, that the x-ray beam is absorbed by the anatomic part rather than penetrating to the recording film or fluoroscopic screen. This must be a carefully selected setting for optimum results both photographically and from the standpoint of hazard to patient or equipment.

(c) The exposure time should be as rapid as possible to avoid the blurring of the image produced by movement in the anatomic part being studied. There may be occasions when movement is employed deliberately in a structure adjoining one which does not move.

(d) Fluoroscopic settings should in general be high kvp (90 to 110) and low milliamperage (2 to 3 ma.), and total fluoroscopic time should not exceed five minutes, with intermittent exposure during fluoroscopy.

(e) The smallest possible target of the x-ray tube should be used to give maximum detail without endangering the x-ray tube for the exposure planned.

(f) There should be a primary filter in the beam just outside the x-ray tube of at least 2 mm. of aluminum (preferably 4 mm. of aluminum), so that those rays which are too weak to penetrate the anatomic part will for the most part be removed prior to their striking the patient.

(g) The x-ray beam should be delimited by a diaphragm and cone to furnish that bare minimum of radiation necessary to cover the anatomic part in question. It is usually a fixed diaphragm over the tube housing aperture, plus a fixed or adjustable cone affixed to the tube housing outside the aperture.

(h) The angulation of the x-ray tube should be carefully chosen to yield maximum information in accordance with the anatomic depiction necessary.

(i) The distance of the x-ray tube from the patient and film should be optimum to diminish distortion and magnification, yet yield the least radiation possible to the patient, and most tolerable exposure to the x-ray machine itself. The distance for purposes of measurement of anatomic parts should usually be 6 feet; for most other radiographic purposes, 40 inches; for close-up detail contact with the patient with the cone may be most desirable; for fluoroscopy, a minimum distance of 18 to 20 inches should be chosen, since closer distances will expose the patient inordinately.

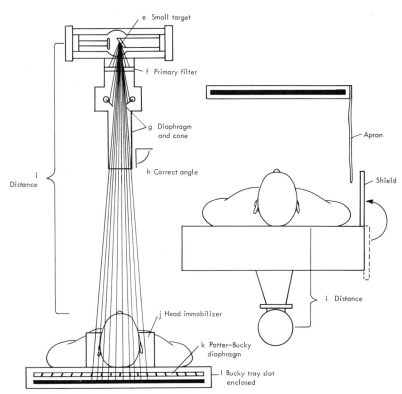

FIGURE 1-19D.   Further protection factors diagrammatically illustrated.

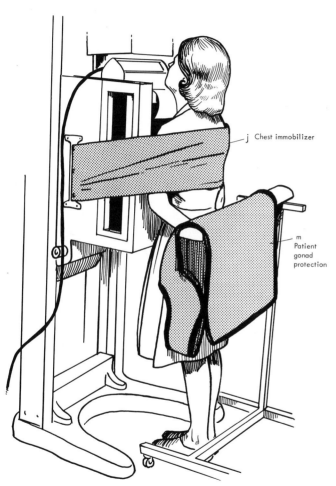

j Chest immobilizer

m
Patient
gonad
protection

(j) Patients should be immobilized as much as is comfortably possible during the exposure to avoid movement during radiography. This may be done with special immobilization devices for both children and adults. A convenient head immobilizer is shown in Figure 1-19D; a good chest immobilizer for children in Figure 1-19B, and for adults in Figure 1-19E.

(k) A Potter-Bucky diaphragm will avoid unnecessary secondary scatter affecting the film, and thus enhance detail—well worth the slight increase in exposure necessary in most instances. The grid type must be carefully chosen for the purposes required.

(l) The x-ray tube housing should be radiation-proof, and the slot containing the Bucky tray in the x-ray table should be enclosed wherever possible to diminish scattered radiation in the x-ray room. An additional lead barrier, hinged to the table, encloses the patient.

(m) The patient's gonads must be protected from radiation wherever possible (see also Figure 1-19A).

FIGURE 1-19E. Further radiation protection factors diagrammatically illustrated.

(n) A lead apron of at least 0.5 mm. lead equivalent should be used beneath the fluoroscopic screen and worn by the technician or any other person in the fluoroscopic room during the procedure; similar lead gloves should also be worn if the hands come anywhere near the patient. Under no circumstances should any part of the technician or physician be exposed to the direct x-ray beam, since these protective devices are designed to protect against scattered radiation only.

(o) When lead-lined aprons are worn, they should protect as much as possible of the technician's skeletal marrow as well as the gonads, and care must be exercised that they are worn properly. For technicians who must be in the room during fluoroscopy, posterior gonad shields should be worn as well as the apron anteriorly, to protect against even the minute amounts of scattered radiation in the room.

(p) Image amplification fluoroscopy should be used with infants if at all possible.

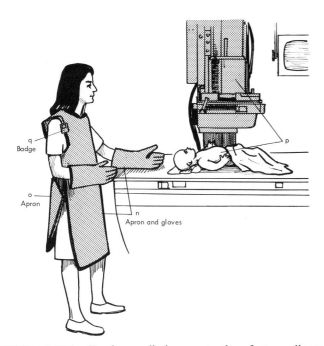

FIGURE 1-19F. Further radiation protection factors diagrammatically illustrated.

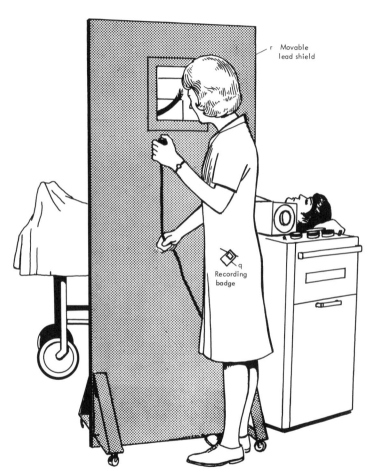

r Movable
   lead shield

q
Recording
badge

FIGURE 1-19G. Further radiation protection factors diagrammatically illustrated.

(q) Technicians should wear exposure recording badges on the critical areas of the body (*outside* the lead protective devices worn) all through the working day. Careful on-going records should be maintained for the life span of the technician (and all personnel exposed) and should be entered accurately at least once every month. Standards for exposure avoidance should be carefully maintained and constantly investigated.

(r) When the mobile x-ray unit is employed, a movable lead shield should also be used to protect the technician during exposure.

(s) Usually, intensifying screen film studies will produce adequate detail and contrast, and will diminish exposure to the patient by a considerable factor. Intensifying screens should be kept clean and in good condition. Nonscreen technique may be employed in special circumstances when a minute foreign body is being sought in the eye, or where calculi or other pathological conditions are being sought around the mouth.

(t) When darkroom fluoroscopy must be employed (in the absence of image amplifiers), at least 20 minutes of accommodation to darkness must be allotted, and specially designed goggles should be worn so that this dark adaptation is retained throughout the time interval when the room is lighted.

In the pages that follow, it is assumed that the instructor will keep the technician student apprised of all necessary adjuncts as just outlined with each area of the body being studied. In this manual, it is not our purpose to repeat further this most important message about protection against the hazards of radiation, since it is assumed that the technician is aware of these first and foremost. Our attention in this manual is primarily devoted to positioning of the patient and tube for anatomic study, and to a demonstration of the film and anatomy so obtained.

Chapter 2 — The Upper Extremity

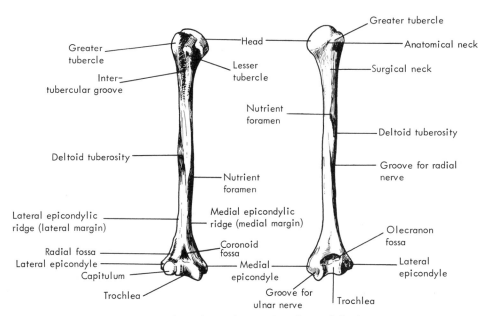

FIGURE 2-1.   Anterior and posterior views of the humerus.

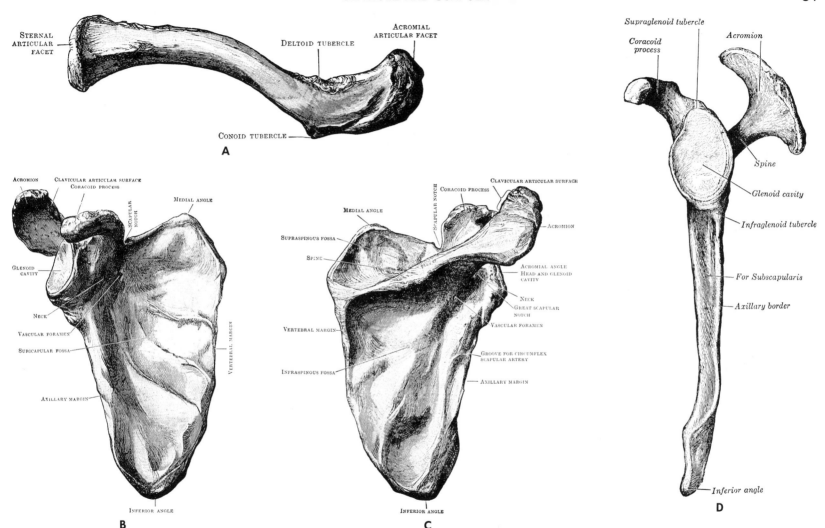

STERNAL ARTICULAR FACET

DELTOID TUBERCLE

ACROMIAL ARTICULAR FACET

CONOID TUBERCLE

A

ACROMION
CLAVICULAR ARTICULAR SURFACE
CORACOID PROCESS
SCAPULAR NOTCH
MEDIAL ANGLE
GLENOID CAVITY
NECK
VASCULAR FORAMEN
SUBSCAPULAR FOSSA
AXILLARY MARGIN
VERTEBRAL MARGIN
INFERIOR ANGLE

B

MEDIAL ANGLE
SUPRASPINOUS FOSSA
SPINE
SCAPULAR NOTCH
CORACOID PROCESS
CLAVICULAR ARTICULAR SURFACE
ACROMION
ACROMIAL ANGLE
HEAD AND GLENOID CAVITY
NECK
GREAT SCAPULAR NOTCH
VASCULAR FORAMEN
GROOVE FOR CIRCUMFLEX SCAPULAR ARTERY
AXILLARY MARGIN
VERTEBRAL MARGIN
INFRASPINOUS FOSSA
INFERIOR ANGLE

C

Supraglenoid tubercle
Coracoid process
Acromion
Spine
Glenoid cavity
Infraglenoid tubercle
For Subscapularis
Axillary border
Inferior angle

D

FIGURE 2-2. **A,** Clavicle viewed from above. (From Cunningham, D. J.: *Textbook of Anatomy,* edited by A. Robinson. Oxford University Press.) **B, C, D,** Anterior, posterior and lateral views of the scapula. (**B** and **C,** From Cunningham, D. J.: *Textbook of Anatomy,* edited by A. Robinson. Oxford University Press. **D,** From Gray, H.: *Gray's Anatomy of the Human Body,* edited by C. W. Goss. Lea & Febiger.)

POINTS OF PRACTICAL INTEREST ABOUT FIGURE 2-3.

1. The patient may be examined either in the erect position or supine as shown, and centered so that the central ray passes midway between the summit of the shoulder and lower margin of the anterior axillary fold.

2. Better contact of the affected shoulder with the film is produced by rotating the opposite shoulder away from the table top approximately 15 to 20 degrees, and supporting the elevated shoulder and hip on sandbags.

3. When looking for faint flecks of calcium in the soft tissues, nonscreen film and technique should be employed unless the shoulder is very muscular, in which case the Potter-Bucky apparatus may be employed in addition. When using the Potter-Bucky diaphragm (or grid cassette) it is best to position the cassette so that the central ray will pass through the center of the cassette and the coracoid process.

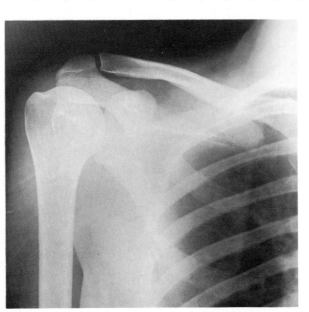

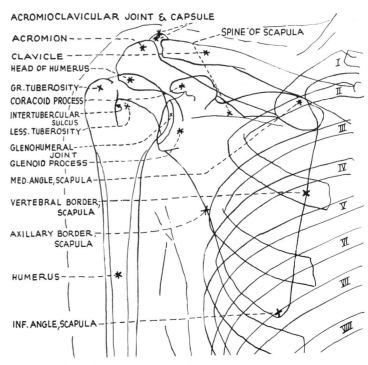

FIGURE 2-3. Neutral anteroposterior view of the shoulder.

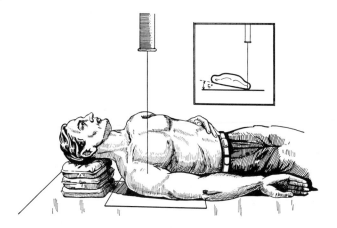

POINTS OF PRACTICAL INTEREST ABOUT FIGURE 2-4

1. One must make certain in this position that the entire humerus is rotated inward in addition to merely the forearm and hand.

2. The central ray may pass through the region of the coracoid process.

3. The angle of rotation of the body may be increased to 15 to 20 degrees instead of 5 degrees as shown. This will produce a slightly better profile view of the glenoid process.

4. It is most important that sandbags be used on the hand and forearm to immobilize the patient. (These have been omitted from the illustration for clarity).

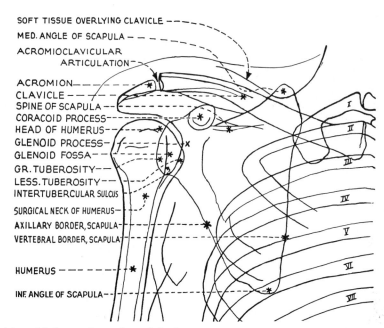

SOFT TISSUE OVERLYING CLAVICLE

MED. ANGLE OF SCAPULA

ACROMIOCLAVICULAR ARTICULATION

ACROMION

CLAVICLE

SPINE OF SCAPULA

CORACOID PROCESS

HEAD OF HUMERUS

GLENOID PROCESS

GLENOID FOSSA

GR. TUBEROSITY

LESS. TUBEROSITY

INTERTUBERCULAR SULCUS

SURGICAL NECK OF HUMERUS

AXILLARY BORDER, SCAPULA

VERTEBRAL BORDER, SCAPULA

HUMERUS

INF. ANGLE OF SCAPULA

FIGURE 2-4. Anteroposterior view of the shoulder with internal rotation of the humerus.

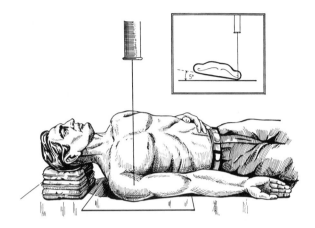

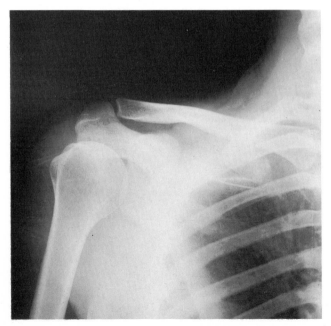

POINTS OF PRACTICAL INTEREST ABOUT FIGURE 2-5.

1. One must make certain to rotate the entire arm externally in addition to the forearm and hand. (Sandbags as indicated for Fig. 2-4.)

2. In order to obtain a slightly better profile view of the glenoid process of the scapula, the angle of rotation may be increased from 5 degrees as shown to 15 or 20 degrees.

3. When looking particularly for small flakes of calcium deposit in the soft tissues of the shoulder, one must use a nonscreen technique with or without the Potter-Bucky diaphragm. The central ray may be directed through the coracoid process rather than as shown in the centering diagram.

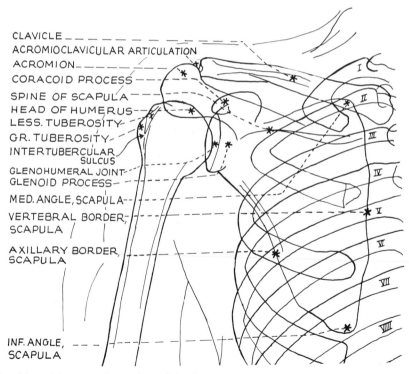

CLAVICLE
ACROMIOCLAVICULAR ARTICULATION
ACROMION
CORACOID PROCESS
SPINE OF SCAPULA
HEAD OF HUMERUS
LESS. TUBEROSITY
GR. TUBEROSITY
INTERTUBERCULAR SULCUS
GLENOHUMERAL JOINT
GLENOID PROCESS
MED. ANGLE, SCAPULA
VERTEBRAL BORDER, SCAPULA
AXILLARY BORDER, SCAPULA
INF. ANGLE, SCAPULA

FIGURE 2-5. Anteroposterior view of the shoulder with external rotation of the humerus.

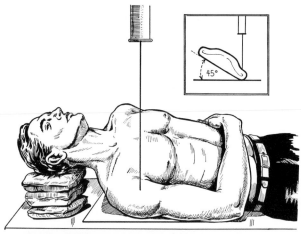

POINTS OF PRACTICAL INTEREST ABOUT FIGURE 2-6

    1. Adjust the degree of rotation to place the scapula parallel with the plane of the film, and the head of the humerus in contact with it. This will usually come to an angle of 45 degrees as shown.

    2. The arm is very slightly abducted and internally rotated, and the forearm is rested against the side of the body.

    3. For a more uniform density, respiration is suspended in the expiratory phase.

    4. The central ray is directed to a point 2 inches medial and 2 inches distal to the upper-outer border of the shoulder.

    5. This view is particularly valuable in cases of suspected chronic dislocation of the shoulder, since in such instances the inferior margin of the glenoid process is frequently eroded or contains spurs rather than having the smooth contour shown.

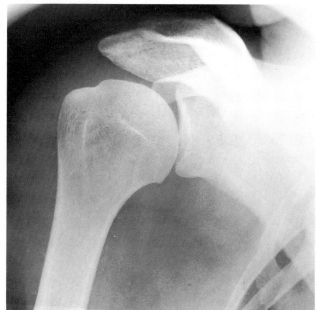

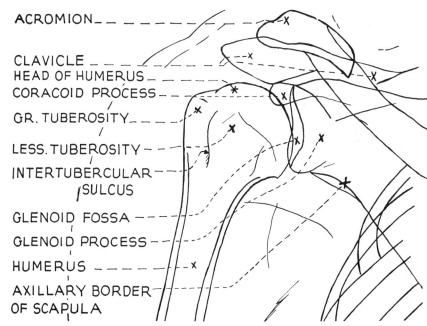

ACROMION

CLAVICLE
HEAD OF HUMERUS
CORACOID PROCESS
GR. TUBEROSITY

LESS. TUBEROSITY

INTERTUBERCULAR
SULCUS

GLENOID FOSSA

GLENOID PROCESS

HUMERUS

AXILLARY BORDER
OF SCAPULA

FIGURE 2-6. View of shoulder for greater detail with reference to the glenoid process (Grashey position).

POINTS OF PRACTICAL INTEREST ABOUT FIGURE 2-7

1. When there is a tear in the acromioclavicular joint capsule, there is a tendency for the distal end of the clavicle to rise above the level of the adjoining acromion process. The two films must be so equivalent in the projection as to make it possible to measure not only the joint space between the clavicle and the acromion process, but also the difference in relation to a horizontal line which would connect the superior margins of the acromion processes.

2. The technique employed should be such as to demonstrate the acromioclavicular joint capsule on each side by soft tissue contrast. Hemorrhage and swelling of the joint capsule may thereby be detected as well.

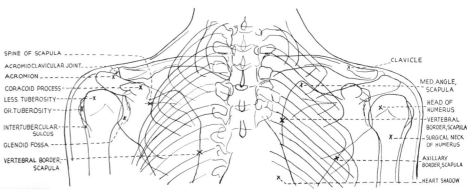

SPINE OF SCAPULA
ACROMIOCLAVICULAR JOINT
ACROMION
CORACOID PROCESS
LESS. TUBEROSITY
GR. TUBEROSITY
INTERTUBERCULAR SULCUS
GLENOID FOSSA
VERTEBRAL BORDER, SCAPULA

CLAVICLE
MED. ANGLE, SCAPULA
HEAD OF HUMERUS
VERTEBRAL BORDER, SCAPULA
SURGICAL NECK OF HUMERUS
AXILLARY BORDER, SCAPULA
HEART SHADOW

FIGURE 2-7. Detection of integrity of the acromioclavicular joint. In small individuals, a single exposure may be sufficient; in larger individuals, two separate exposures may be required with the cone centered over each joint separately without moving the patient. (Pearson position, when projection is posteroanterior instead of anteroposterior as shown.)

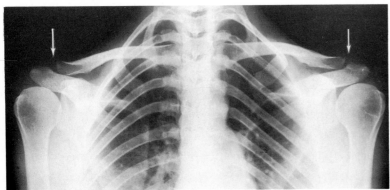

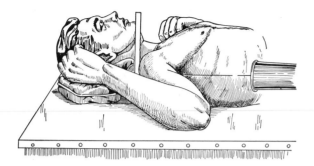

POINTS OF PRACTICAL INTEREST ABOUT FIGURE 2-8

1. The arm is kept in external rotation, while the forearm and hand are adjusted and supported in a comfortable position.

2. The central ray is directed through the axilla to the region of the acromioclavicular joint.

3. The arm should be abducted as nearly as possible to a right angle with respect to the long axis of the body.

4. It is important to push the cassette against the patient's neck as far as possible to obtain maximal visualization of the scapula.

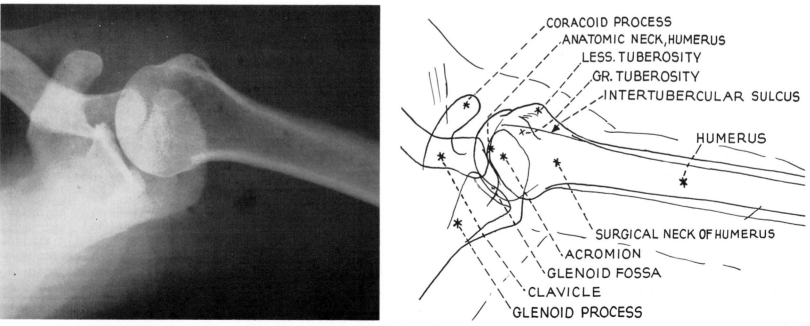

FIGURE 2-8. Lateral view of shoulder with the central horizontal ray projected through the axilla (Lawrence position).

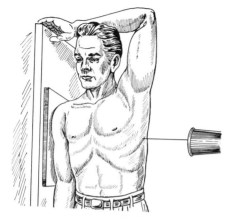

POINTS OF PRACTICAL INTEREST ABOUT FIGURE 2-9

1. For best results one must employ a screen film, with a vertical Potter-Bucky diaphragm, or grid-front cassette.

2. The cassette is centered to the region of the surgical neck of the affected humerus, as is the central ray. The central ray may be angled cephalad 5 to 15 degrees.

3. The patient stands perfectly perpendicular to the film as shown, with the opposite shoulder raised out of the way by resting his forearm upon his head and elevating the opposite scapula.

4. It is best to suspend respiration in full inspiration in this instance so that the air in the lungs will improve the contrast of the bone and decrease the exposure necessary to penetrate the body.

5. This may be the only method of obtaining a lateral view of the upper humerus in the event of a fracture in this location, when the patient is unable to abduct the arm.

6. While the erect position is shown, the recumbent position may also be employed, although it is less desirable.

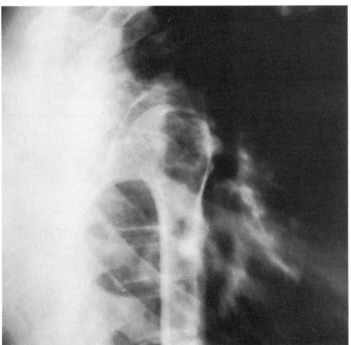

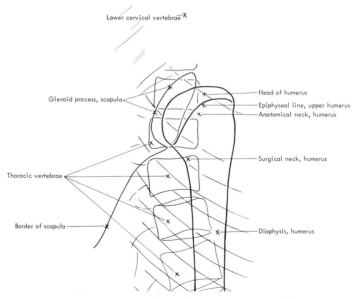

FIGURE 2-9. Lateral view of shoulder with the central horizontal ray projected through the entire body (Lawrence position).

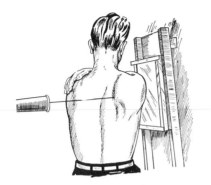

POINTS OF PRACTICAL INTEREST ABOUT FIGURE 2-10

1. The Potter-Bucky diaphragm is necessary to obtain best results with this view.

2. The scapula is placed perpendicular to the film, rotating the opposite shoulder out of view. After palpating it, one centers over the spine of the scapula.

3. To rotate the wing of the scapula outward to its maximum it is best to rest the forearm of the affected side on the opposite shoulder, bringing the arm as close to the anterior chest wall as possible. Although the erect position is preferable, the recumbent position may also be employed in this instance.

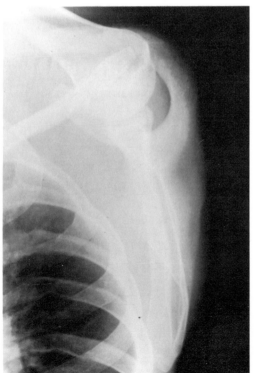

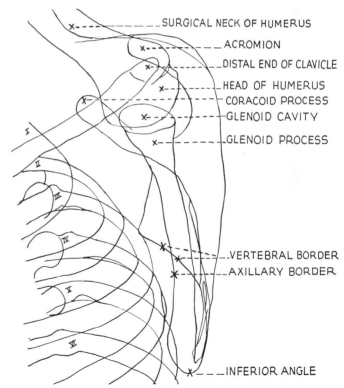

FIGURE 2-10. Lateral view of scapula (modification of Lilienfeld position).

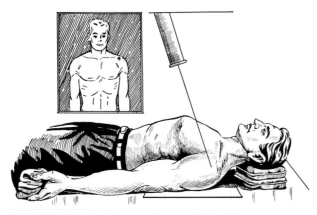

POINTS OF PRACTICAL INTEREST ABOUT FIGURE 2-11

1. A 5 degree angulation of the tube is usually adequate to project the clavicle away from the rest of the thoracic cage in this view.

2. When interpreting this film, the physician must take into account a considerable element of projection and distortion, since the clavicle is a fair distance from the film.

3. The central ray should pass through the middle of the clavicle in this projection, or through the acromioclavicular articulation as shown.

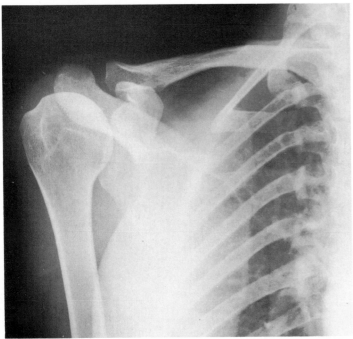

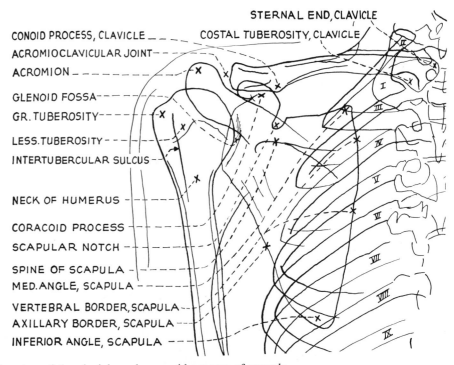

FIGURE 2-11. Special anteroposterior view of the clavicle and coracoid process of scapula.

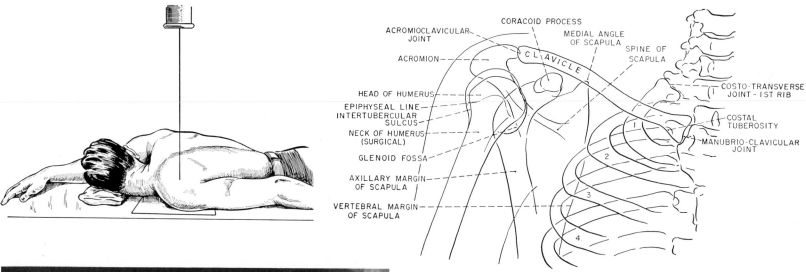

ACROMIOCLAVICULAR JOINT

CORACOID PROCESS

MEDIAL ANGLE OF SCAPULA

SPINE OF SCAPULA

ACROMION

CLAVICLE

COSTO-TRANSVERSE JOINT - 1ST RIB

HEAD OF HUMERUS

EPIPHYSEAL LINE
INTERTUBERCULAR SULCUS

COSTAL TUBEROSITY

NECK OF HUMERUS (SURGICAL)

MANUBRIO-CLAVICULAR JOINT

GLENOID FOSSA

AXILLARY MARGIN OF SCAPULA

VERTEBRAL MARGIN OF SCAPULA

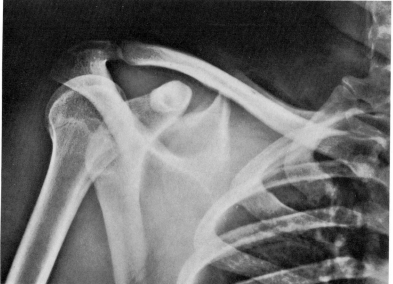

POINTS OF PRACTICAL INTEREST ABOUT FIGURE 2-12

1. This view may be employed with either the erect or the prone position as shown. The erect position is probably more readily obtained in the event of injury to the clavicle.

2. The central ray passes through the center of the clavicle in this instance; an angulation of 10 degrees toward the feet may be employed.

3. Approximately one half of the clavicle is projected over the bony thorax as shown, but there is less distortion and magnification in this view than in Figure 2-11, and hence it is more desirable in some instances.

FIGURE 2-12. Special posteroanterior view of clavicle.

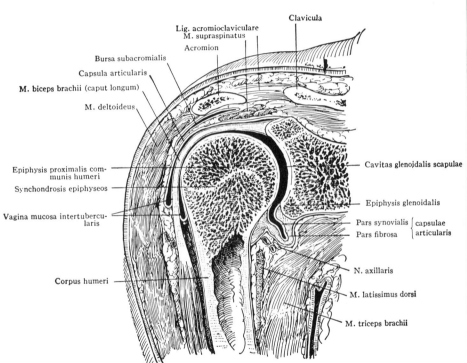

Clavicula

Lig. acromioclaviculare
M. supraspinatus

Acromion

Bursa subacromialis

Capsula articularis

M. biceps brachii (caput longum)

M. deltoideus

Epiphysis proximalis com-
munis humeri

Synchondrosis epiphyseos

Vagina mucosa intertubercu-
laris

Corpus humeri

Cavitas glenoidalis scapulae

Epiphysis glenoidalis

Pars synovialis ⎱ capsulae
Pars fibrosa ⎰ articularis

N. axillaris

M. latissimus dorsi

M. triceps brachii

FIGURE 2-13A. Subdeltoid bursa and its anatomic relationships. (From Anson, B. J., and Maddock, W. G.: *Callender's Surgical Anatomy*, W. B. Saunders Co.)

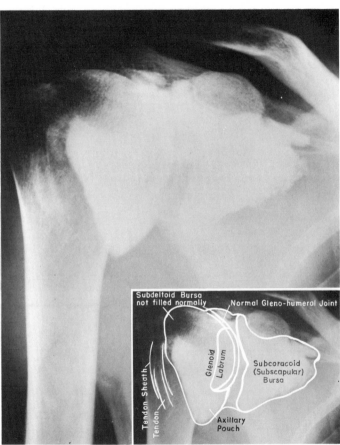

Subdeltoid Bursa
not filled normally

Normal Gleno-humeral Joint

Tendon Sheath

Tendon

Glenoid Labrum

Subcoracoid (Subscapular) Bursa

Axillary Pouch

FIGURE 2-13B. Normal Hypaque arthrogram of an adult's shoulder demonstrating the normal joint, subscapularis bursa and dependent axillary pouch. (From Kernwein, G. A., Roseberg, B., and Sneed, W. R., Jr.: J. Bone & Joint Surg., *39A, 1957.*)

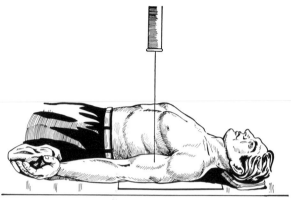

POINTS OF PRACTICAL INTEREST ABOUT
FIGURE 2-14

1. The entire humerus from head to epicondyle should be included if at all possible.

2. One must make certain to supinate the
hand sufficiently so that the epicondyles both lie
flat on the film.

3. The central ray is directed through the
mid-shaft of the humerus.

4. The opposite shoulder may be rotated up
and supported by sandbags in order to facilitate
placing the humerus in better contact with the film.

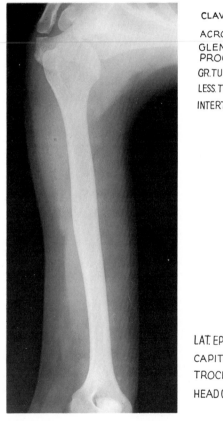

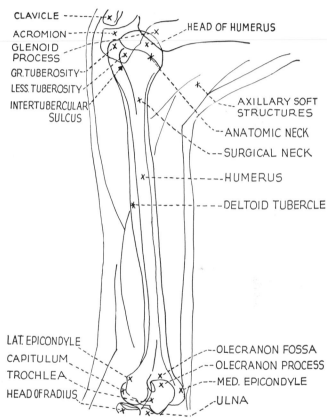

CLAVICLE

ACROMION

GLENOID PROCESS

GR. TUBEROSITY

LESS. TUBEROSITY

INTERTUBERCULAR SULCUS

HEAD OF HUMERUS

AXILLARY SOFT STRUCTURES

ANATOMIC NECK

SURGICAL NECK

HUMERUS

DELTOID TUBERCLE

LAT. EPICONDYLE

CAPITULUM

TROCHLEA

HEAD OF RADIUS

OLECRANON FOSSA

OLECRANON PROCESS

MED. EPICONDYLE

ULNA

FIGURE 2-14. Anteroposterior view of the arm.

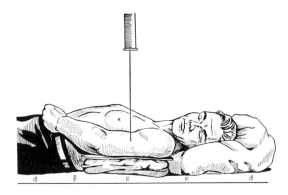

POINTS OF PRACTICAL INTEREST ABOUT FIGURE 2-15

1. One must make certain that the film size chosen is adequate to include the entire shaft of the humerus from head to elbow joint.

2. The two epicondyles must be perfectly superimposed over one another and perpendicular to the film surface. To accomplish this, the physician may have to elevate the film on a sandbag as shown, and flex the forearm, resting the forearm upon the abdomen.

3. An alternative technique allows the patient to sit in a chair and extend the arm across the table. The arm, particularly its lower two-thirds, must be in perfect contact with the film.

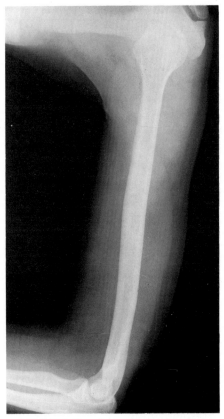

FIGURE 2-15. Lateral view of the arm.

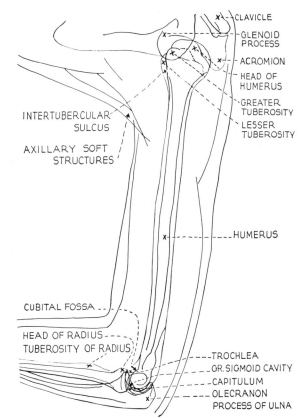

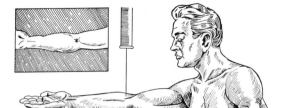

POINTS OF PRACTICAL INTEREST ABOUT FIGURE 2-16

1. Note that the patient is seated low enough to place the shoulder joint and the elbow in approximately the same plane. This assures a good contact between the distal humerus and the film.

2. The anterior surface of the elbow and the plane passing through the epicondyles must be perfectly parallel with the film. To accomplish this the hand must be completely supinated and usually supported in this position by means of a sandbag. Occasionally also the patient must lean somewhat laterally.

3. The olecranon and coronoid fossae of the humerus, being superimposed and merely being a very thin plate of bone, will frequently appear as a foramen rather than as a bony plate, which may be misleading. A foramen in lieu of this bony plate does occur very rarely in anomalous conditions.

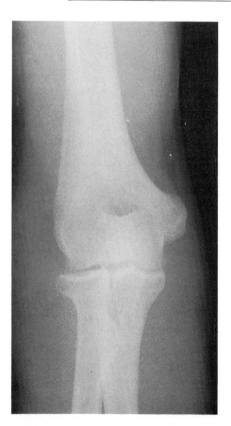

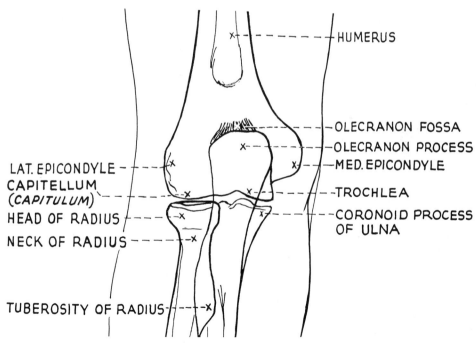

FIGURE 2-16.   Anteroposterior view of elbow.

POINTS OF PRACTICAL INTEREST ABOUT FIGURE 2-17

1. The patient must be seated in such a way as to allow the entire humerus to be placed in good contact with the table top and film.

2. The elbow is flexed as acutely as possible and the hand pronated.

3. It is important in this instance also to obtain a visualization of the soft tissues immediately outside the olecranon process in view of their frequent involvement by inflammatory process and calcium deposit.

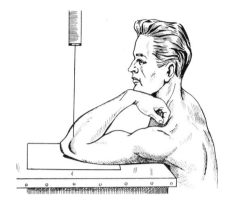

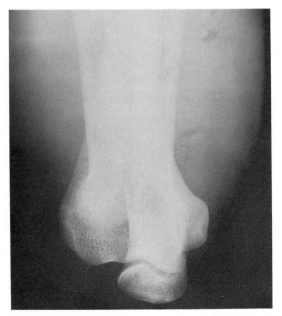

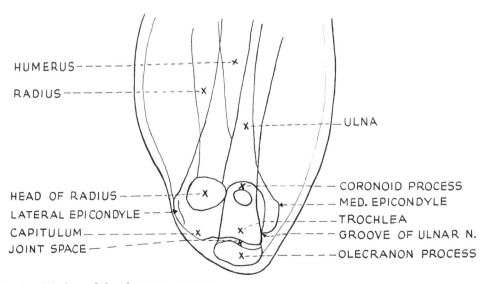

HUMERUS

RADIUS

ULNA

HEAD OF RADIUS

LATERAL EPICONDYLE

CAPITULUM

JOINT SPACE

CORONOID PROCESS

MED. EPICONDYLE

TROCHLEA

GROOVE OF ULNAR N.

OLECRANON PROCESS

FIGURE 2-17.   Special view of the olecranon process.

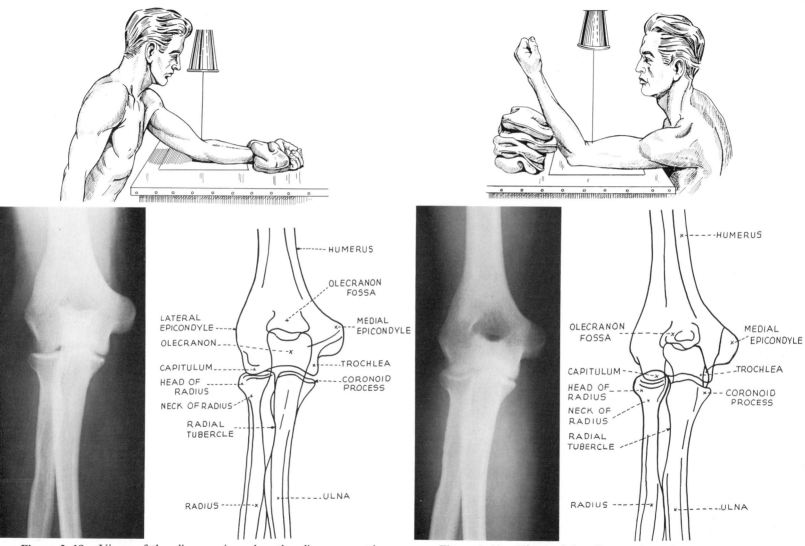

Figure 2–18. Views of the elbow region when the elbow cannot be fully extended. View of the proximal forearm, with a distorted view of the distal humerus.

Figure 2–19. Views of the elbow region when the elbow cannot be fully extended. View of distal humerus, with a distorted view of the proximal forearm.

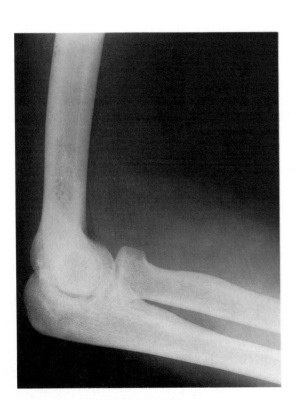

POINTS OF PRACTICAL INTEREST ABOUT FIGURE 2-20

1. The patient is so placed with respect to the table that the arm is at the same levels as the shoulder. Unless this is done the elbow joint proper will not be visualized clearly, and a rather oblique view of the head and neck of the radius will be obtained.

2. The elbow is ordinarily flexed approximately 90 degrees. The center of the film is placed immediately beneath the elbow joint and the central ray passes through the joint and center of the film, the epicondyles of the humerus being superimposed and perpendicular to the latter. The forearm is placed so that the thumb points directly upward and the palm of the hand is perpendicular to the table top surface. The fist may be clenched to facilitate maintenance of position. It is best to immobilize the forearm in this position by means of sandbags.

3. Since fractures of the head and neck of the radius are among those most frequently missed in radiography, one must examine the contour and structure of these regions with extreme care to avoid such an error.

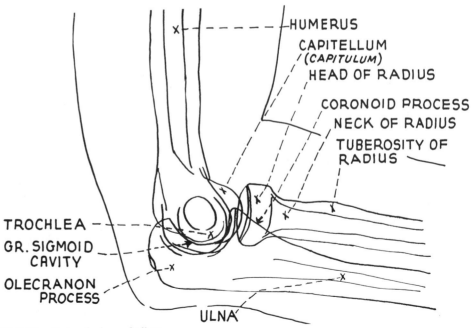

FIGURE 2-20. Lateral view of elbow.

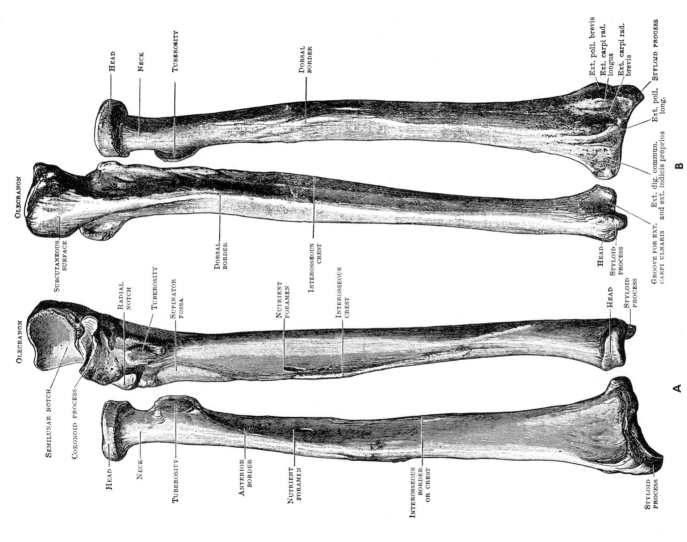

FIGURE 2-21. A, Volar aspect of the radius and ulna; **B,** Dorsal aspect of radius and ulna. (From Cunningham, D. J.: *Textbook of Anatomy,* edited by A. Robinson. Oxford University Press.)

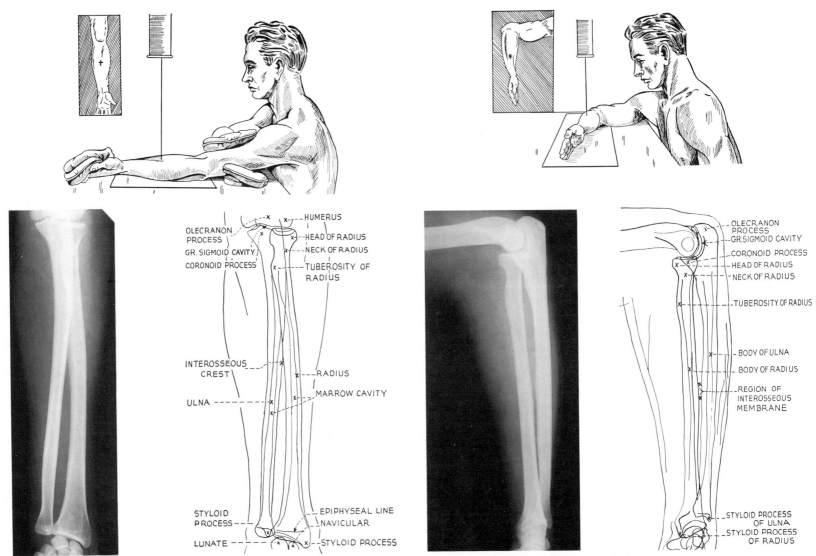

FIGURE 2-22. Anteroposterior view of forearm.

FIGURE 2-23. Lateral view of forearm.

POINTS OF PRACTICAL INTEREST ABOUT FIGURES 2-22 and 2-23

1. When the proximal two-thirds of the forearm are of greatest anatomic interest, the elbow joint is always included. The wrist joint is always included when the major anatomic interest is in the distal one-third of the forearm. Thus, the important technical adjuncts which apply to the elbow joint and wrist also apply here, with the exception that the forearm is always in a supinated position with the volar aspect uppermost in these views.

In any case, it is well to seat the patient low enough to place the shoulder and the elbow in approximately the same plane, to assure good contact between the distal humerus and the film. A platform on the table top, with the patient's arm and the film on the platform, can achieve the same purpose.

2. In both these views, it is important to obtain an accurate concept of the integrity of the interosseous membrane. The ability of the patient to pronate and supinate his forearm depends in greatest measure upon an adequacy of this membrane and the space between the two bones of the forearm throughout their lengths. With injury to the bones of the forearm, there is a tendency for the fragments of the radius and ulna to contact one another and form a bony bridge between them across the interosseous membrane. This bridging must be recognized early and prevented.

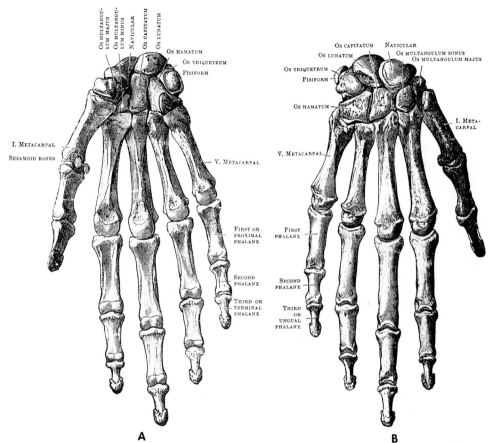

FIGURE 2-24. **A,** Volar aspect of the bones of the right hand and wrist; **B,** Dorsal aspect of the right hand and wrist. (From Cunningham, D. J.: *Textbook of Anatomy,* edited by A. Robinson. Oxford University Press.)

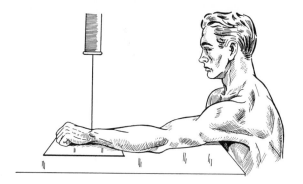

POINTS OF PRACTICAL INTEREST ABOUT FIGURE 2-25

1. The posteroanterior projection of the wrist is usually preferable because it permits better contact between the carpus and the film than is obtained in the reverse projection. In contrast to this, however, the anteroposterior view of the forearm is the more desirable since pronation of the hand would cause the two bones of the forearm to cross one another.

2. The central ray is projected immediately over the navicular carpal bone, midway between the styloid processes.

3. The clenched fist as shown places the wrist at a very slight angulation but the navicular carpal bone is at right angles to the central ray, so that it is usually projected without any superimposition either by itself or by adjoining structures.

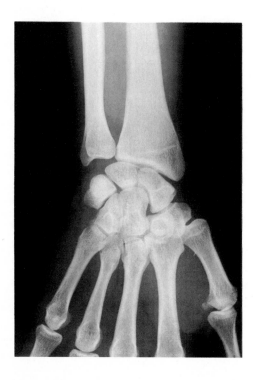

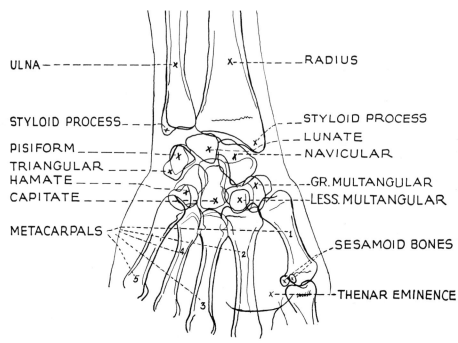

FIGURE 2-25. Posteroanterior view of wrist.

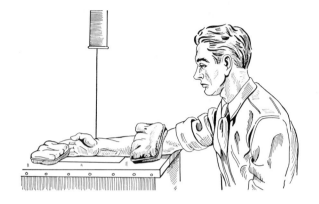

CHART OF RELATED TERMINOLOGY FOR
CARPAL BONES

Scaphoid = Navicular
Lunate
Triquetrum = Triangular Carpal
Pisiform
Multangular majus = Trapezium
Multangular minus = Trapezoid
Capitate
Hamate
Dorsal = posterior
Palmar = anterior (or volar)

The carpal tunnel is filled with tendons and the median nerve passing from the forearm into the palm of the hand. The ulnar vessels and nerve lie on the lateral side of the pisiform bone. The trapezium and part of the scaphoid bone lie in the floor of the "anatomic snuff box."

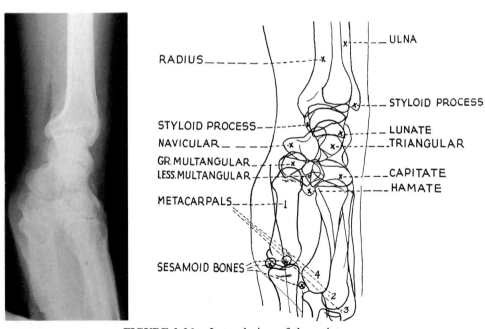

FIGURE 2-26. Lateral view of the wrist.

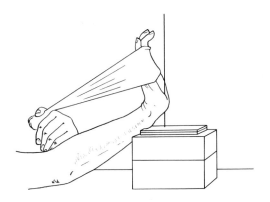

POINT OF PRACTICAL INTEREST ABOUT FIGURE 2-27

If hyperextension of the wrist cannot be maintained as shown, the central ray is directed at an angle of 20 to 30 degrees to the long axis of the hand.

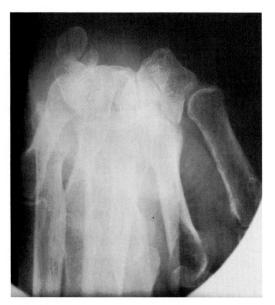

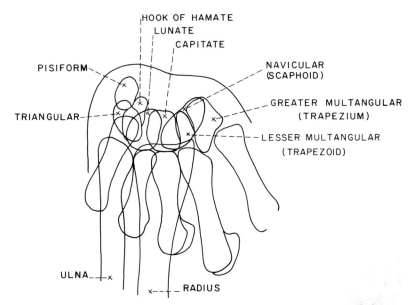

FIGURE 2-27. The carpal tunnel view of the wrist (modification of Gaynor-Hart position, and Templeton and Zim carpal tunnel view).

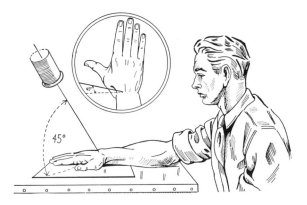

POINTS OF PRACTICAL INTEREST ABOUT FIGURE 2-28

1. This view is an application of the principle of distortion in order to provide increased clarity of a pathologic process within a bony structure. Actually a rather distorted and elongated view of the navicular carpal bone is obtained, but it will be noted that it is completely clear of adjoining structures, for the most part, particularly in the area that is most prone to be fractured, namely its midsection. Also its own structure is not superimposed upon itself.

2. This view is also of some value with reference to the base of the first metacarpal, but is of very little value with reference to the rest of the carpus.

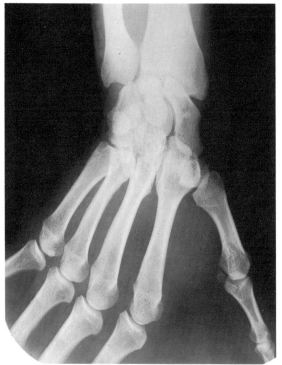

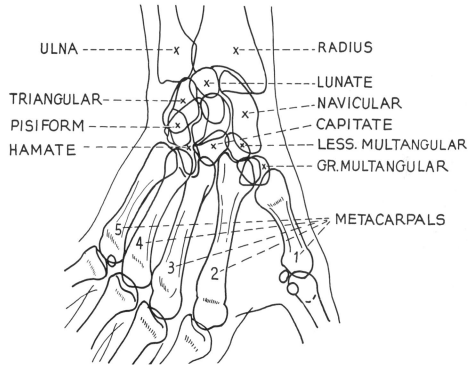

FIGURE 2-28. Special view for demonstrating navicular carpal bone.

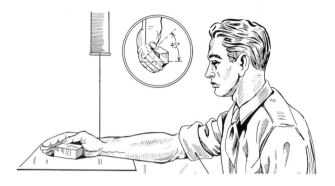

POINTS OF PRACTICAL INTEREST ABOUT FIGURE 2-29

1. The film is placed under the wrist so that the center of the film is approximately 3 to 4 cm. anterior to the carpal bones. This will place it immediately under the navicular carpal bone when the wrist is slightly pronated to about 45 degrees from the lateral position. The hand is supported on a balsa wood block or sandbag as shown, and the forearm may be immobilized by an additional sandbag.

2. The central ray is directed immediately over the navicular carpal bone.

3. This view is also particularly valuable in obtaining a clear perspective of the joint between the greater multangular and the first metacarpal.

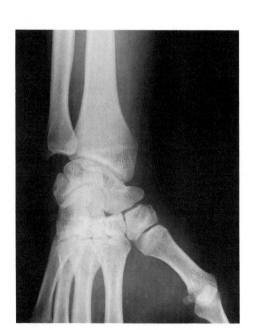

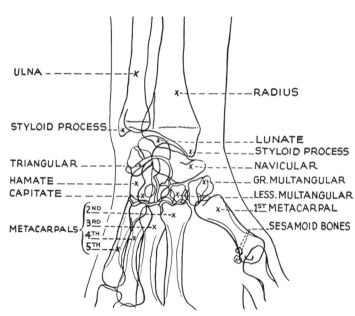

FIGURE 2-29. Oblique view of the wrist.

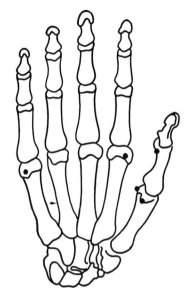

FIGURE 2-30. The most frequent sites of sesamoid bones of the hand.

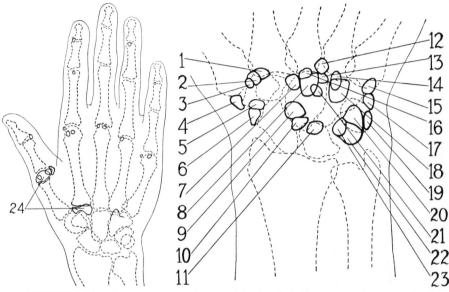

FIGURE 2-31. Supernumerary bones of the hand. 1, Os trapezoides secundarium; 2, trapezium secundarium; 3, pretrapezium; 4, paratrapezium; 5, epitrapezium; 6, radiale externum; 7, styloid; 8, subcapitatum; 9, os centrale; 10, hypolunatum; 11, epilunatum; 12, ossiculum gruberi; 13, os capitatum secondarium; 14, os hamuli proprium; 15, os vesalianum; 16, parastyloid; 17, ulnare externum; 18, hamulare basale; 19, pisiforme proprium; 20, triquetrum ulnare; 21, metastyloid; 22, triquetrum radiale; 23, epipyramis; 24, epiphyses of the head of the first metacarpal and base of the second metacarpal respectively. (From McNeil, C.: *Roentgen Technique,* Charles C Thomas.)

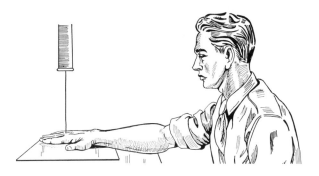

POINTS OF PRACTICAL INTEREST ABOUT FIGURE 2-32

1. The fingers should be spread slightly, and completely extended and in good contact with the film.

2. The central ray should pass through the third metacarpophalangeal joint.

3. It is well to immobilize the forearm just above the wrist by means of a sandbag.

4. The greatest care must be exercised to obtain a clear view, particularly of the tufted ends of the distal phalanges as well as the shafts of the phalanges, since many pathologic processes of a systemic type will produce minute and very important changes in these structures. The student should obtain a very clear mental concept of the normal appearance of the phalanges and metacarpals.

5. If a single finger is in question, a lighter exposure technique is employed and usually four views of that finger from all perspectives are taken.

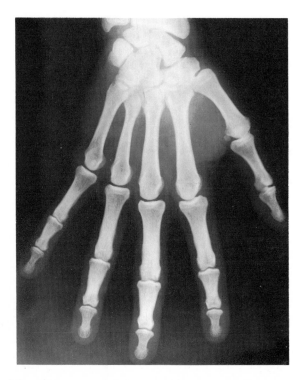

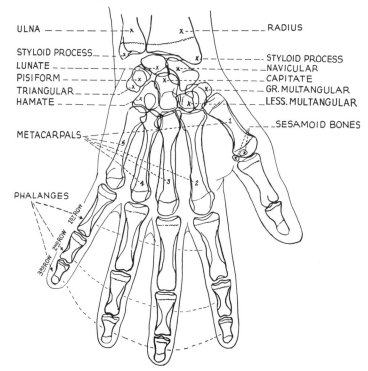

FIGURE 2-32.   Posteroanterior view of the hand.

POINTS OF PRACTICAL INTEREST ABOUT FIGURE 2-33

1. One should adjust the obliquity of the hands so that the metacarpophalangeal joints form an angle of approximately 45 degrees with the film.

2. The central ray is directed vertically through the third metacarpophalangeal joint.

3. Cotton pledgets may be employed to spread the fingers. A 2 inch square of balsa wood placed under the thumb makes an excellent immobilization device.

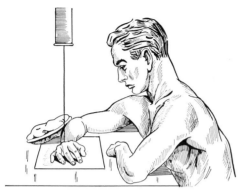

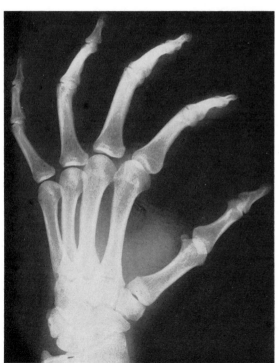

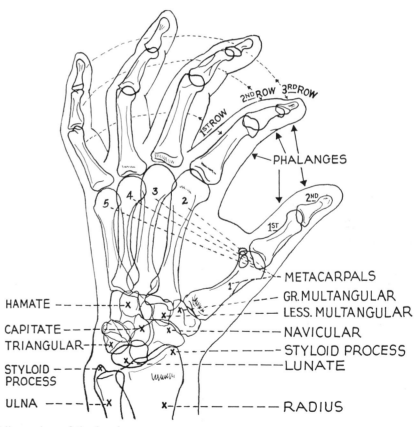

FIGURE 2-33. Oblique view of the hand.

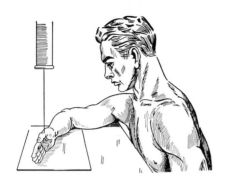

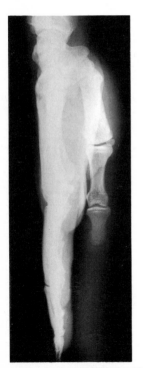

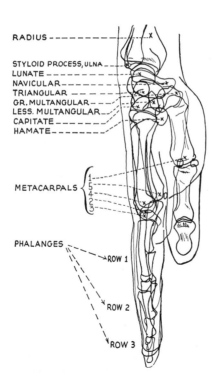

RADIUS

STYLOID PROCESS, ULNA
LUNATE
NAVICULAR
TRIANGULAR
GR. MULTANGULAR
LESS. MULTANGULAR
CAPITE
HAMATE

METACARPALS {
5
4
2
3

PHALANGES
ROW 1

ROW 2

ROW 3

FIGURE 2-34. Straight lateral view of the hand.

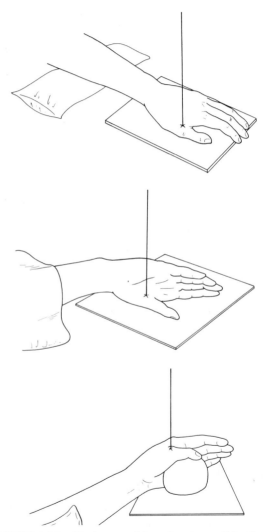

FIGURE 2-35. Various positions for views of the thumb.

Chapter 3 — The Pelvis and Lower Extremity

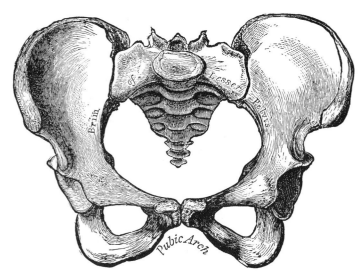

FIGURE 3-1. The bony pelvis (female). (See Chap. 8 for significance in relation to obstetrical radiology.) (From Gray, H.: *Gray's Anatomy of the Human Body*, edited by C. M. Goss. Lea & Febiger.)

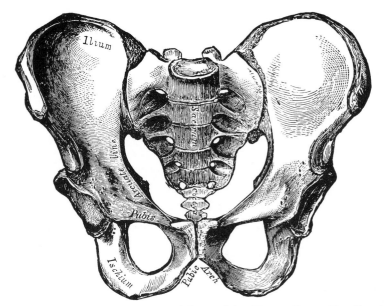

FIGURE 3-2. The bony pelvis (male). (From Gray, H.: *Gray's Anatomy of the Human Body*, edited by C. M. Goss. Lea & Febiger.)

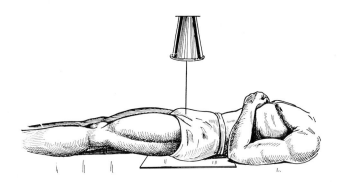

POINTS OF PRACTICAL INTEREST ABOUT FIGURE 3-3

1. Center the patient to the median line of the table with the center of a 14 x 17 inch cassette placed crosswise 1½ inches above the superior margin of the pubic symphysis. This will place the upper border of the film above the iliac crest and the lower border of the film well below the lesser trochanters of the femurs.

2. In order to project the necks of the femurs in their full length it is well to invert the feet about 15 degrees and immobilize them with sandbags in this position.

3. The entire pelvis must be symmetrical. This may necessitate placing a folded sheet or balsa wood block under one side.

4. There are various special views for the ilium, the acetabulum, the anterior pelvic bones and the pubes which have not been included in this text. These special views need be employed only on rare occasions.

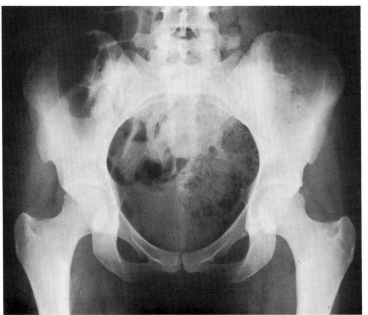

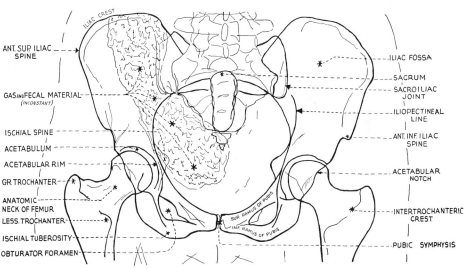

FIGURE 3-3.   Anteroposterior view of the pelvis.

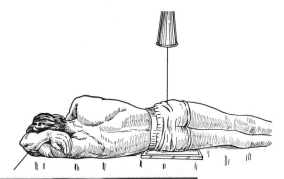

POINTS OF PRACTICAL INTEREST ABOUT FIGURE 3-4

1. The patient is placed in the lateral position, either erect or recumbent, and the film is placed in the Potter-Bucky diaphragm. The knees and hips are slightly flexed to facilitate maintenance of position.

2. The gluteal cleft is placed parallel with the film.

3. Immobilization with a compression band is frequently very helpful. This is applied across the trochanteric region of the pelvis.

4. Center in the midaxillary plane over the depression between the iliac crest and the greater trochanter of the femur.

5. There should be almost perfect superposition of the ischial spines as well as the acetabula in this projection.

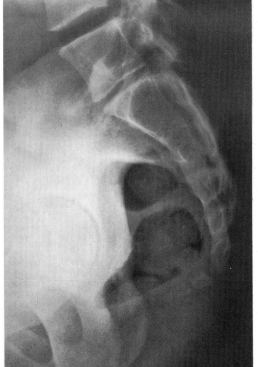

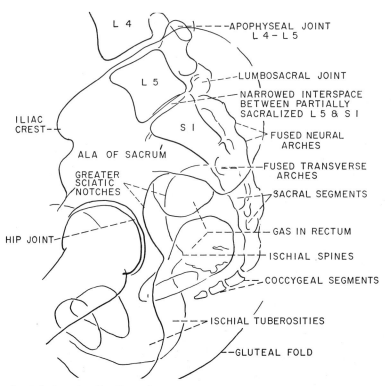

FIGURE 3-4.   Lateral view of pelvis for visualization of sacrum.

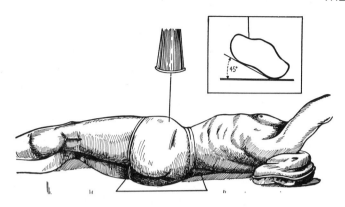

POINTS OF INTEREST ABOUT FIGURE 3-5

1. Elevate the side being examined approximately 45 degrees and support the shoulder and the upper thigh on sandbags, making certain that the sandbags do not appear on the radiograph.

2. The sacroiliac joint which is farthest from the film will appear most clearly and this is the one which is being examined. The two articular surfaces of the sacroiliac joint closest to the film are superimposed over one another, and hence this point is not shown to best advantage.

3. A somewhat similar oblique view of the sacroiliac joints may be obtained in the posteroanterior projection by placing the patient obliquely prone instead of supine as just noted.

4. Oblique views of both sacroiliac joints are always obtained because one joint offers some comparison for analysis of the other.

5. The central ray may be angled 5 degrees cephalad. In some patients this improves visualization of the sacroiliac and lumbar apophyseal joints.

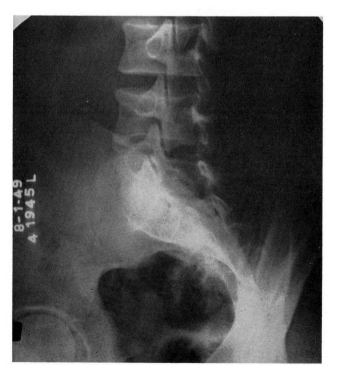

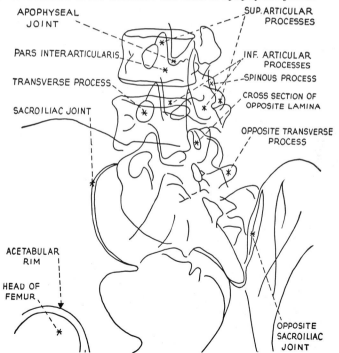

FIGURE 3-5. Oblique view of the sacroiliac joints and lower lumbar spine.

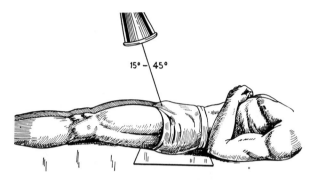

POINTS OF PRACTICAL INTEREST ABOUT FIGURE 3-6

1. For more marked distortion angulation up to 45 degrees of the tube cephalad may be employed.

2. The central ray is adjusted so that it enters the body just above the pubic symphysis and so that it will leave the body at approximately the upper margin of the sacrum or at the level of the fifth lumbar segment. Care is exercised to center the x-ray film to the central ray of the x-ray tube, otherwise one will not obtain the anatomic structures depicted.

3. This view is particularly valuable for demonstrating sacralization of the last lumbar transverse processes as is indicated in the accompanying diagram. Also defects in the neural arch of the fifth lumbar vertebra are well demonstrated in this view.

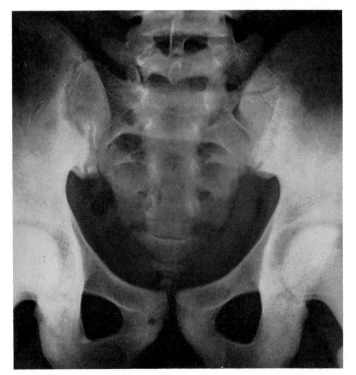

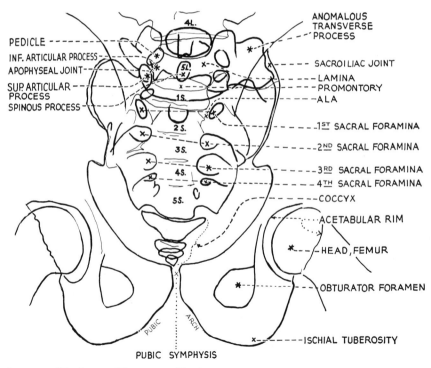

FIGURE 3-6. Distorted view of sacrum (Taylor, or Meese, position).

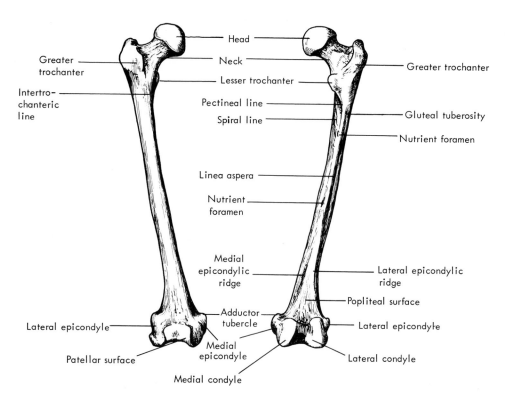

Head

Greater
trochanter

Neck

Greater trochanter

Lesser trochanter

Intertro-
chanteric
line

Pectineal line

Spiral line

Gluteal tuberosity

Nutrient foramen

Linea aspera

Nutrient
foramen

Medial
epicondylic
ridge

Lateral epicondylic
ridge

Popliteal surface

Lateral epicondyle

Adductor
tubercle

Lateral epicondyle

Patellar surface

Medial
epicondyle

Lateral condyle

Medial condyle

Anterior Aspect

Posterior Aspect

FIGURE 3-7. Diagram of anterior and posterior aspects of femur.

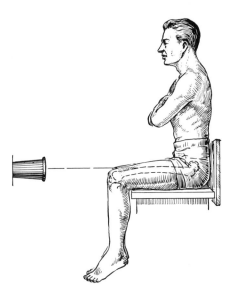

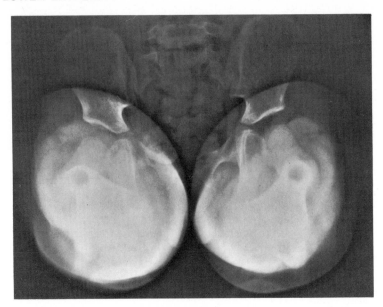

FIGURE 3-8. Special view designed to measure the degree of anteversion of the neck of the femur with respect to the shaft. Note that the patient is positioned so that the central ray strikes the middle of the shaft of the femur, and not the knee joint proper. The shaft of the femur arches posteriorly. It is the *proximal* one-half of the femoral shaft which is horizontal and actually the distal one-half of the femur dips downward toward the floor slightly. It is this expedient which will permit a diagnostic film to be obtained using lumbosacral spine technical factors. Otherwise, the detail procured will be inadequate for measurement. In the film so obtained (shown intensified), the detail is poor, but adequate to draw the angle of anteversion as indicated in the tracing. One line is drawn along the inferior margins of the femoral condyles; the other is drawn through the axis of the neck of the femur. The angle between may then be measured.

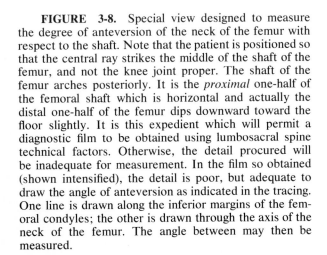

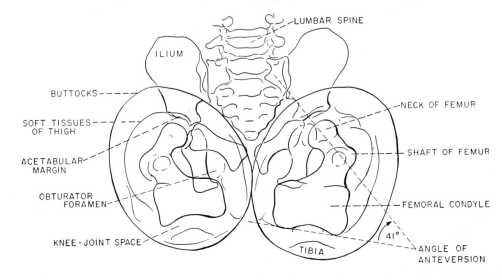

TABLE 3-1.   Normal Degrees of Anteversion of the Femoral Neck*

Age	Anteversion (in degrees)
Birth to 1 year	30-50
2 years	30
3-5	25
6-12	20
12-15	17
16-20	11
Greater than 20	8

*Averages adapted from Billing, L.: Acta radiol. Supp. *110*:1-80, 1954; and Budin, E., and Chandler, E.: Radiology *69*:209-213, 1951.

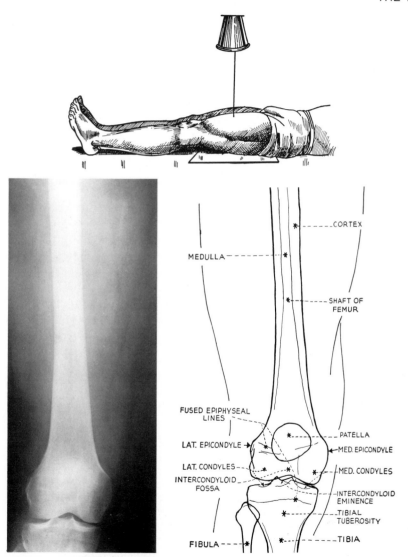

FIGURE 3-9.   Routine anteroposterior view of femur.

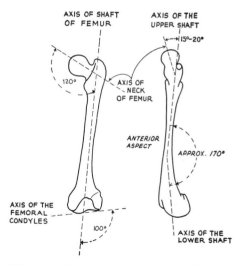

FIGURE 3-10.   Axial relationships of the shaft of the femur. (Angles are approximations and not invariable.)

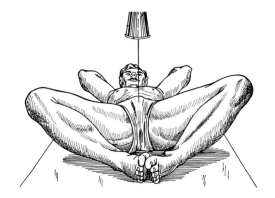

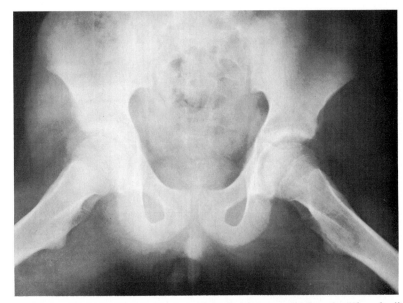

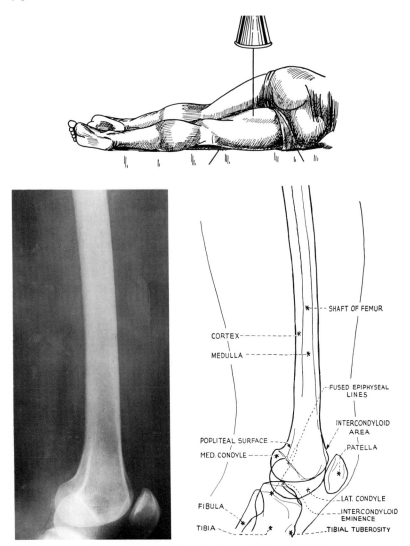

SHAFT OF FEMUR

CORTEX

MEDULLA

FUSED EPIPHYSEAL
LINES

INTERCONDYLOID
AREA

POPLITEAL SURFACE

MED. CONDYLE

PATELLA

FIBULA

LAT. CONDYLE

INTERCONDYLOID
EMINENCE

TIBIA

TIBIAL TUBEROSITY

FIGURE 3-11. Routine lateral view of thigh.

FIGURE 3-12. Lateral view of both hips, employing the "frog-leg" (Cleaves) position. (See Fig. 3-14 for anatomic tracing of one side.)

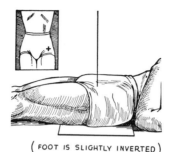

(FOOT IS SLIGHTLY INVERTED)

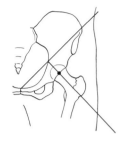

POINTS OF PRACTICAL INTEREST ABOUT FIGURE 3-13

1. The patient is placed in the perfectly supine position. The entire pelvis must be symmetrical even though only one side is considered.

2. *For maximum elongation and detail of the femoral neck, the foot is inverted approximately 15 degrees and immobilized in that position by means of a small sandbag.*

3. A line is drawn between the anterior-superior iliac spine and the superior margin of the pubic symphysis. The centering point is 1 inch distal to the midpoint of this line. Ordinarily, this will fall immediately over the hip joint proper.

4. If the foot is everted instead of inverted, the lesser trochanter will be shown in maximum detail and the neck of the femur will be completely foreshortened.

5. For maximum detail of both the greater and the lesser trochanter the foot should point directly upward and remain perpendicular to the table top at the time the film is obtained.

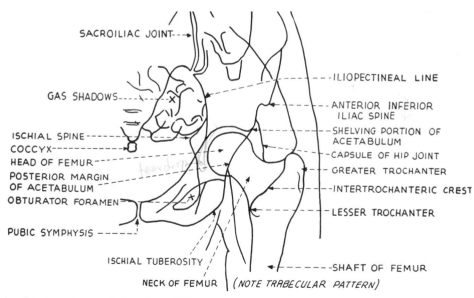

SACROILIAC JOINT

GAS SHADOWS

ISCHIAL SPINE
COCCYX
HEAD OF FEMUR
POSTERIOR MARGIN
OF ACETABULUM
OBTURATOR FORAMEN

PUBIC SYMPHYSIS

ISCHIAL TUBEROSITY

NECK OF FEMUR

ILIOPECTINEAL LINE

ANTERIOR INFERIOR
ILIAC SPINE

SHELVING PORTION OF
ACETABULUM

CAPSULE OF HIP JOINT

GREATER TROCHANTER

INTERTROCHANTERIC CREST

LESSER TROCHANTER

SHAFT OF FEMUR

(NOTE TRABECULAR PATTERN)

FIGURE 3-13. Route anteroposterior view of hip.

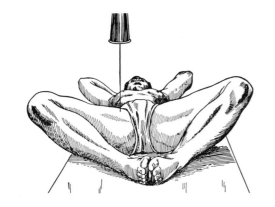

POINTS OF PRACTICAL INTEREST ABOUT FIGURE 3-14

1. The "frog-leg" lateral view of the hip is actually a useful but imperfect lateral perspective of the head, neck and upper shaft of the femur. The acetabulum remains in an anteroposterior relationship, and the normal anteversion of the neck of the femur with respect to the shaft is not shown. Moreover, this technique cannot be employed following most injuries in which the hip joint motion is very limited and painful. Nevertheless, it is particularly useful in analysis of suspected hip abnormalities in children, and when acetabular lateral perspectives are unnecessary. Technically, this view is easier to obtain than is the true lateral shown in Figure 3-15.

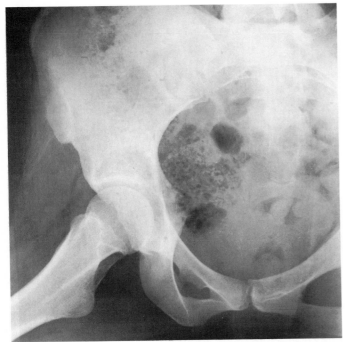

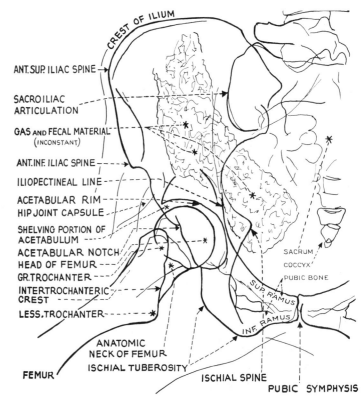

CREST OF ILIUM

ANT. SUP. ILIAC SPINE

SACROILIAC ARTICULATION

GAS AND FECAL MATERIAL (INCONSTANT)

ANT. INF. ILIAC SPINE

ILIOPECTINEAL LINE

ACETABULAR RIM

HIP JOINT CAPSULE

SHELVING PORTION OF ACETABULUM

ACETABULAR NOTCH

HEAD OF FEMUR

GR. TROCHANTER

INTERTROCHANTERIC CREST

LESS. TROCHANTER

ANATOMIC NECK OF FEMUR

ISCHIAL TUBEROSITY

FEMUR

ISCHIAL SPINE

PUBIC SYMPHYSIS

SACRUM

COCCYX

PUBIC BONE

SUP. RAMUS

INF. RAMUS

FIGURE 3-14. Lateral view of one hip, employing the "frog-leg" position (Cleaves position).

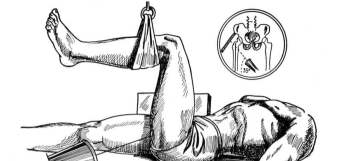

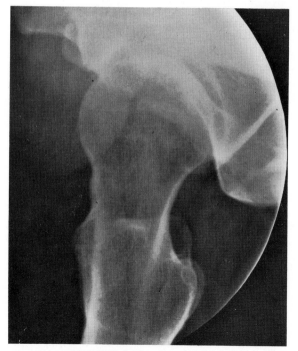

POINTS OF PRACTICAL INTEREST ABOUT FIGURE 3-15

1. The patient is placed in a supine position and the pelvis is elevated on a firm pillow or folded sheets, sufficiently to raise the ischial tuberosity approximately 3 cm. from the table top. This support of the gluteus must not extend beyond the lateral margin of the body so that it will not interfere with the placement of the cassette directly on the table top.

2. To localize the long axis of the femoral neck: (a) Draw a line between the anterior-superior iliac spine and the upper border of the pubic symphysis and mark its center point. (b) Next draw a line approximately 4 inches long perpendicular to this midpoint, extending down to the anterior surface of the thigh. This latter line represents the long axis of the femoral neck.

3. Adjust the central ray so that it is perpendicular to the midpoint of this long axis and adjust the film perpendicular to the table top so that the projection of this long axis will fall entirely upon the film.

4. If the foot is maintained in a vertical position the anteversion of the neck with respect to the shaft of the femur will be demonstrated. If the foot of the affected side is inverted approximately 15 degrees the plane of the neck will be parallel with the film and form a straight line with the axis of the shaft of the femur.

5. The unaffected side may be supported over the x-ray tube or by a sling from above as shown.

6. The thickness of the part traversed by the central ray is comparable with that of a lateral lumbar spine, and the same technical factors as for a lateral lumbar spine film should ordinarily be employed.

7. A grid cassette is a very desirable adjunct for this projection.

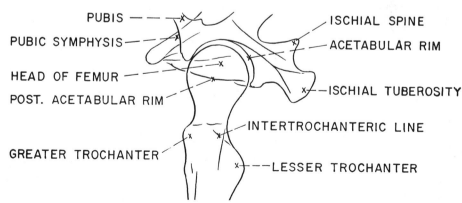

FIGURE 3-15. Routine lateral view of hip, employing a horizontal x-ray beam (Danelius-Miller Modification of Lorenz position).

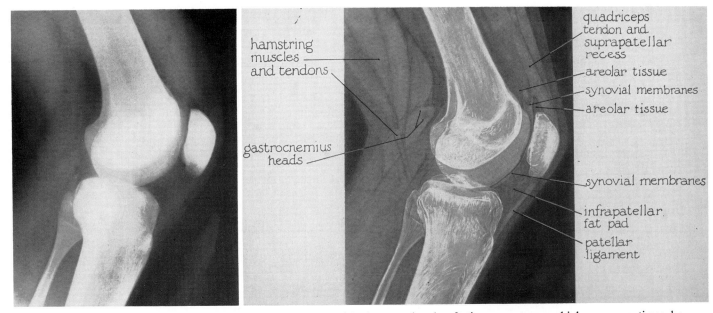

FIGURE 3-16. A normal lateral view of the knee with the associated soft tissue anatomy which can sometimes be identified by either routine views or viewing the film with a bright light. (From Lewis, R. W.: Am. J. Roentgenol. *65*, 1951.)

POINTS OF PRACTICAL INTEREST ABOUT FIGURE 3-17.

1. The knee should be completely extended with the patient in the supine position. If this cannot be done, the posteroanterior projection is preferable.

2. Alternately, if the knee cannot be fully extended, the cassette should be elevated on sandbags to bring it into closer contact with the popliteal space. If the degree of flexion of the knee is great, a curved cassette or curved film holder should be employed.

3. The leg is adjusted in the true anteroposterior position and the distal apex of the patella is noted.

4. Center the cassette and the central ray of the x-ray tube approximately 1 cm. below the patellar apex.

5. When radiographing the joint space it may be helpful to tilt the tube approximately 5 degrees cephalad. This expedient will help give a clear view of the knee joint space because it superimposes the anterior and posterior margins of the tibial plateau somewhat more satisfactorily.

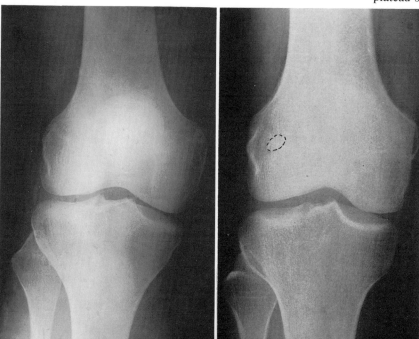

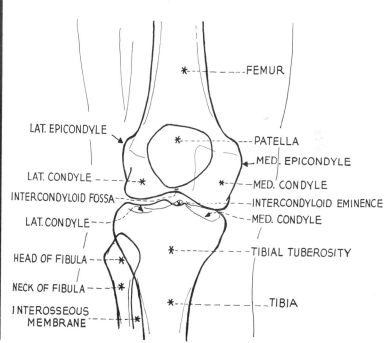

FIGURE 3-17. Routine anteroposterior view of knee. Radiograph at right demonstrates fabella; labeled tracing is of radiograph at left.

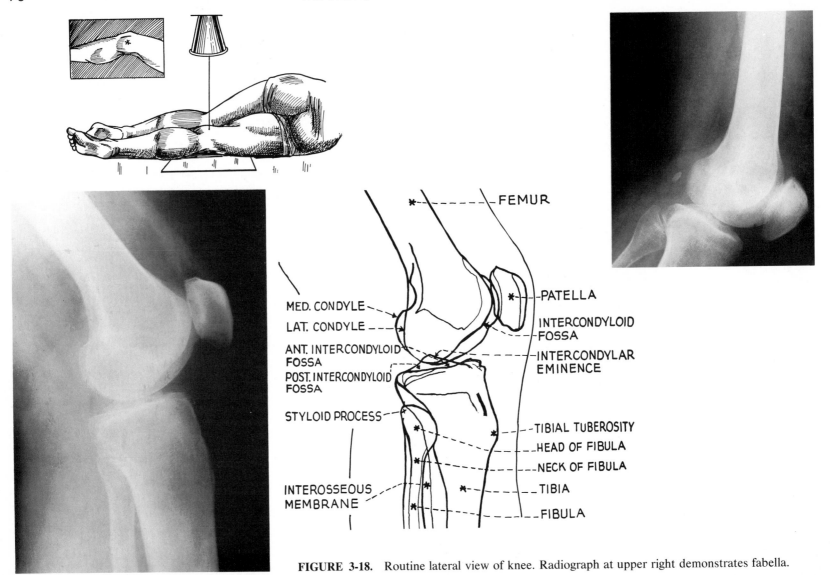

MED. CONDYLE

LAT. CONDYLE

ANT. INTERCONDYLOID
FOSSA

POST. INTERCONDYLOID
FOSSA

STYLOID PROCESS

INTEROSSEOUS
MEMBRANE

FEMUR

PATELLA

INTERCONDYLOID
FOSSA

INTERCONDYLAR
EMINENCE

TIBIAL TUBEROSITY

HEAD OF FIBULA

NECK OF FIBULA

TIBIA

FIBULA

FIGURE 3-18. Routine lateral view of knee. Radiograph at upper right demonstrates fabella.

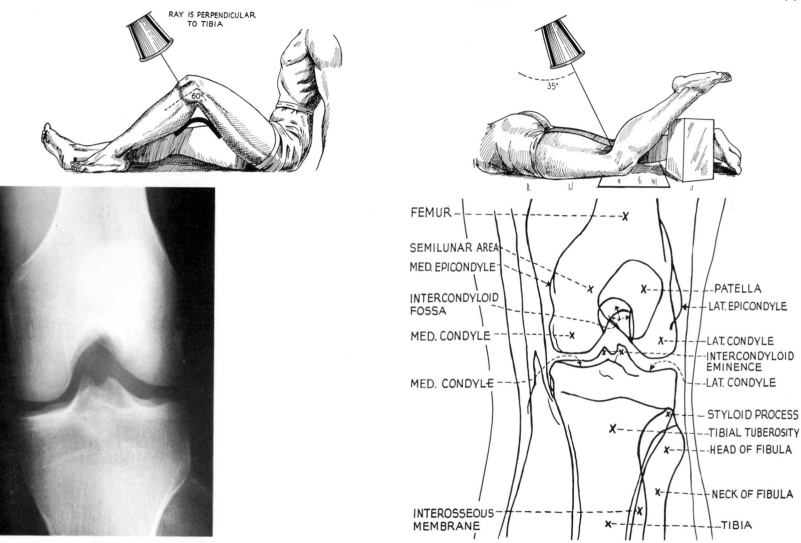

RAY IS PERPENDICULAR TO TIBIA

60°

35°

FEMUR — — — — — — — — — — — — X

SEMILUNAR AREA

MED. EPICONDYLE

INTERCONDYLOID FOSSA

MED. CONDYLE — — — — — — X

MED. CONDYLE — — — —

INTEROSSEOUS MEMBRANE

PATELLA

LAT. EPICONDYLE

LAT. CONDYLE

INTERCONDYLOID EMINENCE

LAT. CONDYLE

STYLOID PROCESS

TIBIAL TUBEROSITY

HEAD OF FIBULA

NECK OF FIBULA

TIBIA

FIGURE 3-19. Special view of intercondyloid fossa of femur. Very similar radiographs are obtained with alternate methods of positioning the patient. (Camp-Coventry position with patient prone; Béclère position with patient sitting.)

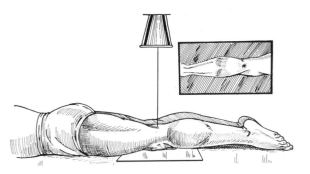

POINTS OF PRACTICAL INTEREST ABOUT FIGURE 3-20

1. The patient is placed in the prone position with the ankles and the feet usually supported by sandbags.

2. The film is centered to the patella and the central ray so adjusted as to pass through the center of the patella. The heel may have to be rotated outward slightly to accomplish this.

3. Ordinarily, it is desirable to use a telescopic cone and bring the cone fairly close to the knee in order to produce a distortion of the superimposed femoral condyles and a clearer concept of the patella, which lies next to the film.

4. This view definitely gives better detail of the patella than can be obtained in the anteroposterior projection.

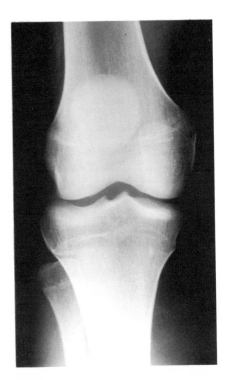

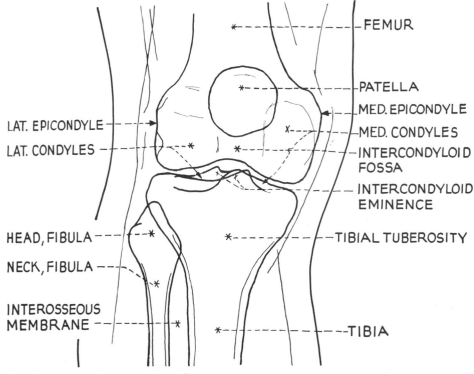

FIGURE 3-20. Posteroanterior view of patella.

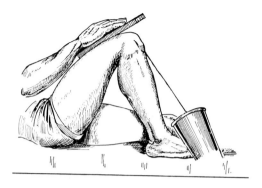

POINTS OF PRACTICAL INTEREST ABOUT FIGURE 3-21

1. This view may be obtained with the patient either prone or supine. In the prone position, the thigh is placed flat against the table and the leg flexed by means of a band wrapped around the ankle and the ends held by the patient's hand. If the patient is supine, the film is placed along the distal aspect of the thigh as shown.

2. The central ray is directed at right angles to the joint space between the patella and the femoral condyles; the degree of central ray angulation depends upon the degree of flexion of the knee. Ordinarily the central ray should be parallel to the articular margin of the patella.

3. The outer margin of the patella as projected in this view frequently presents a rather serrated and irregular appearance which must not be interpreted as abnormal. This serrated appearance is due to points of tendinous attachments to the bony substance of the patella, as well as to penetration by nutrient vessels.

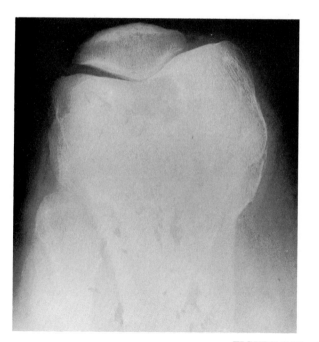

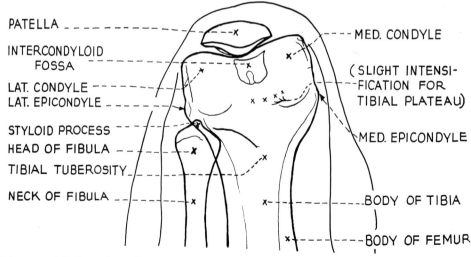

FIGURE 3-21. Special tangential view of patella (Settegast position).

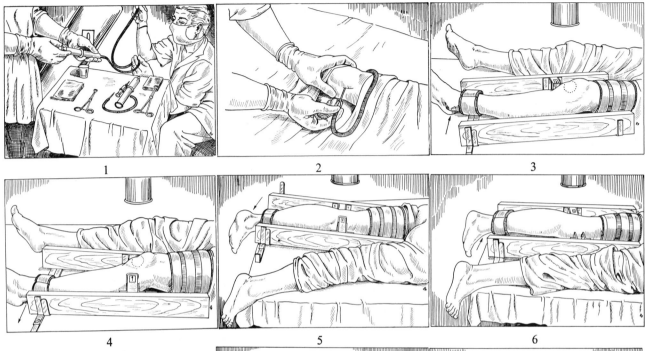

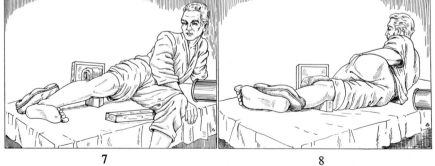

FIGURE 3-22. Routine technique of pneumoarthrography of the knee. **1,** Method of loading the 50 cc. syringes from the oxygen tank under sterile technique. **2,** Method of inserting needle under the superior margin of the patella into the suprapatellar bursa where 80 to 120 cc. of oxygen is thereafter injected. **3,** Method of positioning the patient for the anteroposterior view of the lateral meniscus. Note the lateral side of the knee joint is being spread by the special spreader device. **4,** Method of positioning patient for the anteroposterior view of the medial meniscus, spreading the medial side of the knee joint. **5,** Method of positioning patient for posteroanterior view of the lateral meniscus. **6,** Method of positioning patient for posteroanterior view of the medial meniscus. **7,** Method of positioning patient for a horizontal or decubitus view of the lateral meniscus in the anteroposterior projection. **8,** Method of positioning patient employing a horizontal x-ray beam spreading the medial joint space.

In both of these latter projections the oxygen rises to the top, giving one a maximum delineation of the topmost portion of the knee, still obtaining a spread visualization of the knee.

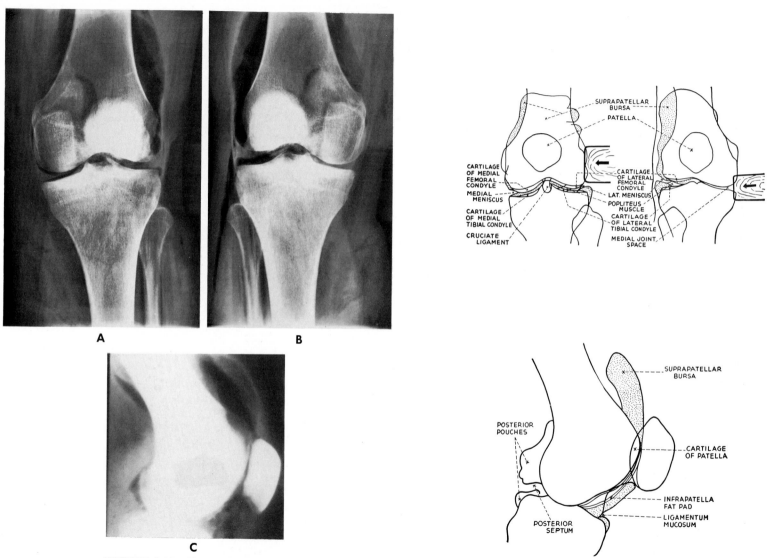

FIGURE 3-23.   Pneumoarthrography of the knee. Radiographs **A** and **B** were obtained in the posteroanterior projection, first with the medial knee joint spread, and next with the lateral knee joint spread; **C** shows the knee in a straight lateral projection.

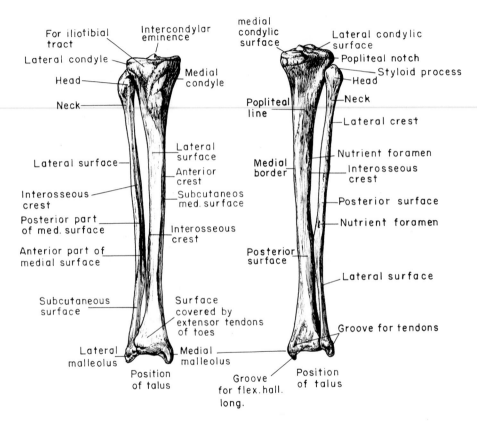

Anterior Aspect   Posterior Aspect

FIGURE 3-24.   Tibia and fibula, anterior and posterior aspects.

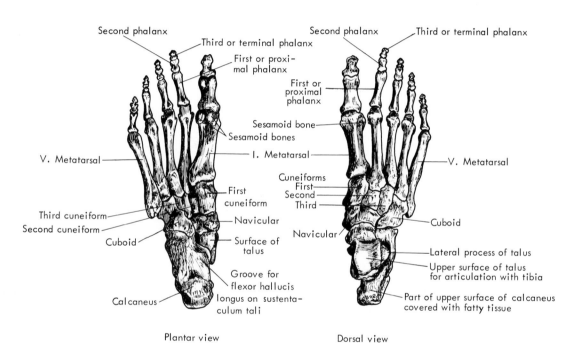

Second phalanx

Third or terminal phalanx

First or proximal phalanx

Sesamoid bones

V. Metatarsal

First cuneiform

Third cuneiform

Second cuneiform

Cuboid

Navicular

Surface of talus

Groove for flexor hallucis longus on sustentaculum tali

Calcaneus

Plantar view

Second phalanx

Third or terminal phalanx

First or proximal phalanx

Sesamoid bone

I. Metatarsal

Cuneiforms
First
Second
Third

Navicular

V. Metatarsal

Cuboid

Lateral process of talus

Upper surface of talus for articulation with tibia

Part of upper surface of calcaneus covered with fatty tissue

Dorsal view

FIGURE 3-25. Plantar and dorsal views of foot.

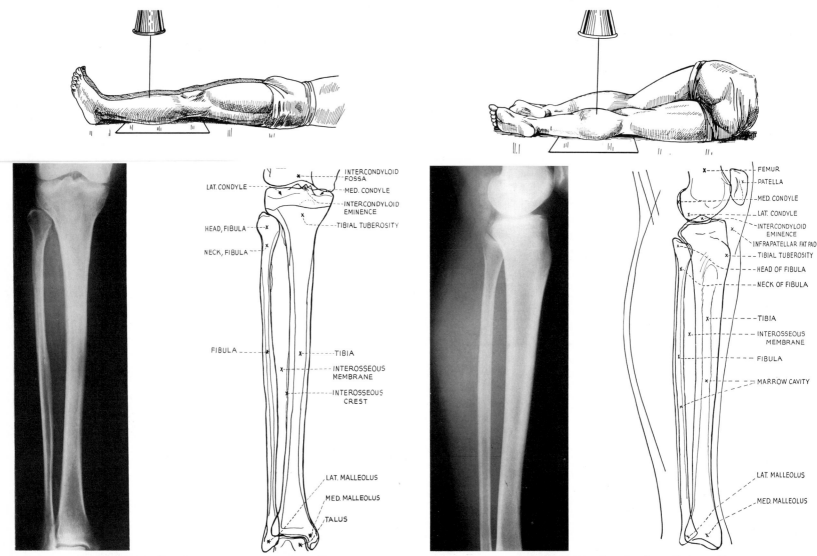

FIGURE 3-26.   Routine anteroposterior view of leg.

FIGURE 3-27.   Routine lateral view of leg.

POINTS OF PRACTICAL INTEREST ABOUT FIGURE 3-28

1. If less overlapping of the distal tibia and fibula is desired, the foot should be inverted slightly. This expedient will increase the clarity of the lateral malleolus particularly, but will interfere with the measurement of the distance between the talal articular margin and the malleoli.

2. In young individuals, in whom the distal epiphyses of the tibia and fibula are not yet united to their respective shafts, it is particularly important to obtain comparison films of the opposite normal side. It may otherwise be very difficult to be certain of the absence of a slight fracture through the epiphyseal disk.

3. Although the ligaments around the ankle are not visualized radiographically, it is important to know their relationships accurately. Often the more important aspect of injury to the ankle concerns the ligamentous rather than the bony abnormality.

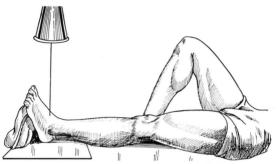

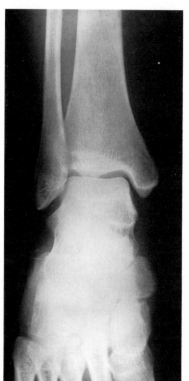

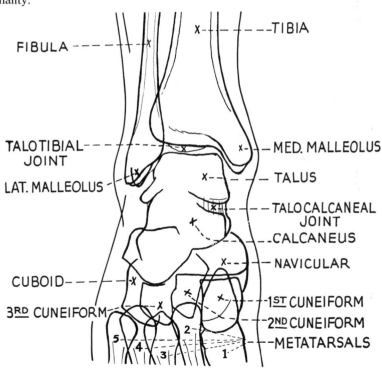

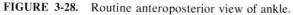

FIGURE 3-28.   Routine anteroposterior view of ankle.

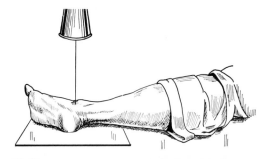

POINTS OF PRACTICAL INTEREST ABOUT FIGURE 3-29

1. The affected leg and ankle are so placed that the sagittal plane of the leg is perfectly parallel with the table top and film. The film holder and central ray are centered to a point approximately 2 cm. proximal to the tip of the lateral malleolus. A sandbag or balsa wood block placed under the distal one-third of the foot facilitates true alignment.

2. The unaffected side is sharply flexed and placed in a comfortable position forward so that there will be no movement during the x-ray exposure.

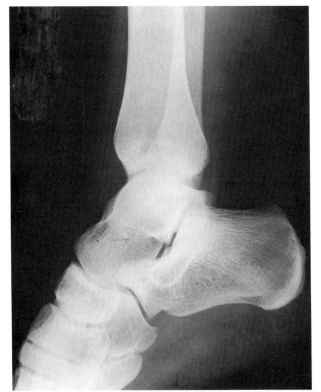

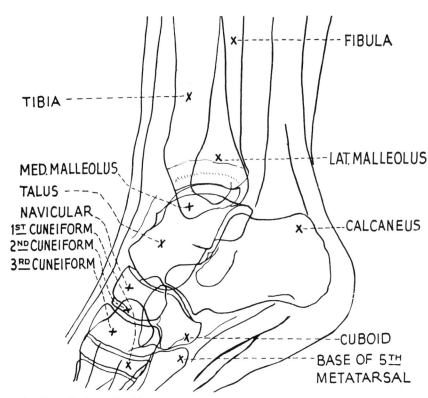

FIGURE 3-29. Routine lateral view of ankle.

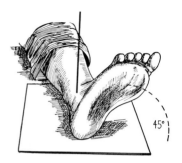

POINTS OF PRACTICAL INTEREST ABOUT FIGURE 3-30

1. As much as possible, keep the leg in the anteroposterior position while inverting the foot approximately 45 degrees. Immobilize with sandbags placed across the leg and against the plantar surface of the foot.

2. The central ray is directed to the middle of the talotibial joint.

3. This view permits an unobstructed projection of the lateral malleolus and of the space between the talus and malleolus where so frequently injury may be manifest.

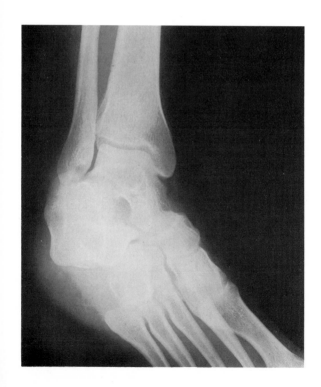

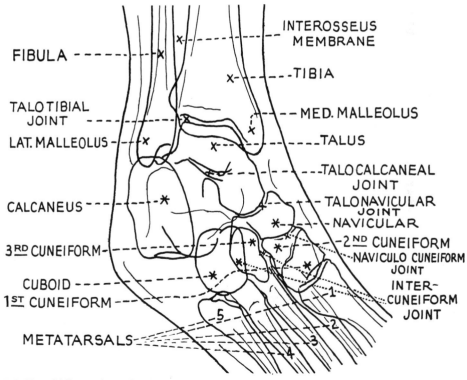

FIGURE 3-30. Oblique view of ankle.

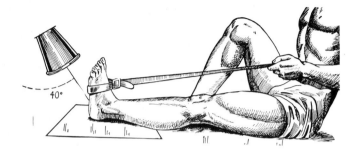

POINTS OF PRACTICAL INTEREST ABOUT FIGURE 3-31

1. The ankle is placed over the film so that the talotibial joint falls over the central portion of the film.

2. The plantar surface of the foot should be at as near to a right angle with the table top and film as possible in acute flexion.

3. The central ray should be centered to the midpoint of the film. It will usually enter the plantar surface at the level of the bases of the fifth metatarsals and emerge in the region of the upper tarsus.

4. Ordinarily all portions of the calcaneus are included between the tuberosity and the sustentaculum tali.

5. An alternate view may be obtained by placing the patient prone, film perpendicular to the table top in contact with the sole of the foot, and directing the central ray through the heel with 45 degree caudad angulation.

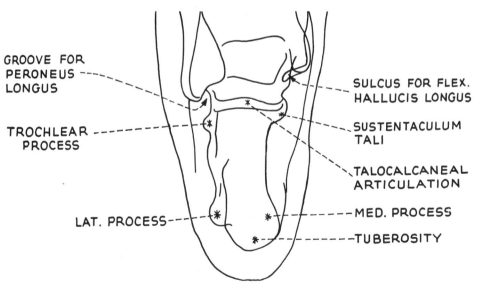

FIGURE 3-31. Special tangential view of calcaneus.

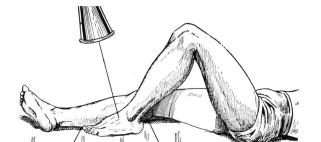

POINTS OF PRACTICAL INTEREST ABOUT FIGURE 3-32

1. It will be noted that for visualization of the entire tarsus, both this view and the anteroposterior view of the ankle (Fig. 3-28) are necessary. The talus is not shown to good advantage in this projection, whereas the more distal tarsal bones are not presented clearly in the anteroposterior view of the ankle.

2. For special problems, this view may also be required with the patient standing and bearing his weight.

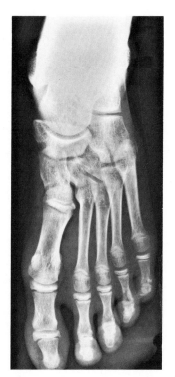

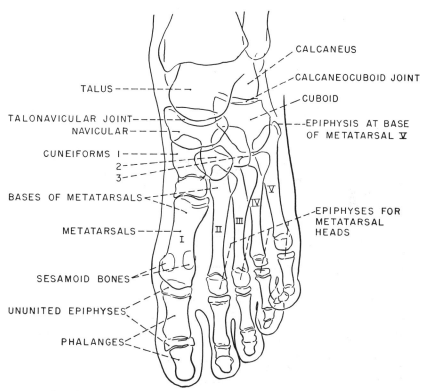

FIGURE 3-32. Anteroposterior view of foot.

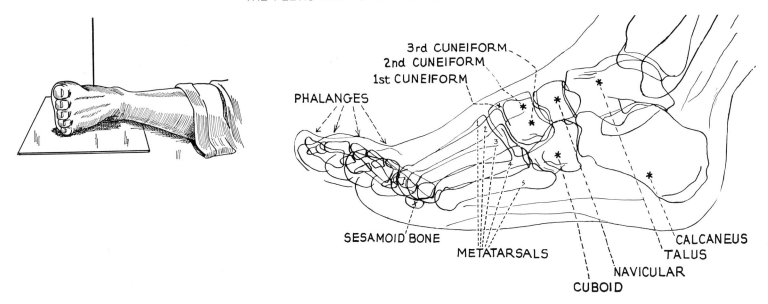

3rd CUNEIFORM
2nd CUNEIFORM
1st CUNEIFORM

PHALANGES

SESAMOID BONE

METATARSALS

CUBOID

NAVICULAR

CALCANEUS
TALUS

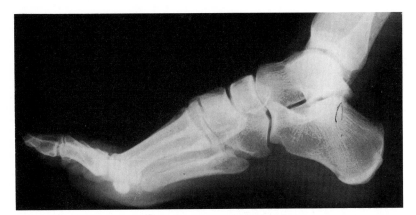

FIGURE 3-33. Lateral view of foot.

POINTS OF PRACTICAL INTEREST ABOUT FIGURE 3-33

1. The knee may be elevated slightly on a sandbag so that the sagittal plane of the foot is perfectly parallel with the table top and film. The center of the tarsus is placed over the center of the film.

2. The ankle is immobilized by means of a sandbag.

3. The recumbent position is utilized to demonstrate the bony structure particularly. If one is desirous of showing the longitudinal arch under weight-bearing conditions, an erect film is obtained with the patient standing, but in rather similar fashion.

4. If a coned-down lateral view of the body of the calcaneus is desired, the foot is positioned similarly, but the central ray passes through the central portion of the calcaneus rather than through the center of the tarsus. The latter view of the calcaneus is particularly valuable for demonstration of Boehler's critical angle.

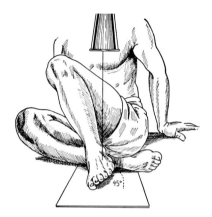

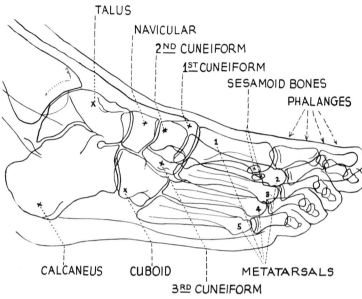

TALUS
NAVICULAR
2ND CUNEIFORM
1ST CUNEIFORM
SESAMOID BONES
PHALANGES

CALCANEUS   CUBOID   METATARSALS
3RD CUNEIFORM

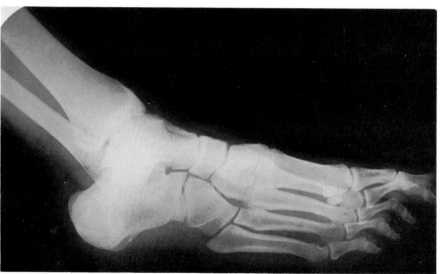

FIGURE 3-34.   Oblique view of foot.

POINTS OF PRACTICAL INTEREST ABOUT FIGURE 3-34

1. This view is particularly valuable *(a)* to demonstrate the intertarsal joints; *(b)* to outline the various tarsal bones more clearly; *(c)* to demonstrate the joint between the tarsus and the fourth and fifth metatarsals as well as the structural detail of the base of the fifth metatarsal.

2. This oblique projection is employed when structural detail of the bones of the foot is of paramount interest. It is ordinarily employed along with the anteroposterior projection of the foot. When, however, we desire to localize a foreign body accurately, it is the true lateral projection of the foot which is employed instead of this oblique projection.

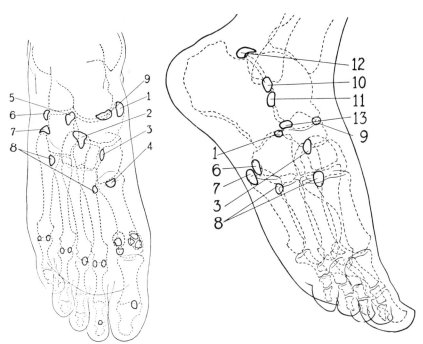

FIGURE 3-35. Schematic diagram to show sesamoid bones and supernumerary bones of the foot. 1, Os tibiale externum; 2, processus uncinatus; 3, intercuneiforme; 4, pars peronea metatarsalia I; 5, cuboides secundarium; 6, os peroneum; 7, os vesalianum; 8, intermetatarseum; 9, accessory navicular; 10, talus accessorius; 11, os sustentaculum; 12, os trigonum; 13, calcaneus secundarius. The most common of these are: 1, 6, 7, 9 and 12. (From McNeill, C.: *Roentgen Technique,* Charles C Thomas.)

KITE POSITIONS FOR CONGENITAL CLUBFOOT STUDIES

Kite positions are exactly positioned dorsoplantar and lateral projections for radiography of the congenital clubfoot. No attempt is made to change the unusual relationship of the bones when placing the foot on the film or cassette.

The dorsoplantar projection demonstrates the degree of adduction of the forefoot and the degree of inversion of the calcaneus. The central ray must be directed exactly vertical to the tarsus.

The lateral view demonstrates the anterior talar subluxation and the degree of plantar, equinus flexion. The central ray is directed vertically to the midtarsal area.

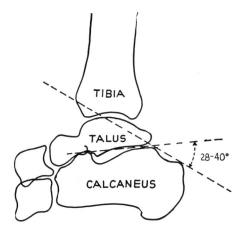

FIGURE 3-36. The criteria for a normal calcaneus (Boehler).

Chapter 4 — The Skull

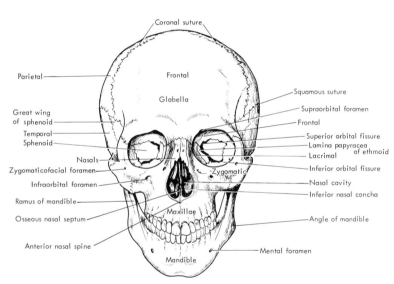

FIGURE 4-1A. Skull viewed from its frontal aspect.

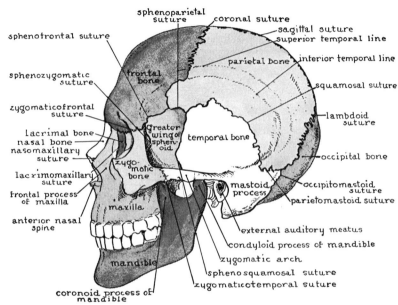

FIGURE 4-1B. Lateral view of the skull showing the bones of the calvarium, face and mandible. (From Pendergrass, E. P., Schaeffer, J. P., and Hodes, P. J.: *The Head and Neck in Roentgen Diagnosis*. Charles C Thomas.)

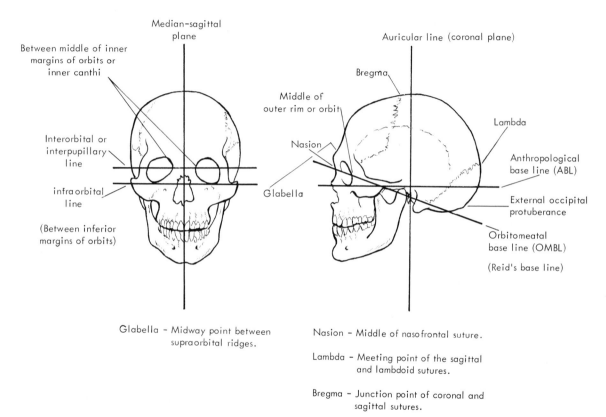

Median-sagittal plane

Between middle of inner margins of orbits or inner canthi

Interorbital or interpupillary line

infraorbital line

(Between inferior margins of orbits)

Auricular line (coronal plane)

Bregma

Middle of outer rim or orbit

Nasion

Glabella

Lambda

Anthropological base line (ABL)

External occipital protuberance

Orbitomeatal base line (OMBL)

(Reid's base line)

Glabella – Midway point between supraorbital ridges.

Nasion – Middle of nasofrontal suture.

Lambda – Meeting point of the sagittal and lambdoid sutures.

Bregma – Junction point of coronal and sagittal sutures.

FIGURE 4-2. Commonly used reference points and lines on skull. Reid's base line, originally described as a line from the infraorbital rim to the external auditory meatus, is seldom used as a reference line because the canthomeatal line, from the outer canthus of the eye to the external auditory meatus, is more clearly defined on the patient.

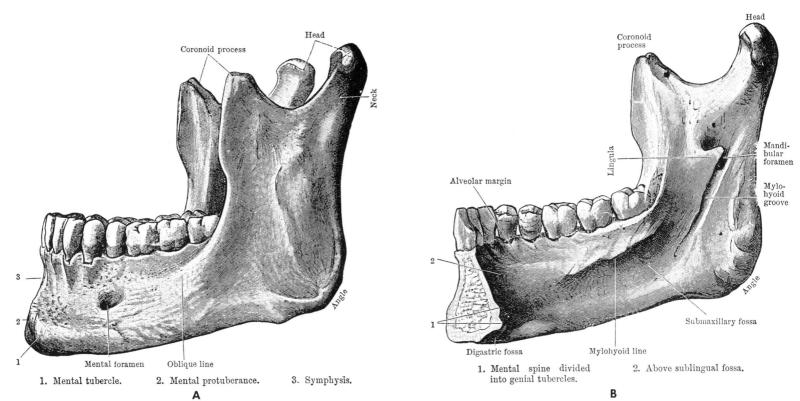

1. Mental tubercle.   2. Mental protuberance.   3. Symphysis.

A

1. Mental spine divided   2. Above sublingual fossa.
   into genial tubercles.

B

FIGURE 4-3.   A, Mandible, seen from the left side. **B,** Medial surface of the right half of the mandible. (From Cunningham, D. J.: *Textbook of Anatomy,* edited by A. Robinson. Oxford University Press.)

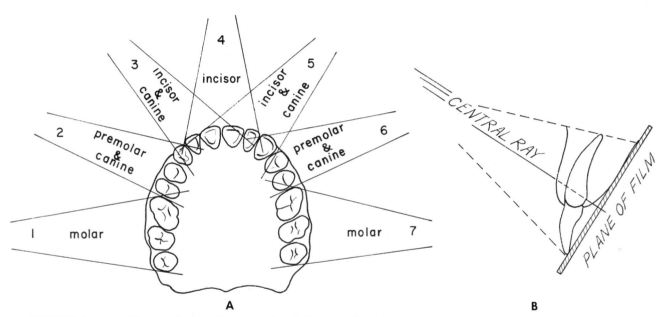

4

3

5

incisor

incisor
&
canine

incisor
&
canine

2

premolar
&
canine

6

premolar
&
canine

1   molar

molar   7

A

CENTRAL RAY

PLANE OF FILM

B

FIGURE 4-4.   A, The usual seven intraoral dental films obtained for each dental arch. **B,** The angulation of the central ray with respect to the tooth and film. ("Bite-wing films" for demonstration of crown cavities are not illustrated. Refer to dental x-ray technique manuals.)

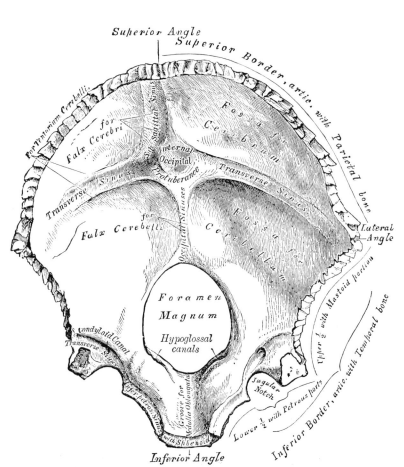

FIGURE 4-5. The occipital bone, inner surface. (From Gray, H.:
Gray's Anatomy of the Human Body, edited by C. M. Goss. Lea & Febiger.

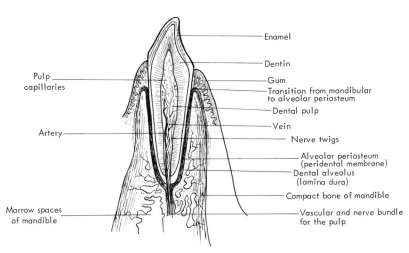

FIGURE 4-6. Vertical section of inferior canine tooth in situ.

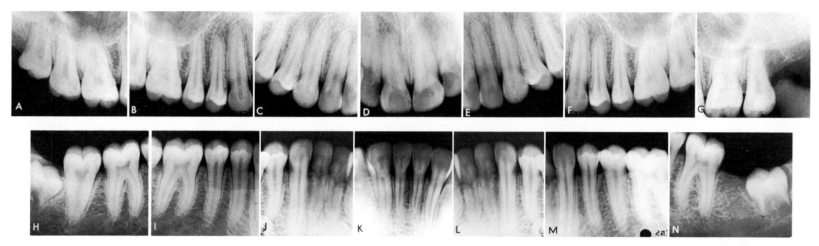

FIGURE 4-7. Representative intraoral dental films: **A**, Right upper molar area; **B**, right upper bicuspid area; **C**, right upper cuspid area; **D**, upper incisor area; **E**, left upper cuspid area; **F**, left upper bicuspid area; **G**, left upper molar area; **H**, right lower molar area; **I**, right lower bicuspid area; **J**, right lower cuspid area; **K**, lower incisor area; **L**, left lower cuspid area; **M**, left lower bicuspid area; **N**, left lower molar area.

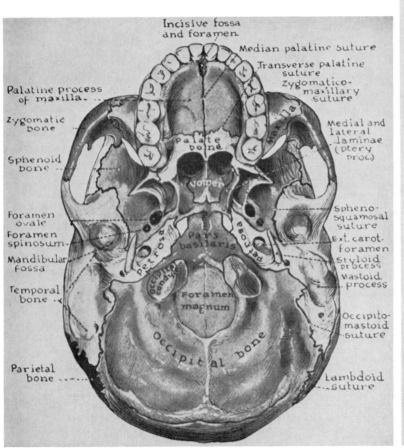

FIGURE 4-8. The skull viewed from below. (From Pendergrass, E. P., Schaeffer, J. P., and Hodes, P. J.: *The Head and Neck in Roentgen Diagnosis*. Charles C Thomas.)

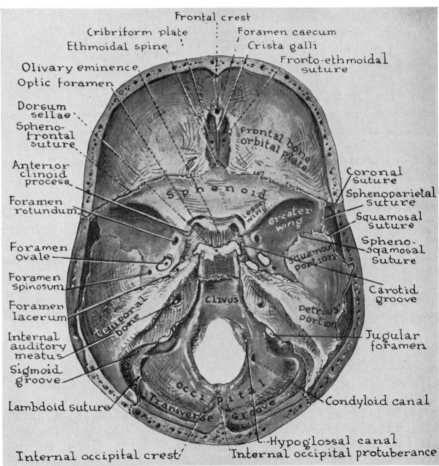

FIGURE 4-9. Internal aspect of the base of the skull. (From Pendergrass, E. P., Schaeffer, J. P., and Hodes, P. J.: *The Head and Neck in Roentgen Diagnosis*. Charles C Thomas.)

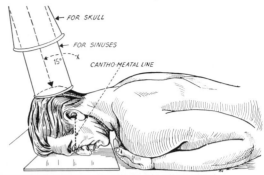

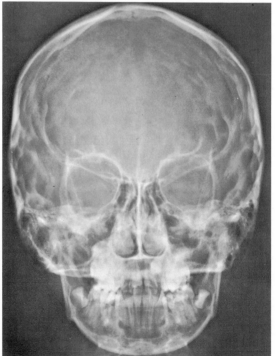

POINTS OF PRACTICAL INTEREST ABOUT FIGURE 4-10

1. The patient's head is adjusted so that the sagittal plane is perfectly perpendicular to the table top and so that the canthomeatal line (outer canthus of the eye to the tragus of the ear or external acoustic meatus) is perpendicular to the plane of the film also. It may be necessary to support the patient's chin on either his fist or a folded towel.

2. The central ray is centered to the glabella and angled toward the feet approximately 15 degrees with respect to the canthomeatal line.

3. It will be noted that in this view the petrous ridges are projected near the inferior margins of the orbits, and hence a clearer concept of the orbits is obtained than would be possible without the 15 degree angulation. Also the lesser and greater wings of the sphenoid bone are projected in the orbits. In the straight postero-anterior view of the skull these are obscured by the petrous ridges, which are for the most part projected into the orbits.

4. If the frontal bone in itself is the point of major interest, a straight postero-anterior view of the frontal bone is obtained without angulation of the tube.

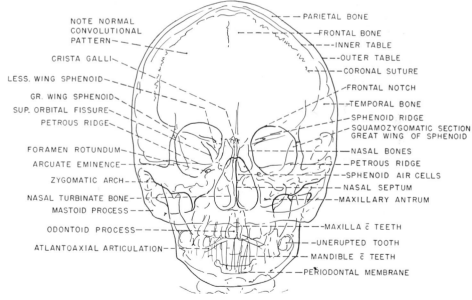

FIGURE 4-10. Caldwell's projection of the skull: Note that patient is positioned so that the canthomeatal line is perpendicular to the film. (The original Caldwell projection for sinuses was 23 degrees with respect to the glabellomeatal line, which is the same as 15 degrees with respect to the canthomeatal line, but more variable and hence a less accurate designation.)

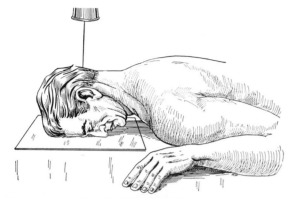

POINTS OF PRACTICAL INTEREST ABOUT FIGURE 4-11

1. It will be noted that this view differs from the Caldwell position in that the central ray of the x-ray tube is perpendicular to the film and coincides with the canthomeatal line. It will be noted that the petrous ridges are projected into the orbits, completely obscuring the orbital contents. The sphenoid ridges are projected over the petrous ridges and likewise are considerably obscured.

2. The posterior instead of the anterior cells of the ethmoidal sinuses are shown, and the dorsum sellae is seen as a curved line extending between the orbits just above the ethmoids.

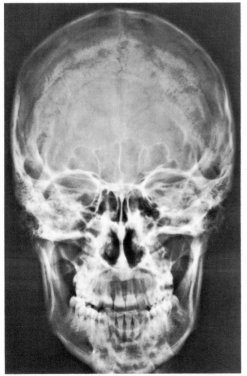

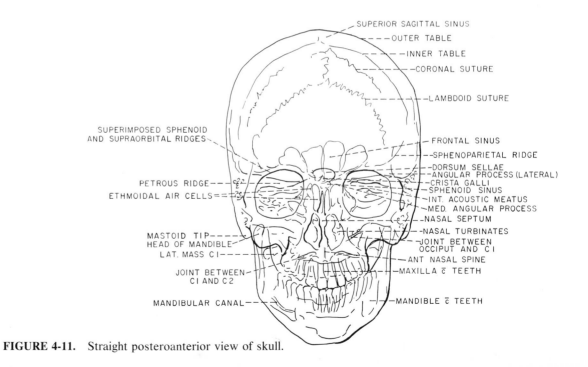

FIGURE 4-11.   Straight posteroanterior view of skull.

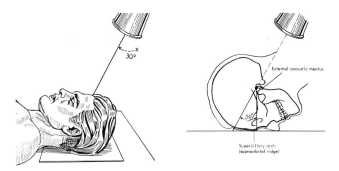

POINTS OF PRACTICAL INTEREST ABOUT FIGURE 4-12

1. The sagittal plane of the patient is placed perpendicular to the table top and along the midline of the table.

2. The head is adjusted so that the canthomeatal line is approximately perpendicular to the table top. This will require that the chin be somewhat depressed upon the neck.

3. The central ray is adjusted at an angle of 30 degrees toward the feet so that it enters the forehead ordinarily at the hairline, and leaves the posterior portion of the cranium in the region of the external occipital protuberance.

4. For better projection of the dorsum sellae into the foramen magnum a somewhat greater angle than 30 degrees may be employed (up to 45 degrees).

5. A view of similar value may be obtained with the patient prone and the tube angled 30 degrees toward the head rather than toward the feet. In the latter instance the central ray enters the head in the region of the external occipital protuberance and leaves the forehead approximately 4 cm. above the superciliary arches. This is called the *reverse Towne's projection*, nuchofrontal projection or Haas position.

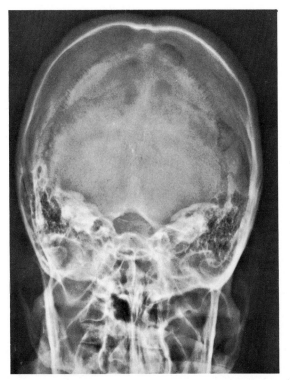

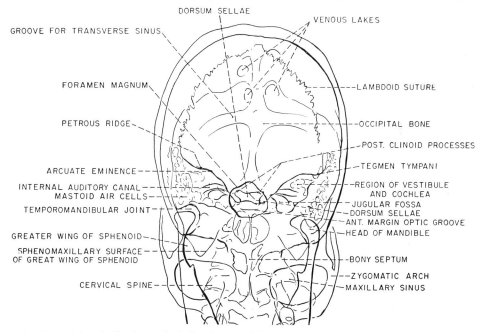

FIGURE 4-12.   Towne's projection of the skull, also called Grashey position.

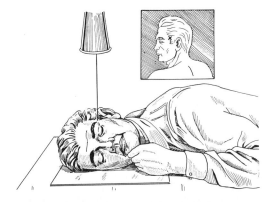

POINTS OF PRACTICAL INTEREST ABOUT FIGURE 4-13

1. The position of the head is adjusted so that its sagittal plane is parallel with the table top and with the film. Its coronal plane is centered to the longitudinal axis of the table. The film is placed transversely in the Potter-Bucky diaphragm beneath the skull.

2. A support is placed under the chin; usually the clenched fist of the patient is adequate in this regard.

3. The central ray passes through a point one inch above the midpoint of the line joining the outer canthus of the eye with the tragus of the ear (canthomeatal line). This will ordinarily fall immediately over the sella turcica.

4. To evaluate a good lateral projection the two halves of the mandible should be almost perfectly superimposed over one another. If the two rami of the mandible are obliquely projected at fair distances from each other, the projection of the skull is too oblique and should be repeated.

5. It is to be noted that a rather oblique and distorted view of the upper cervical spine is obtained in this lateral view of the skull. This view must not be used routinely for examination of this segment of cervical spine.

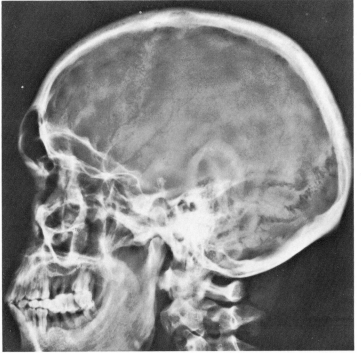

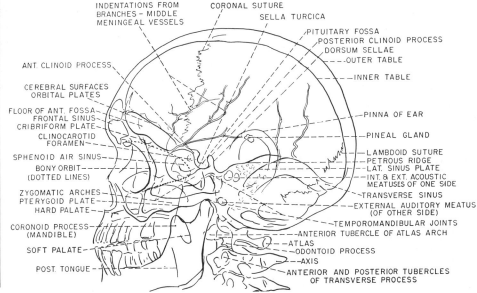

FIGURE 4-13.   Lateral view of skull.

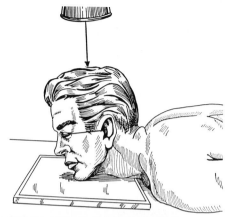

POINTS OF PRACTICAL INTEREST ABOUT FIGURE 4-14

1. The head should be rested on the fully extended chin. The more nearly perpendicular the line of the face is to the film, the more satisfactory will be this projection.

2. If possible, the canthomeatal line should be parallel with the table top and film.

3. The central ray should pass through the sagittal plane of the skull perpendicular to the canthomeatal line at its midpoint. It may be necessary to angle the central ray caudally to maintain this relationship if the patient is unable to extend the chin sufficiently.

4. This view is particularly valuable for visualization of the facial bones in tangential projection. It is used along with the frontal view of the facial bones in every instance.

5. This view is also of value for visualization of the posterior ethmoid and sphenoid cells.

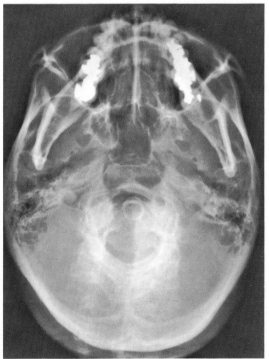

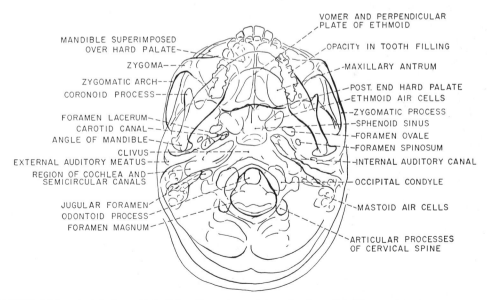

FIGURE 4-14.   Axial view of skull (verticosubmental projection; Schüller position).

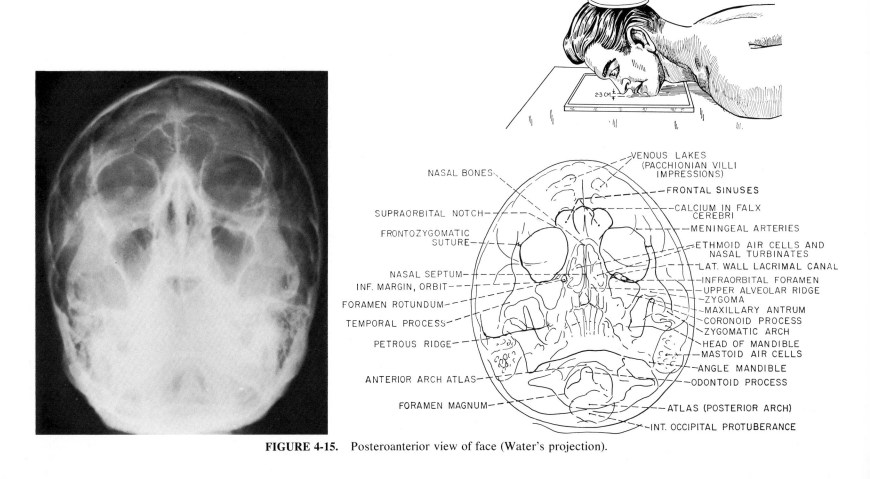

for Skull

for Sinuses

2-3 CM

VENOUS LAKES
(PACCHIONIAN VILLI
IMPRESSIONS)

NASAL BONES

FRONTAL SINUSES

CALCIUM IN FALX
CEREBRI

SUPRAORBITAL NOTCH

MENINGEAL ARTERIES

FRONTOZYGOMATIC
SUTURE

ETHMOID AIR CELLS AND
NASAL TURBINATES

LAT. WALL LACRIMAL CANAL

NASAL SEPTUM

INFRAORBITAL FORAMEN

INF. MARGIN, ORBIT

UPPER ALVEOLAR RIDGE

ZYGOMA

FORAMEN ROTUNDUM

MAXILLARY ANTRUM

CORONOID PROCESS

TEMPORAL PROCESS

ZYGOMATIC ARCH

HEAD OF MANDIBLE

PETROUS RIDGE

MASTOID AIR CELLS

ANGLE MANDIBLE

ANTERIOR ARCH ATLAS

ODONTOID PROCESS

ATLAS (POSTERIOR ARCH)

FORAMEN MAGNUM

INT. OCCIPITAL PROTUBERANCE

FIGURE 4-15.   Posteroanterior view of face (Water's projection).

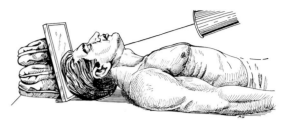

POINTS OF PRACTICAL INTEREST ABOUT FIGURE 4-16

1. The film and the patient's head are placed so that the canthomeatal line is parallel with the surface of the film.

2. The central ray is directed perpendicular to the midpoint of the canthomeatal line in the sagittal plane of the patient's skull.

3. A similar view may be obtained in the sitting posture with the patient's head leaned backward against a firm support; or in the supine position by placing a pillow under the upper back. Wherever possible a grid cassette or Potter-Bucky diaphragm should be employed.

4. In this view a clearer concept of the anterior ethmoidal cells is obtained and ordinarily the facial bones and mandible are projected over one another.

5. This view is also of value for visualization of the zygomatic arches, since they are thrown into bold relief by means of this projection. However, a lighter exposure technique must be employed for this purpose.

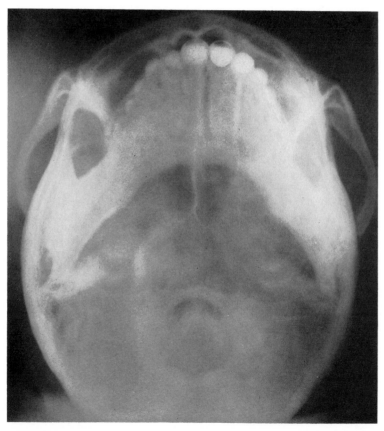

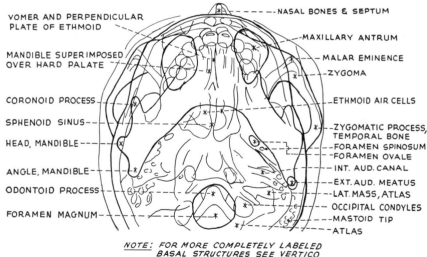

FIGURE 4-16. Axial view of face (submentovertical view): Using a slightly "lighter" exposure technique, this view is utilized for visualization of the zygomatic arches in the inferosuperior projection.

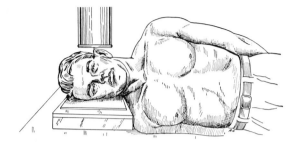

POINTS OF PRACTICAL INTEREST ABOUT FIGURE 4-17

1. The sagittal plane of the head is adjusted so that it is perfectly parallel with the film and the table top.

2. The cassette may be placed directly under the head without utilizing the Potter-Bucky diaphragm provided that the extended cone is likewise placed directly in contact with the opposite side of the head.

3. Center to the region of the sella turcica over a point 2.5 cm. anterior to and 2 cm. above the external acoustic meatus. Alternately one may center at a point about 2 cm. above the midpoint of the canthomeatal line.

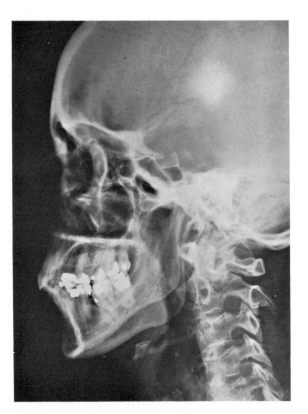

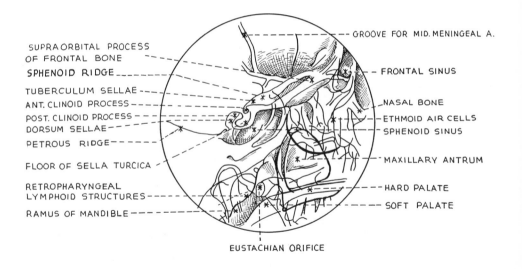

SUPRAORBITAL PROCESS OF FRONTAL BONE	GROOVE FOR MID. MENINGEAL A.
SPHENOID RIDGE	FRONTAL SINUS
TUBERCULUM SELLAE	
ANT. CLINOID PROCESS	NASAL BONE
POST. CLINOID PROCESS	ETHMOID AIR CELLS
DORSUM SELLAE	SPHENOID SINUS
PETROUS RIDGE	
FLOOR OF SELLA TURCICA	MAXILLARY ANTRUM
RETROPHARYNGEAL LYMPHOID STRUCTURES	HARD PALATE
RAMUS OF MANDIBLE	SOFT PALATE

EUSTACHIAN ORIFICE

FIGURE 4-17.   Lateral view of face.

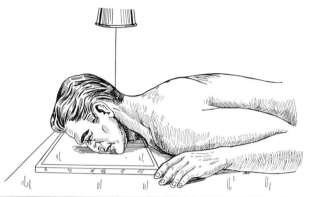

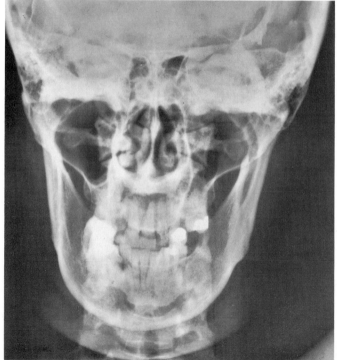

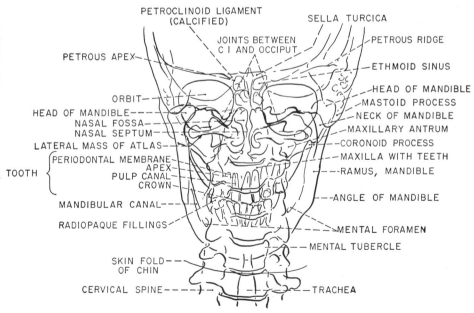

PETROCLINOID LIGAMENT
(CALCIFIED)

SELLA TURCICA

JOINTS BETWEEN
C I AND OCCIPUT

PETROUS RIDGE

PETROUS APEX

ETHMOID SINUS

ORBIT

HEAD OF MANDIBLE

HEAD OF MANDIBLE

MASTOID PROCESS

NASAL FOSSA

NECK OF MANDIBLE

NASAL SEPTUM

MAXILLARY ANTRUM

LATERAL MASS OF ATLAS

CORONOID PROCESS

PERIODONTAL MEMBRANE

MAXILLA WITH TEETH

APEX

RAMUS, MANDIBLE

TOOTH

PULP CANAL

CROWN

ANGLE OF MANDIBLE

MANDIBULAR CANAL

RADIOPAQUE FILLINGS

MENTAL FORAMEN

MENTAL TUBERCLE

SKIN FOLD
OF CHIN

CERVICAL SPINE

TRACHEA

FIGURE 4-18. Posteroanterior view of mandible.

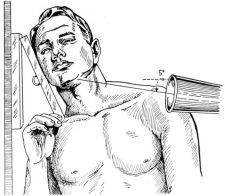

POINTS OF PRACTICAL INTEREST ABOUT FIGURE 4-19

1. The film is placed against the patient's cheek at an angle of approximately 15 degrees from the vertical.

2. The broad surface of the mandibular body is placed parallel to the plane of the film.

3. To avoid distortion a long target-to-film distance may be employed.

4. For better detail of the ramus of the mandible, the central ray may be directed inward, centering over the ramus, which may be brought into a position more directly parallel with the plane of the film.

5. If more information is desired regarding the body of the mandible near the symphysis, the head is rotated so that this area is nearer the film.

6. It is ordinarily easier to obtain an erect position of the injured mandible than the recumbent, although the recumbent view may be obtained in somewhat similar fashion.

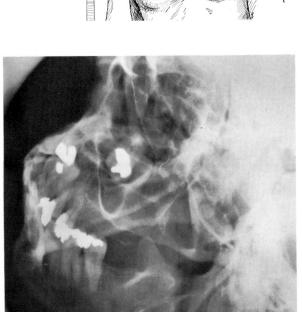

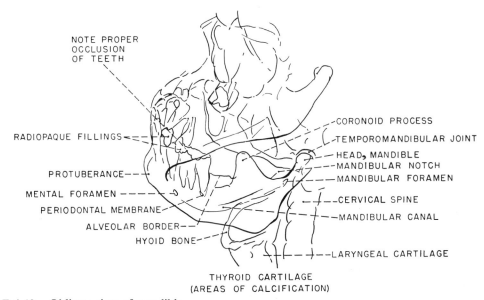

NOTE PROPER OCCLUSION OF TEETH

RADIOPAQUE FILLINGS

PROTUBERANCE

MENTAL FORAMEN

PERIODONTAL MEMBRANE

ALVEOLAR BORDER

HYOID BONE

CORONOID PROCESS

TEMPOROMANDIBULAR JOINT

HEAD, MANDIBLE

MANDIBULAR NOTCH

MANDIBULAR FORAMEN

CERVICAL SPINE

MANDIBULAR CANAL

LARYNGEAL CARTILAGE

THYROID CARTILAGE (AREAS OF CALCIFICATION)

FIGURE 4-19. Oblique view of mandible.

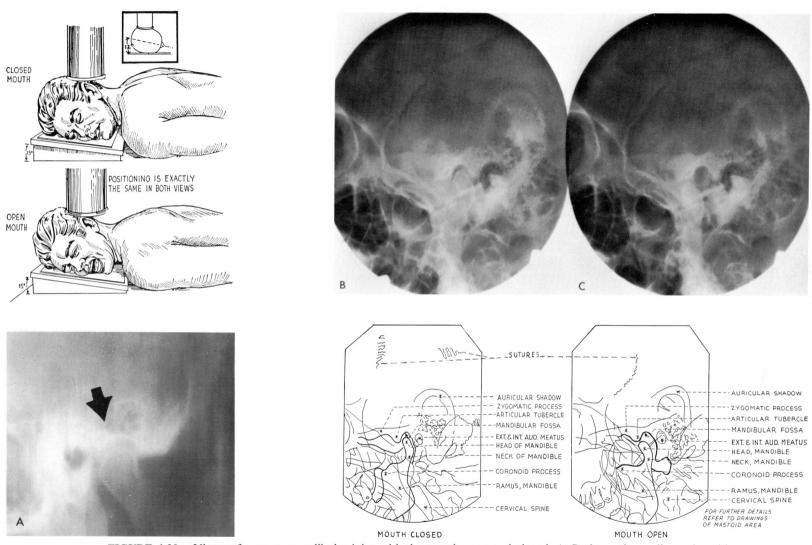

FIGURE 4-20. Views of temporomandibular joint with the mouth open and closed. **A,** Body-section radiography with mouth closed; B, and **C,** LogEtronic prints of radiographs.

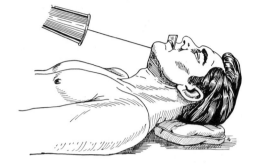

NOTES ABOUT USE OF OCCLUSAL FILMS AROUND THE MOUTH

These are frequently used for detection of calculi in salivary glands and ducts, and in conjunction with oblique and lateral films of the face in "sialograms"—radiographs of the salivary ducts and glands following the injection of iodized oil into the appropriate duct.

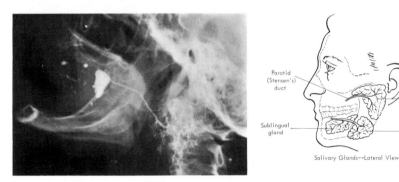

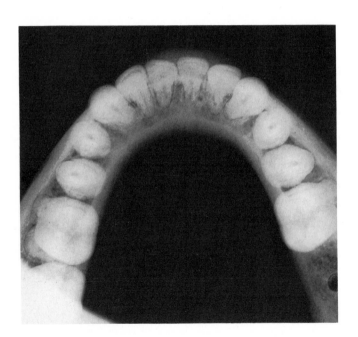

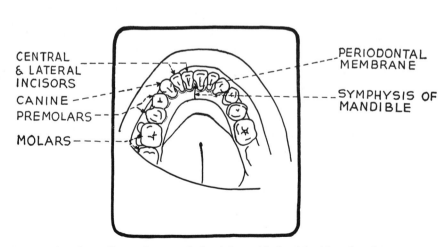

FIGURE 4-21. Occlusal view of mandible (intraoral) and sialogram showing salivary ducts and gland (parotid gland in this example).

FIGURE 4-23. Lateral view of nasolacrimal system: *a,* lacrimal puncta; *b,* canaliculi; *c,* lacrimal sac; *d,* lacrimal duct. Contrast medium, 1 to 2 cc. warmed Beck's bismuth and oil paste. (From Pendergrass, E. P., Schaeffer, J. P., and Hodes, P. J.: *The Head and Neck in Roentgen Diagnosis.* Charles C Thomas.)

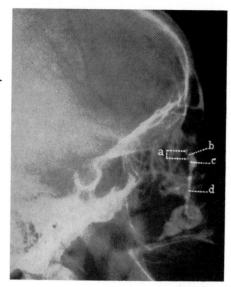

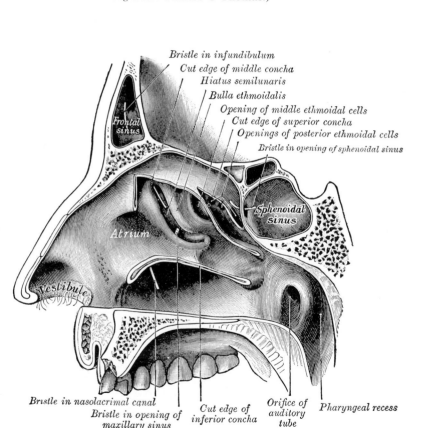

FIGURE 4-22. Lateral wall of nasal cavity to demonstrate apertures leading into it. (From Gray, H.: *Gray's Anatomy of the Human Body,* edited by C. M. Goss. Lea & Febiger.)

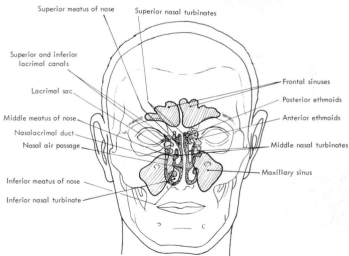

FIGURE 4-24. Frontal diagram of face showing position of nasal air passages and related frontal and maxillary paranasal sinuses.

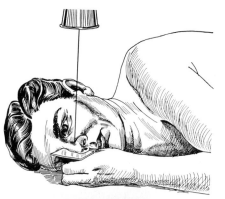

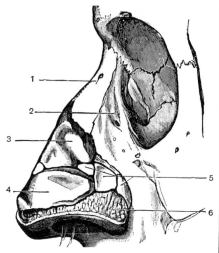

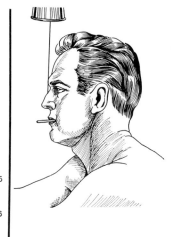

FIGURE 4-25. Diagram to illustrate bones and cartilages of external nose. *1.* Nasal bone: *2,* frontal processes of maxilla; *3,* lateral cartilage; *4,* greater alar cartilage; *5,* lesser alar cartilage; *6,* fatty tissue of ala nasi. (From C. M. West in Cunningham, D. J.: *Textbook of Anatomy.* Oxford University Press.)

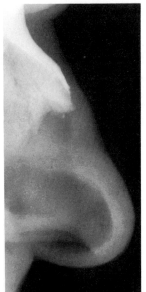

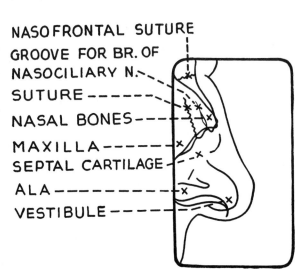

NASOFRONTAL SUTURE
GROOVE FOR BR. OF
NASOCILIARY N.
SUTURE
NASAL BONES
MAXILLA
SEPTAL CARTILAGE
ALA
VESTIBULE

FIGURE 4-26. Lateral view of nasal bones.

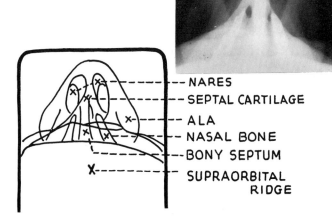

NARES
SEPTAL CARTILAGE
ALA
NASAL BONE
BONY SEPTUM
SUPRAORBITAL RIDGE

FIGURE 4-27. Tangential superoinferior view of nasal bones.

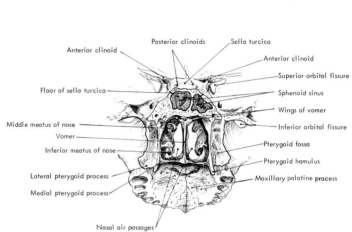

FIGURE 4-28. Coronal section through nasopharynx viewed from posterior aspect and showing osseous posterior nasal apertures.

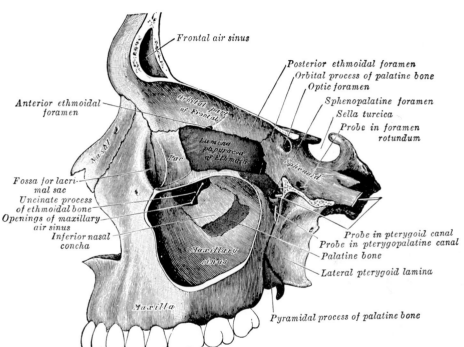

FIGURE 4-29. Left maxillary sinus opened from lateral side. (From Gray, H.: *Gray's Anatomy of the Human Body,* edited by C. M. Goss. Lea & Febiger.)

POINTS OF PRACTICAL INTEREST ABOUT FIGURE 4-30

1. In this view, the petrous ridge is projected along the inferior margin of the orbit. The anatomic structures of major interest here are: the frontal sinuses; the ethmoid sinuses; the bony nasal septum; and the orbital contents, not including the optic foramina, however. The superior orbital fissure, with the bony structures immediately surrounding it, is seen to maximum advantage. These margins must be clearly identified.

2. Although the maxillary antra can be delineated here, they are not seen to good advantage because they are obscured by the projection of the petrous ridges.

3. The degree of aeration of the nasal air passages is also of importance, and can be evaluated in this projection. The middle and superior nasal turbinates can usually be identified. When these latter structures are swollen or hypertrophied, interference with aeration may result.

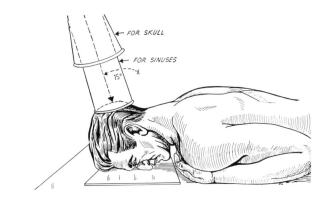

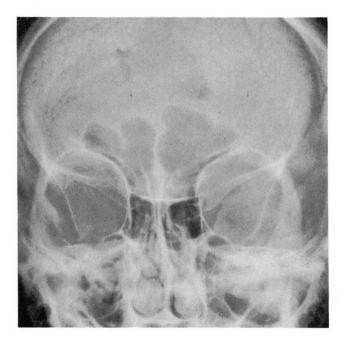

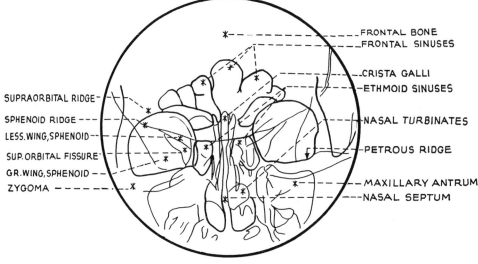

FIGURE 4-30.   Caldwell's projection for the paranasal sinuses.

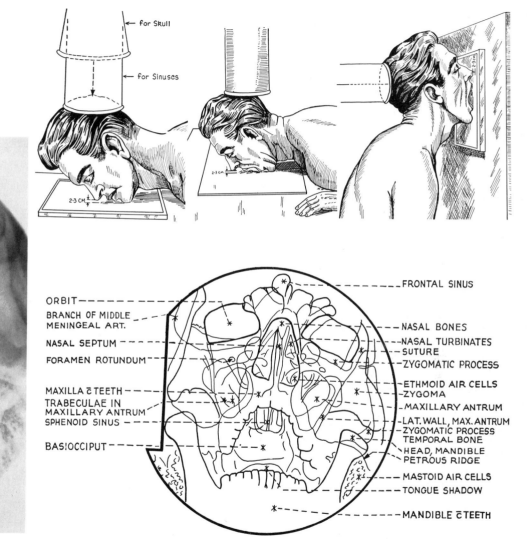

ORBIT
BRANCH OF MIDDLE
MENINGEAL ART.
NASAL SEPTUM
FORAMEN ROTUNDUM

MAXILLA c̄ TEETH
TRABECULAE IN
MAXILLARY ANTRUM
SPHENOID SINUS

BASIOCCIPUT

FRONTAL SINUS

NASAL BONES
NASAL TURBINATES
SUTURE
ZYGOMATIC PROCESS
ETHMOID AIR CELLS
ZYGOMA
MAXILLARY ANTRUM
LAT. WALL, MAX. ANTRUM
ZYGOMATIC PROCESS
TEMPORAL BONE
HEAD, MANDIBLE
PETROUS RIDGE
MASTOID AIR CELLS
TONGUE SHADOW
MANDIBLE c̄ TEETH

for Skull
for Sinuses

FIGURE 4-31. Water's projection for the paranasal sinuses. Drawings show positioning of patient with mouth closed, with mouth open, and for erect film; radiograph and tracing show mouth open. The view through the open mouth to show the sphenoid sinuses is also called the Pirie transoral projection.

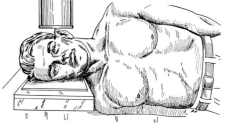

POINTS OF PRACTICAL INTEREST ABOUT FIGURE 4-32

1. The structures which must be clearly identified in this view are: the frontal sinuses; the sphenoid sinuses; the sella turcica; the retropharyngeal lymphoid structures and adjoining air space.

2. The maxillary antra and ethmoids may have confusing appearances, since so many anatomic structures are projected over one another in these planes. The nasal turbinates especially may simulate the appearance of a tumor within the maxillary antra.

3. The walls of the orbits are considerably obscured, but some effort should be made to delineate these as well as is possible.

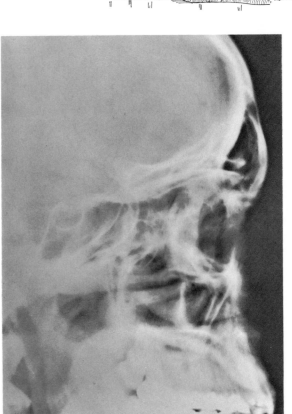

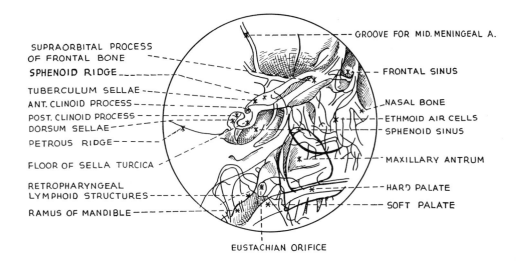

SUPRAORBITAL PROCESS OF FRONTAL BONE
SPHENOID RIDGE
TUBERCULUM SELLAE
ANT. CLINOID PROCESS
POST. CLINOID PROCESS
DORSUM SELLAE
PETROUS RIDGE
FLOOR OF SELLA TURCICA
RETROPHARYNGEAL LYMPHOID STRUCTURES
RAMUS OF MANDIBLE

GROOVE FOR MID. MENINGEAL A.
FRONTAL SINUS
NASAL BONE
ETHMOID AIR CELLS
SPHENOID SINUS
MAXILLARY ANTRUM
HARD PALATE
SOFT PALATE

EUSTACHIAN ORIFICE

FIGURE 4-32.   Lateral projection of paranasal sinuses.

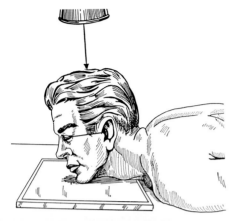

POINTS OF PRACTICAL INTEREST ABOUT FIGURE 4-33

In contrast with the similar view for visualization of the base of the skull, the cassette may be placed immediately beneath the patient's chin, at table-top level, rather than in the Bucky tray with Bucky technique. Under these circumstances, a cylindrical cone is placed directly on the patient's head, with the central ray perpendicular to Reid's base line. If the patient's neck cannot be sufficiently extended, the edge of the cassette farthest from the chin may be raised on a towel, so that it will be closely applied to the lower jaw, and the central ray may be angled so that it is at least perpendicular to the infraorbital meatal line.

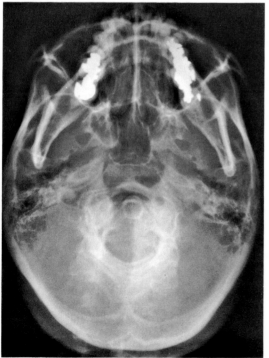

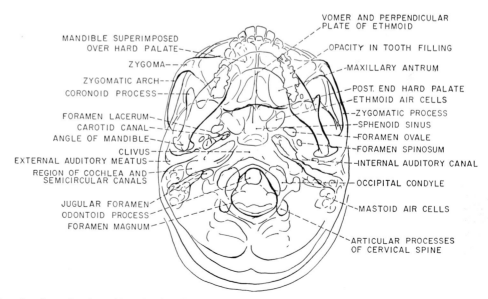

VOMER AND PERPENDICULAR PLATE OF ETHMOID
MANDIBLE SUPERIMPOSED OVER HARD PALATE
OPACITY IN TOOTH FILLING
ZYGOMA
MAXILLARY ANTRUM
ZYGOMATIC ARCH
CORONOID PROCESS
POST. END HARD PALATE
ETHMOID AIR CELLS
ZYGOMATIC PROCESS
FORAMEN LACERUM
SPHENOID SINUS
CAROTID CANAL
FORAMEN OVALE
ANGLE OF MANDIBLE
FORAMEN SPINOSUM
CLIVUS
INTERNAL AUDITORY CANAL
EXTERNAL AUDITORY MEATUS
REGION OF COCHLEA AND SEMICIRCULAR CANALS
OCCIPITAL CONDYLE
JUGULAR FORAMEN
MASTOID AIR CELLS
ODONTOID PROCESS
FORAMEN MAGNUM
ARTICULAR PROCESSES OF CERVICAL SPINE

FIGURE 4-33. Verticosubmental view of skull for visualization of sphenoid and ethmoid paranasal sinuses (modified Schüller position).

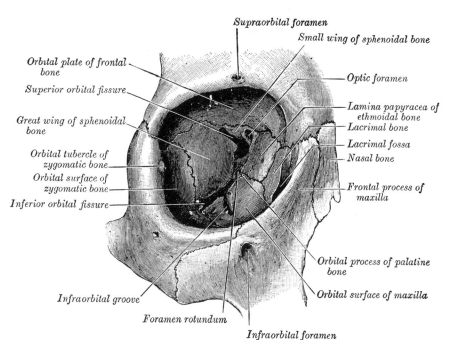

FIGURE 4-34. The anatomy of the orbit. (From Gray, H.: *Gray's Anatomy of the Human Body,* edited by C. M. Goss. Lea & Febiger.)

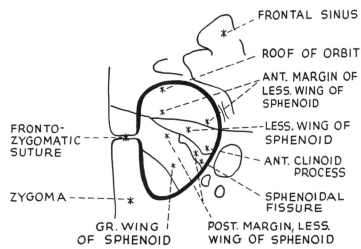

FIGURE 4-35. Tracing of orbital projection obtained by Caldwell's position.

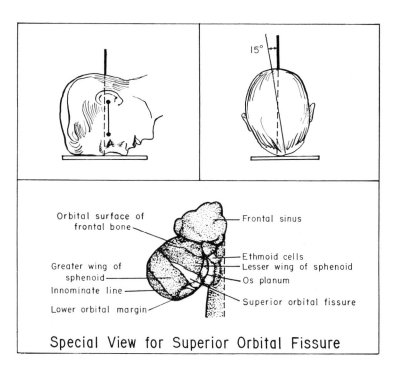

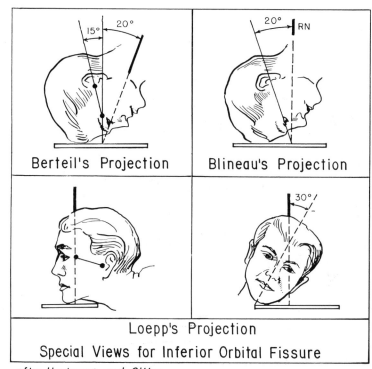

after Hartmann and Gilles

FIGURE 4-36. Special techniques for examination of the orbit, apart from the usual views of the facial bones previously demonstrated.

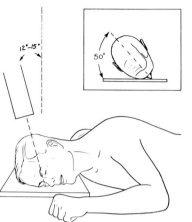

POINTS OF PRACTICAL INTEREST ABOUT FIGURE 4-37

1. The position of the patient in this view is identical to that of Stenvers' view of the petrous ridges. The central ray of the x-ray beam, however, is directed 12 degrees *toward the feet,* if the angulated beam is employed, instead of 12 degrees *toward the head* (Stenvers' view).

2. When one studies optic foramina, the two sides are compared with one another; hence, equivalent views of the two sides must be obtained.

3. The ethmoid air cells are also clearly delineated here to best advantage.

4. In the Rhese position, the patient's head is angled 53°, and the central ray is not angled.

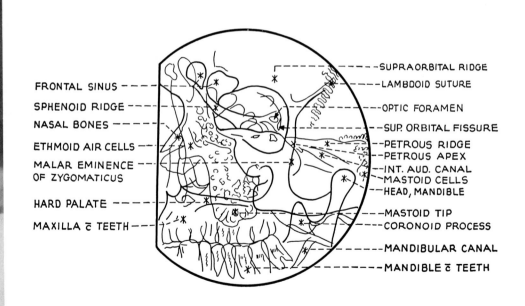

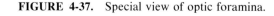

FIGURE 4-37. Special view of optic foramina.

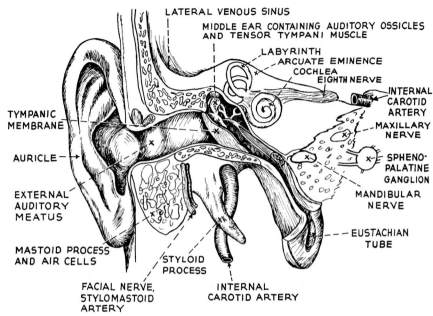

FIGURE 4-38. Anatomy of the temporal bone.

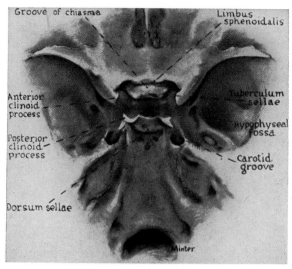

FIGURE 4-39. A common type of sella turcica. (From Pendergrass, E. P., Schaeffer, J. P., and Hodes, P. J.: *The Head and Neck in Roentgen Diagnosis.* Charles C Thomas.)

LINE OF DIAPHRAGMA SELLAE

ANT. CLINOID PROCESSES

POSTERIOR CLINOID PROCESSES

TUBERCULUM SELLAE

DORSUM SELLAE

SPHENOID

A-B = GREATEST ANTERO-POSTERIOR DIAMETER

C-D = GREATEST DEPTH

E-F = POSITION OF DIAPHRAGMA SELLAE

A

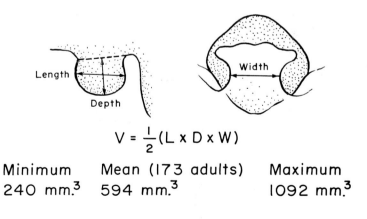

$$V = \frac{1}{2}(L \times D \times W)$$

Minimum
240 mm.^{3}

Mean (173 adults)
594 mm.^{3}

Maximum
1092 mm.^{3}

B

FIGURE 4-40. **A,** Method of measuring sella turcica (Camp). **B,** Volume of sella turcica (Di Chiro and Nelson method).

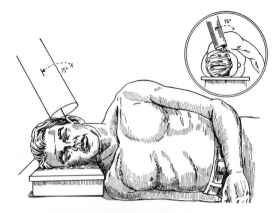

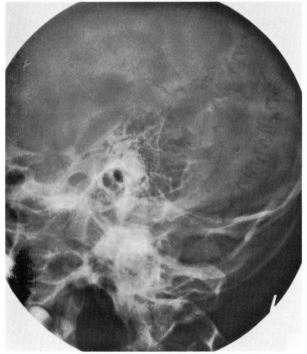

POINTS OF PRACTICAL INTEREST ABOUT FIGURE 4-41

1. There are actually two different ways of obtaining this projection—both acceptable. The alternative to the one shown is by placing a 15 degree angle board under the patient's head and utilizing a central ray that is perpendicular to the table top and centered to the mastoid process which is closest to the film. Thus, instead of angling the tube as shown here, the patient's head is angled an equivalent amount instead.

2. The routine recommended for study of this projection is as follows:

   (a) Note the degree of pneumatization, and whether the cells are diploic, small, mixed or large.

   (b) Note the relative radiolucency of the cells, and the integrity of their walls.

   (c) Trace the integrity of the lateral sinus plate.

   (d) Locate and state the size of the emissary vein.

   (e) Study the auditory meatuses for erosion or enlargement.

   (f) Note the integrity of the temporomandibular joint.

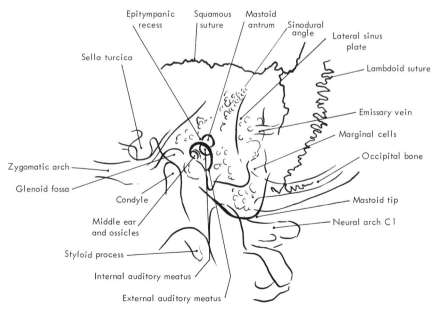

FIGURE 4-41. Lateral projection of mastoid process (Law's position).

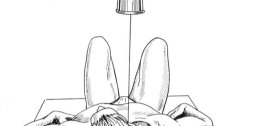

POINTS OF PRACTICAL INTEREST ABOUT FIGURE 4-42

    1. The auricles of the ears should be folded forward to avoid the projection of the pinna over the mastoid structures.

    2. The smallest possible cone should be employed at a fairly close target-to-film distance (25 to 30 inches). The head is rotated 45 degrees away from the side being radiographed, and the tube is angled 15 degrees caudally, centering over the midpoint of the canthomeatal line.

    3. In this view the mastoid process is projected away from the rest of the calvarium, and the mastoid cells in the tip of the process are shown to best advantage. A rather light exposure technique must be employed to gain this view. This same projection, however, may also be used to visualize the petrous portion of the temporal bone if a somewhat heavier exposure technique is employed.

    4. Comparison films between the two mastoids are always obtained.

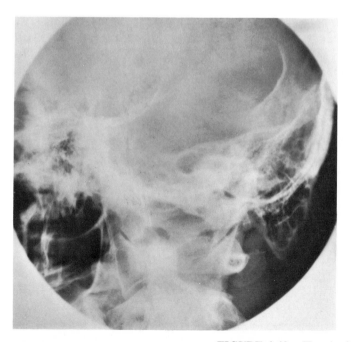

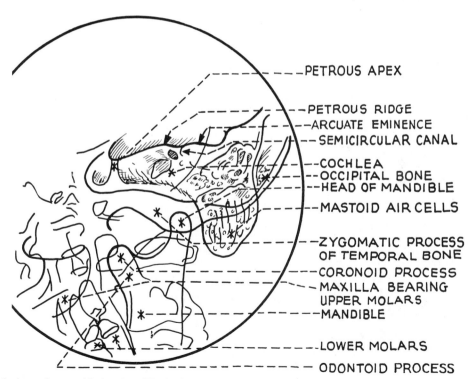

FIGURE 4-42. Tangential view of mastoid tips (modified Hickey position).

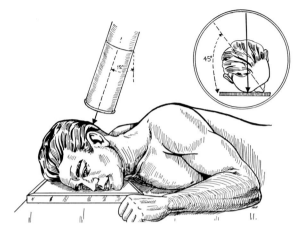

POINTS OF PRACTICAL INTEREST ABOUT FIGURE 4-43

1. Position the patient's head so that the tip of the nose, the point of the chin, and the outer canthus of the eye are all in contact with the plane of the film. This will place the head at an angle of approximately 45 degrees with respect to the film.

2. Adjust the central ray so that it passes to the midpoint of the film at an angle of 12 degrees.

3. In this position the petrous ridge is parallel with the plane of the film and its longest axis is shown to best advantage.

4. This view may also be utilized for visualization of the tips of the mastoid cells if a lighter exposure technique is employed. However, when satisfactory exposure factors are utilized to see the innermost aspect of the petrous ridge, the mastoid air cells and the tips of the mastoids will not be seen to good advantage except in an extremely bright light.

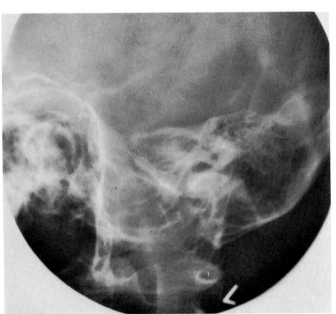

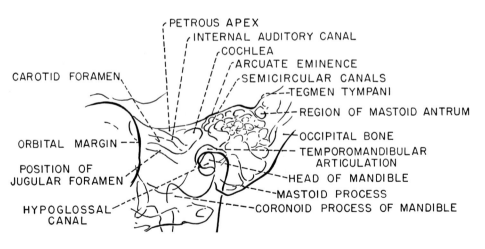

FIGURE 4-43. Stenvers' view of petrous ridge.

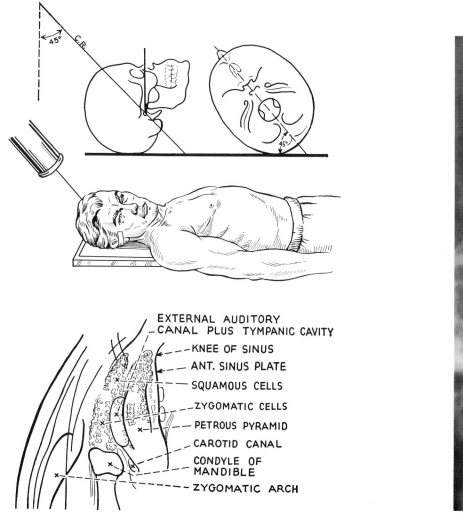

EXTERNAL AUDITORY
CANAL PLUS TYMPANIC CAVITY
— KNEE OF SINUS
— ANT. SINUS PLATE
— SQUAMOUS CELLS
— ZYGOMATIC CELLS
— PETROUS PYRAMID
— CAROTID CANAL
CONDYLE OF
MANDIBLE
— ZYGOMATIC ARCH

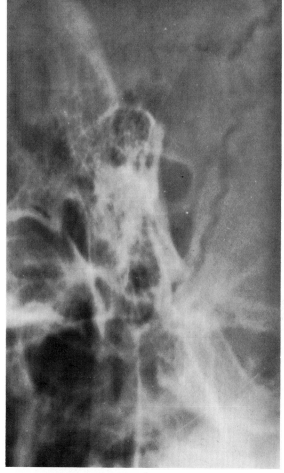

FIGURE 4-44. Mayer's position for examination of petrous ridge and mastoids. Schematic drawing made from a radiograph.

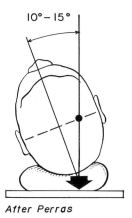

10° – 15°

25° – 30°

—Plane of Virchow

After Perras

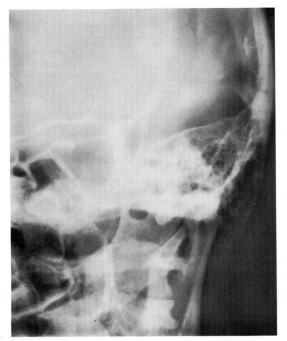

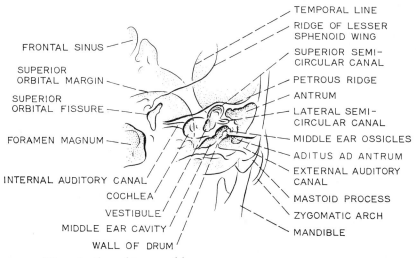

TEMPORAL LINE

RIDGE OF LESSER
SPHENOID WING

SUPERIOR SEMI-
CIRCULAR CANAL

FRONTAL SINUS

PETROUS RIDGE

SUPERIOR
ORBITAL MARGIN

ANTRUM

SUPERIOR
ORBITAL FISSURE

LATERAL SEMI-
CIRCULAR CANAL

MIDDLE EAR OSSICLES

FORAMEN MAGNUM

ADITUS AD ANTRUM

EXTERNAL AUDITORY
CANAL

INTERNAL AUDITORY CANAL

COCHLEA

MASTOID PROCESS

VESTIBULE

ZYGOMATIC ARCH

MIDDLE EAR CAVITY

MANDIBLE

WALL OF DRUM

FIGURE 4-45. Chaussee III projection of temporal bone.

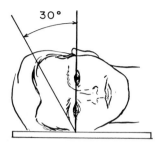

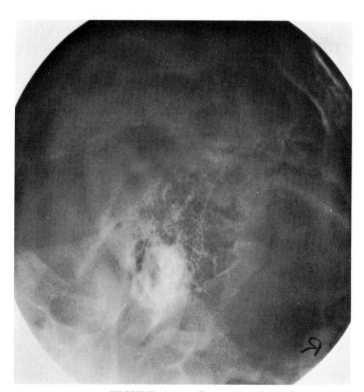

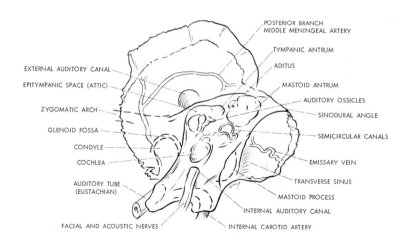

POSTERIOR BRANCH
MIDDLE MENINGEAL ARTERY

TYMPANIC ANTRUM

EXTERNAL AUDITORY CANAL — ADITUS

EPITYMPANIC SPACE (ATTIC) — MASTOID ANTRUM

AUDITORY OSSICLES

ZYGOMATIC ARCH — SINODURAL ANGLE

SEMICIRCULAR CANALS

GLENOID FOSSA —

CONDYLE —

COCHLEA — EMISSARY VEIN

TRANSVERSE SINUS

AUDITORY TUBE
(EUSTACHIAN) — MASTOID PROCESS

INTERNAL AUDITORY CANAL

FACIAL AND ACOUSTIC NERVES — INTERNAL CAROTID ARTERY

FIGURE 4-46.   Runström view of mastoid. The positions of some vital adjoining structures, such as facial and acoustic nerves, internal carotid arteries and auditory tube are shown for clarification of anatomy.

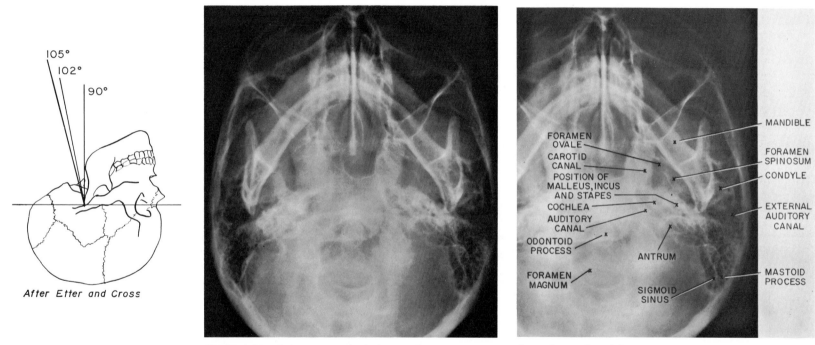

FIGURE 4-47.   Submentovertical view to demonstrate tympanic cavity, and ossicles.

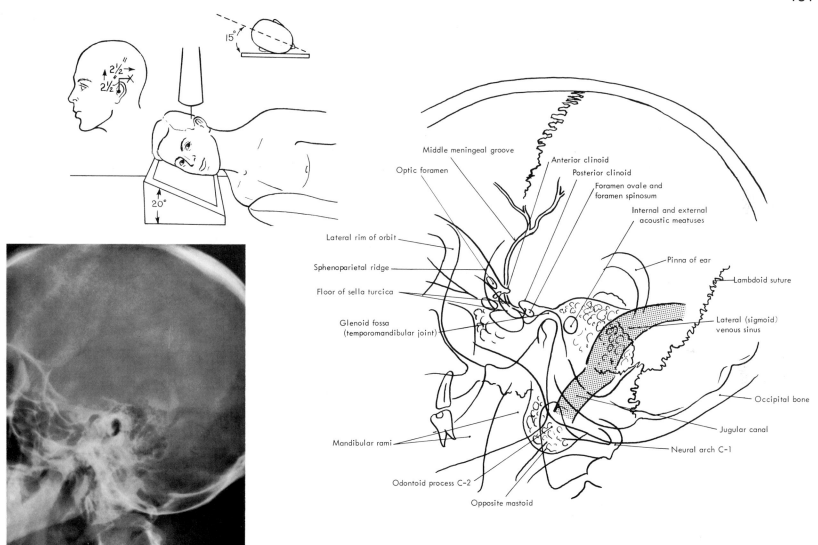

FIGURE 4-48. Special view for jugular canal.

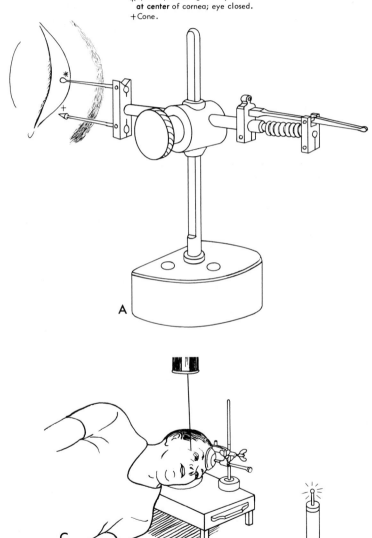

*Sphere pressed against eyelid **at center** of cornea; eye closed.
+Cone.

A

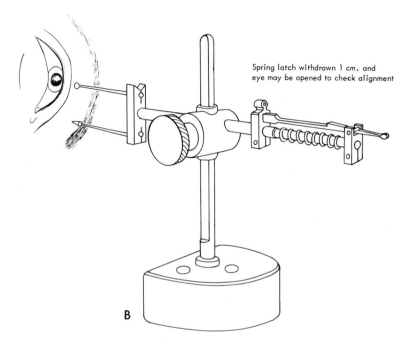

Spring latch withdrawn 1 cm. and eye may be opened to check alignment

B

C

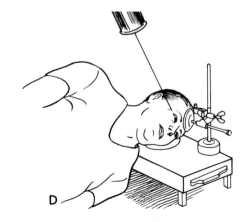

D

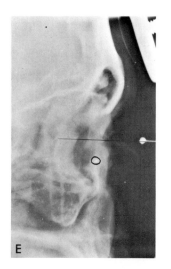
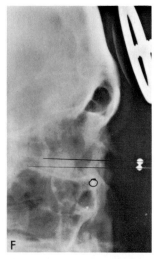
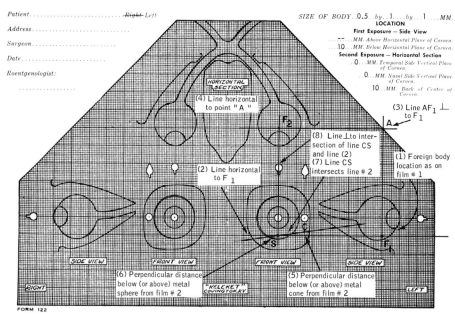

FIGURE 4-49. Sweet method for localization of foreign bodies in the eye. The patient's head is placed upon a slide tunnel so constructed that one-half of an 8 by 10 inch cassette is protected while the other half is being exposed. **A,** The indicator ball of the localizer apparatus is adjusted to the center of the eye with the eyelid closed. The cone-shaped metal tip lies directly below the ball. **B,** Upon release of the trigger, both the cone and ball rebound a carefully calibrated distance of 10 millimeters. **C,** The first exposure is made with the central ray of the x-ray beam perpendicular to the plane of the film and parallel to the patient's eyes, passing through both corneas and superimposing the shadows of the indicator ball and cone and their supporting stems. During exposure, the patient is asked to fix his gaze on a small light source or mark on the wall, eyes open, looking straight forward. **D,** For the second exposure the x-ray tube is shifted toward the patient's feet 4 to 5 inches and tilted so that the central ray passes through the ball of the localizer making an angle of some 10 to 15 degrees with the vertical; the cassette tray is moved to its second position. The films obtained are shown in **E** and **F**.

The method of transferring data from the films to the localizer chart: (1) From straight lateral film #1 the foreign body is indicated in its exact relationship to the superimposed metal ball and cone (F1); (2) a line is drawn horizontally with respect to F1; (3) a line is drawn perpendicularly from F1 to derive point A; (4) a horizontal line is drawn through A and crossing the horizontal plane depiction; (5) from film #2 the perpendicular distance below (or above) the metal cone is measured and plotted (point C); (6) from film #2 the perpendicular distance below (or above) the metal sphere is measured and plotted (point S); (7) line CS is drawn (note here that CS intersects horizontal line #2); (8) line is drawn perpendicular to intersection of line CS and line #2.

Point F1 indicates position of foreign body behind the center of the cornea and below the horizontal plane. Point F2 indicates the position of the foreign body medial or lateral to the center of the cornea, and thus all three dimensions are noted.

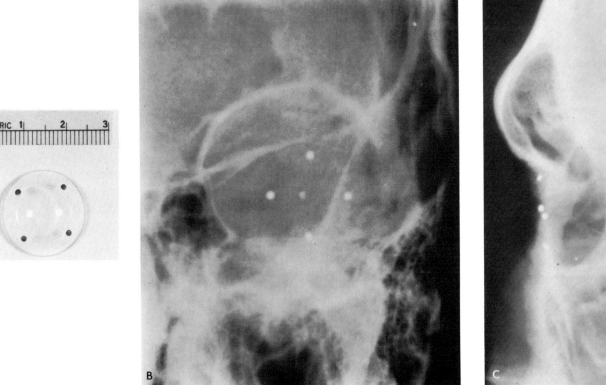

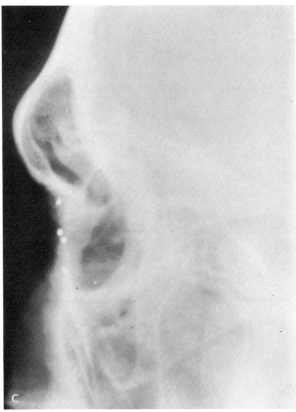

FIGURE 4-50.   Foreign body localization in the eye with the aid of the Thorpe plastic lens. The conjunctiva is anesthetized by the physician, and the lens placed into proper position over the cornea of the eye. Straight posteroanterior and lateral views of the eye are then obtained. **A,** Photograph of the lens; **B,** posteroanterior radiograph of the eye with the lens in place over the cornea; **C,** lateral view. The position of the foreign body is noted and measured with respect to the lead markers on the lens. This is a modification of the Pfeiffer-Comberg method. (The plastic lens was obtained from the House of Vision, Inc., Chicago, Illinois–Catalogue No. XP 3611.)

Chapter 5 — The Brain

RADIOGRAPHIC STUDY OF THE BRAIN

The radiographic methods of investigating the brain include: plain film studies (for physiologic or abnormal areas of calcification or radiolucency, i.e., lipomas of the corpus callosum); special studies with radioisotopes (outside the scope of the present text); and pneumoencephalography, ventriculography and cerebral angiography. Pneumoencephalography involves the injection into the subarachnoid space in the spinal region of a gaseous contrast medium that replaces the cerebrospinal fluid so that the ventricles of the brain and the subarachnoid space surrounding it may be visualized. In ventriculography, the contrast medium (usually gaseous) is injected directly into the ventricles of the brain through burr holes in the calvarium or through the space afforded by sutures of the skull. Cerebral angiograms are produced by injecting a contrast medium (opaque and of a type readily excreted by the urinary tract) directly into the arterial system supplying the brain, and immediately thereafter obtaining films during the arterial, capillary and venous phases in at least two perpendicular projections. Ideally, these are obtained simultaneously and rapidly, as will be described, so that the arterial and venous anatomy can be studied as accurately as possible.

PNEUMOENCEPHALOGRAMS AND VENTRICULOGRAMS

Some Technical Aspects

Our emphasis in this text is on the elementary aspects studied from the viewpoint of the radiographer and the interested medical trainee. Greater detail may be obtained from texts devoted exclusively to this subject (Taveras and Wood).

The gas most frequently employed is air filtered through sterile cotton, although many others have also been used.

The pneumoencephalographic examination is begun with the patient in a sitting position, and the air is introduced by lumbar puncture. The first fraction of 5 to 8 ml. is injected without withdrawal of a significant amount of cerebrospinal fluid, and the air is trapped in the posterior fossa by carefully flexing the head (90 degrees as shown in Figure 5-11). Ideally, at this juncture, fluoroscopy with the aid of image amplification and closed circuit television will indicate whether the position is optimum. Films are obtained in posteroanterior and lateral perspectives. As the degree of flexion of the head is carefully diminished (Fig. 5-11), air may be seen to rise above the tentorium cerebelli into the third and lateral ventricles. The intermittent injection of small amounts of air (following withdrawal of similar amounts of cerebrospinal fluid) will often permit radiographic visualization of important anatomic detail otherwise obscured by superimposed gas shadows.

If the head is immobilized and the patient is strapped in a suitable "tumbling" chair, and if the passage of the air is monitored by closed circuit television, the best positions of the head for optimum filling of the ventricles and subarachnoid space surrounding the brain can be achieved with maximum efficiency. If much cerebrospinal fluid must be drained off, approximately 80 ml. of air may be utilized in the course of the study.

In some instances, for reasons usually difficult to explain, the air will enter the subdural rather than the subarachnoid space. Since this has little diagnostic value, the needle should be repositioned.

Descriptive Terms for Positions and Views

Anteroposterior (A-P): Beam traverses head from front to back, parallel to Reid's base line.
Posteroanterior (P-A): Beam traverses from back to front.
Half axial: May be either P-A, or A-P. Beam is at an angle with respect to Reid's base line, usually between 12 and 35 degrees, although, in the initial pneumoencephalographic films, this may be as much as 90 degrees.

Axial: The beam traverses the skull from base to vertex or vice versa, usually perpendicular to Reid's base line.

Decubitus: The central x-ray beam is in the horizontal plane, and the patient is lying down, *prone* if facing downward, and *supine* if on his back and facing upward.

Brow up, Brow down: Face up or face down respectively.

Lateral: Side view, named by the side closest to the film.

Oblique: The sagittal axis of the body is turned at an angle to the film; view is named by the side closest to the film. The angle is usually 45 degrees unless otherwise specified.

The positions are illustrated in the ensuing pages. In every instance, unless the projection is oblique, *the central x-ray beam must be absolutely perpendicular to the sagittal or coronal plane of the head and the film.* A minimum of two views, perpendicular to one another, is usually obtained in each position of the head, as the air shifts from one area to another. These views are illustrated with respect to the position of both the head and the central ray so that radiograph and related anatomy can be properly understood.

Anyone who would attempt radiography of this area must have some basic understanding of the anatomy of the brain. The anatomic sketches included herein are minimal in this respect, although admittedly radiographers probably need fewer reference points of anatomy than do physicians.

Usual Sequence of Head Positions and Views Obtained

1. Patient sitting, head half axial at 90 degrees, 65 degrees or 45 degrees; posteroanterior and lateral views (Fig. 5-11).

2. Patient sitting, head erect; anteroposterior and lateral views (Fig. 5-12).

3. Patient sitting, head erect; Towne's views, 15 to 35 degrees, as in Figure 5-14, but erect.

4. Patient prone, brow down; posteroanterior and lateral views (Fig. 5-16). (half-axial view may also be obtained.)

5. Patient supine, brow up; anteroposterior and lateral views, (Fig. 5-13), and half axial views if desired, in Towne's projection (Fig. 5-14).

6. Patient prone again, but head turned first to one side and then the other; in each of these two positions, posteroanterior and lateral views are obtained, the posteroanterior views utilizing a horizontal beam (Fig. 5-15).

7. Body-section radiographs and tomograms are utilized whenever a clearer view of a given anatomic part is desired. Tomography is a technique whereby the patient's head is slowly rotated on its vertical axis during a lateral exposure, especially of the midline structures such as the cerebral aqueduct or fourth ventricle. This is virtually routine with us as an adjunct to step 1.

GROSS ANATOMY OF THE BRAIN AS RELATED TO RADIOGRAPHY

The Meninges

Figure 5-1 demonstrates the arrangement of the three meningeal layers: (1) The dura mater, which is the endosteum or inner fibrous lining of the inner table of the calvarium; (2) the pia mater,

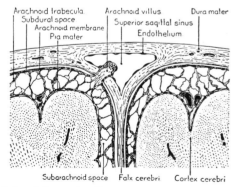

FIGURE 5-1. Schematic diagram of coronal section of meninges and cortex (From Gray, H.: *Gray's Anatomy of the Human Body*, edited by C. M. Goss. Lea & Febiger.)

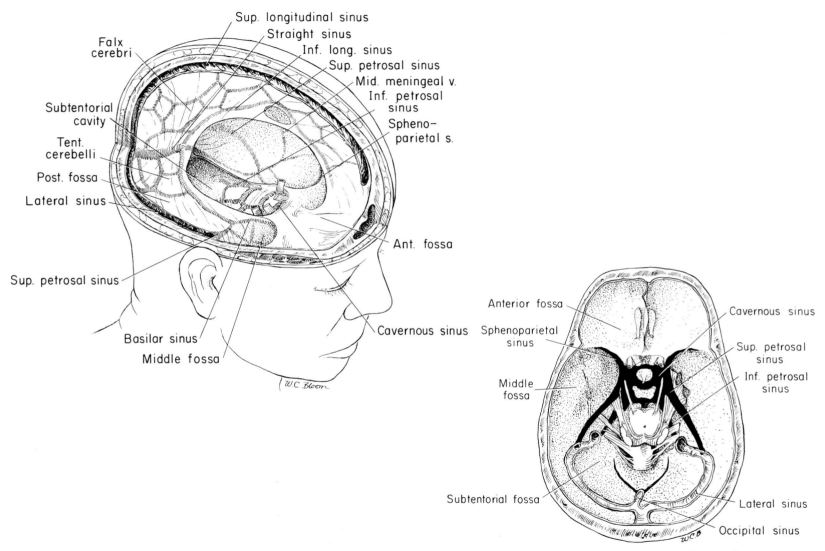

FIGURE 5-2. Major dural sinuses surrounding the brain. (Modified from Bailey, P.: *Intracranial Tumors*. Charles C Thomas, 1933.)

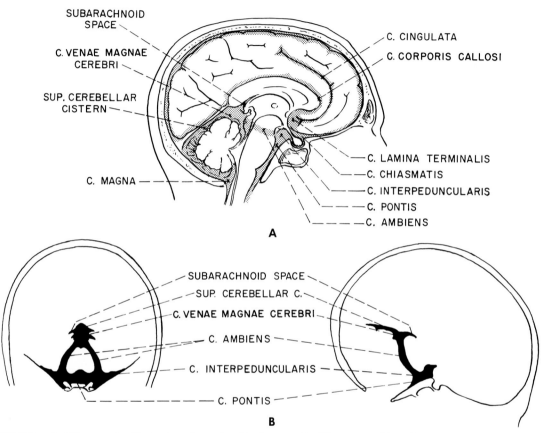

SUBARACHNOID
SPACE

C. VENAE MAGNAE
CEREBRI

SUP. CEREBELLAR
CISTERN

C. MAGNA

C. CINGULATA

C. CORPORIS CALLOSI

C. LAMINA TERMINALIS

C. CHIASMATIS

C. INTERPEDUNCULARIS

C. PONTIS

C. AMBIENS

A

SUBARACHNOID SPACE

SUP. CEREBELLAR C.

C. VENAE MAGNAE CEREBRI

C. AMBIENS

C. INTERPEDUNCULARIS

C. PONTIS

B

FIGURE 5-3.   A, Diagram to illustrate subarachnoid cisterns. **B,** Cisterna ambiens in Towne's and lateral projections. (Modified from Robertson, E. G.: *Pneumoencephalography.* Charles C Thomas.)

which is adherent to the surface of the brain and follows its convolutions closely; and (3) the arachnoid membrane, which lies between the two and is connected by a network of loose strands or trabeculae to the pia mater.

The dura mater splits in certain areas (the major venous sinuses, which are illustrated in Fig. 5-2) and it projects into the cranial cavity to form: (1) the falx cerebri, which projects between the two cerebral hemispheres; (2) the tentorium cerebelli, which arches over the cerebellum and supports much of the cerebrum; (3) the falx cerebelli, which extends between the tentorium cerebelli and the occipital bone; and (4) the diaphragma sellae, which roofs over the sella turcica.

Between the dura mater and the arachnoid, is the subdural space, which normally contains only a small amount of fluid.

Between the arachnoid and the pia mater is the subarachnoid space, which contains the cerebrospinal fluid removed at the time of pneumoencephalography. In certain areas, the subarachnoid space is quite wide and forms lakes called cisterns. These are illustrated in Figure 5-3.

In pneumoencephalography, the air is introduced into the subarachnoid space of the lumbar region and will circulate in this space almost exclusively. Sometimes, however, it will enter the subdural space, either overlying the brain or beneath the tentorium cerebelli, and produce a tent-shaped appearance here. Occasionally, air will enter the subdural space exclusively, with virtually no visualization of the subarachnoid space. This variation has no abnormal significance, and upon repeating the examination a more satisfactory result is usually obtained. Subdural air overlying the brain may at times be confused with cerebral or cortical atrophy, unless the examiner is aware of this possibility.

Not infrequently after the introduction of air in the lumbar subarachnoid space, only the sulci surrounding the brain are visualized, and the ventricles are not. This appearance will be described more fully later.

Subdivisions of the Brain

The brain is divided into five principal parts (Figs. 5-4, 5-5): (1) the cerebrum, composed of two cerebral hemispheres, lying above a plane drawn between the internal occipital protuberance, the petrous ridges and the floor of the anterior cranial fossa; (2) the cerebellum, composed of two hemispheres and a small central portion called the vermis, lying in the posterior fossa; (3) the midbrain, which lies between the cerebral hemispheres above, and the hindbrain below; (4) the pons, lying beneath the fourth ventricle between the cerebral peduncles above and the medulla oblongata below; and (5) the medulla oblongata, which lies immediately above the spinal cord above the level of the foramen magnum.

The Convolutions of the Brain, Gyri, Sulci and Fissures, Lateral Aspect

The cerebral hemispheres have numerous folds that follow a rather definite pattern and are called gyri or convolutions; these are separated from each other by grooves, called sulci if they are relatively shallow and fissures when they are deep (Figs. 5-4, 5-5, 5-6). The brain is subdivided into lobes by the fissures, as illustrated in the same figures.

The central lobe, or island of Reil, lies deep within the lateral (Sylvian) fissure. Also, the frontal, parietal, occipital and temporal lobes are identified above the tentorium cerebelli, and the cerebellar lobes, the vermis of the cerebellum, the pons and the medulla oblongata below the tentorium cerebelli.

The Ventricular System

The ventricles of the brain are a series of communicating cavities, lined by ependymal epithelium and containing cerebrospinal fluid, which communicate with the subarachnoid space surrounding the brain and the spinal cord and with the central canal of the cord (Figs. 5-7 and 5-8).

The lateral ventricles, one in each cerebral hemisphere, communicate with one another and with the third ventricle via the interventricular foramina. Each consists of a body and three horns — the frontal, the occipital and the temporal.

The third ventricle is a midline slitlike cavity, 2 to 8 mm. wide and about 3 cm. long. Anteriorly, there is an extension from its floor toward the sella turcica (infundibulum, optic recess and hypothalamic extension). Posteriorly, there is a narrow midline channel extending from the floor that connects the third with the fourth ventricle and is called the cerebral aqueduct (aqueduct of Sylvius). This is an arched structure with a radius of 3.5 to 3.8 cm. with respect to the dorsum sellae, measuring about 1.5 cm. in length and about 2 to 3 mm. in diameter.

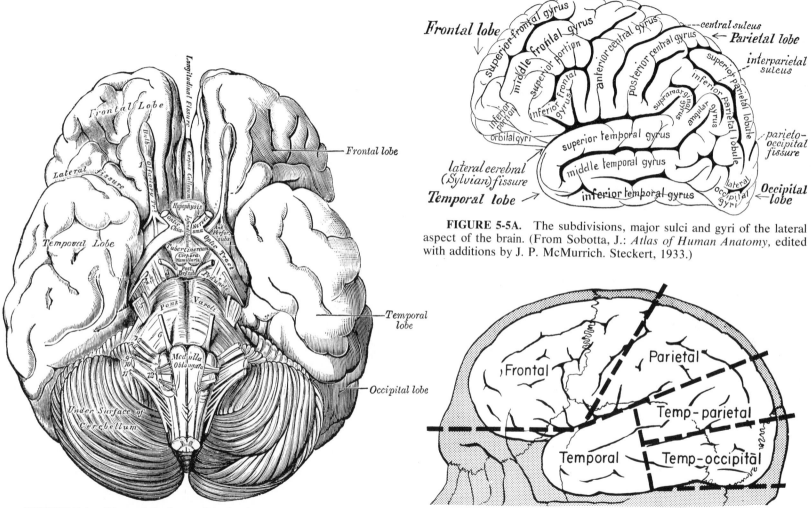

FIGURE 5-4. View of the base of the brain. (From Gray, H.: *Gray's Anatomy of the Human Body,* edited by C. M. Goss. Lea & Febiger.)

FIGURE 5-5A. The subdivisions, major sulci and gyri of the lateral aspect of the brain. (From Sobotta, J.: *Atlas of Human Anatomy,* edited with additions by J. P. McMurrich. Steckert, 1933.)

FIGURE 5-5B. Diagram showing the position of the various subdivisions of the brain as considered clinically and radiologically (supratentorial.)

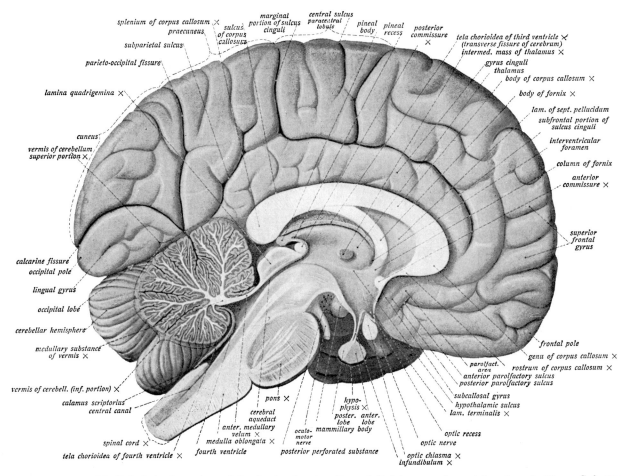

FIGURE 5-6. Medial sagittal section of the brain showing the subdivisions, major sulci and gyri. (From Sobotta, J.: *Atlas of Human Anatomy,* edited with additions by J. P. McMurrich. Steckert, 1933.)

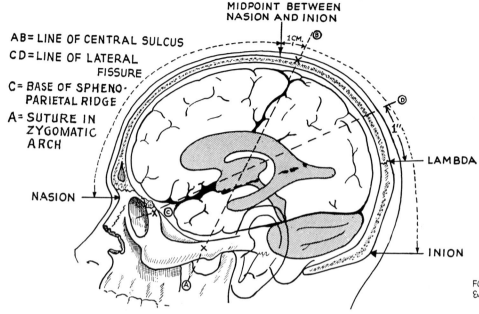

AB = LINE OF CENTRAL SULCUS
CD = LINE OF LATERAL FISSURE
C = BASE OF SPHENO-PARIETAL RIDGE
A = SUTURE IN ZYGOMATIC ARCH

MIDPOINT BETWEEN NASION AND INION

LAMBDA

NASION

INION

FIGURE 5-7. Diagram of the brain: relationship of the central sulcus and lateral fissure to the ventricles and skull.

The fourth ventricle is a midline cavity, diamond-shaped in frontal projection and triangular in lateral cross section. It communicates anteroinferiorly with the central canal of the medulla oblongata. There are outpouchings laterally (lateral recesses or foramina of Luschka) which communicate with the cisterna magna. Anterior to the choroid plexus of the fourth ventricle, there is a midline foramen (foramen of Magendie) which connects this ventricle with the cisterna cerebellomedullaris. The average measurements of the fourth ventricle are: superoinferiorly, 4 cm.; and from the apex in the roof (fastigium) to the floor, 1.6 cm.

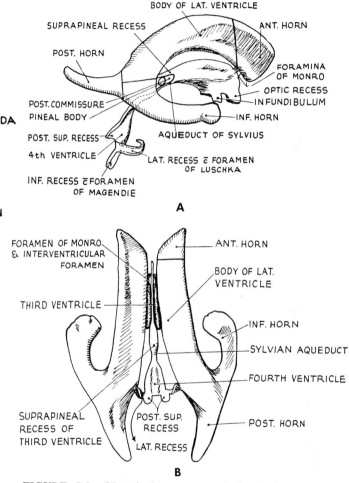

BODY OF LAT. VENTRICLE
SUPRAPINEAL RECESS
POST. HORN
ANT. HORN
FORAMINA OF MONRO
OPTIC RECESS
INFUNDIBULUM
POST. COMMISSURE
PINEAL BODY
INF. HORN
POST. SUP. RECESS
4th VENTRICLE
AQUEDUCT OF SYLVIUS
LAT. RECESS ē FORAMEN OF LUSCHKA
INF. RECESS ē FORAMEN OF MAGENDIE

A

FORAMEN OF MONRO & INTERVENTRICULAR FORAMEN
ANT. HORN
BODY OF LAT. VENTRICLE
THIRD VENTRICLE
INF. HORN
SYLVIAN AQUEDUCT
FOURTH VENTRICLE
SUPRAPINEAL RECESS OF THIRD VENTRICLE
POST. SUP. RECESS
LAT. RECESS
POST. HORN

B

FIGURE 5-8. Ventricular system of the brain. **A,** Lateral projection; **B,** superior projection.

The Subarachnoid Cisterns

The important cisterns are illustrated in Figure 5-3. These appear as lakelike structures on pneumoencephalograms and are helpful in detecting space-occupying lesions.

The fissures and sulci can also on occasion be identified and offer clues to disease processes. When excessively wide, they point toward atrophy. When displaced from a normal relationship, a space-occupying lesion may be suspected.

Cerebrospinal Fluid

It is probable that the cerebrospinal fluid is produced in the three following regions (Fig. 5-10): the *choroid plexuses* (1) of the ventricles, which produce most of the fluid; the *ependyma* of the central canal of the spinal cord (7), lending a small current of fluid which tends to go cephalad; and the *perivascular linings* of the blood vessels that enter and leave the brain in close proximity with the subarachnoid spaces.

The intraventricular fluid flows down the ventricles (2 to 5) to the fourth ventricle (6), and thereafter flows out of the fourth ventricle through the foramina of Magendie and Luschka into the subarachnoid space (8 to 13). There is probably no other communication between the intraventricular fluid and the subarachnoid fluid.

The fluid then distributes itself in the subarachnoid space underlying and covering the brain (8 to 13), and is ultimately absorbed by diffusion through the arachnoid villi (or granulations) into the great dural sinuses (14). There is also a small amount of absorption through the perineural lymphatics.

It is probable that the fluid in the subdural space is produced locally by its own mesothelial cells, but the exact relationship of this fluid to the cerebrospinal fluid is not known.

(Text continues on page 154.)

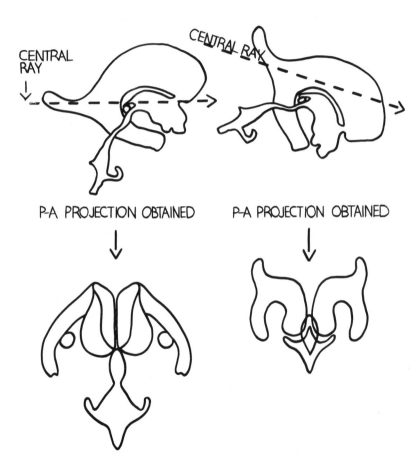

FIGURE 5-9. Radiographic appearance of ventricles in frontal and lateral perspectives, with appropriate tilted or angled views.

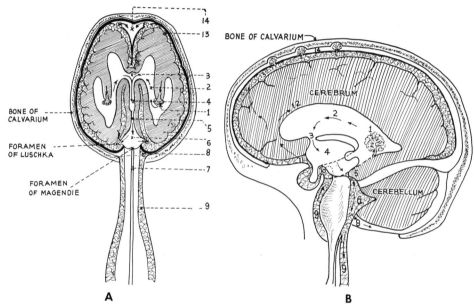

FIGURE 5-10. Diagrams to illustrate the circulation of the cerebrospinal fluid. **A,** Frontal projection; **B,** lateral projection. (See text for explanation.)

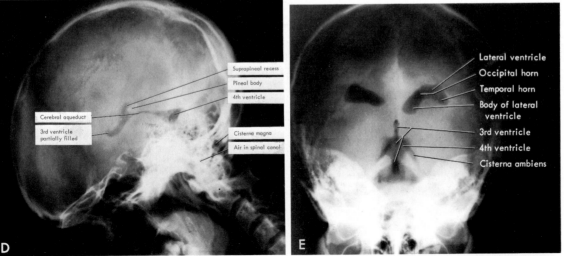

FIGURE 5-11. **A**, **B**, and **C**, The relationship of posture to the distribution of gas in the cadaver. In **A**, the flexion is 90 degrees; in **B**, 65 degrees; in **C**, 45 degrees. (From Robertson, E. G.: *Pneumo-encephalography*. Charles C Thomas.) **D** and **E**, Radiographs (intensified) obtained by the Robertson-Lindgren technique in posteroanterior and lateral projections (not identical).

Labels in D:
Suprapineal recess
Pineal body
4th ventricle
Cerebral aqueduct
3rd ventricle partially filled
Cisterna magna
Air in spinal canal

Labels in E:
Lateral ventricle
Occipital horn
Temporal horn
Body of lateral ventricle
3rd ventricle
4th ventricle
Cisterna ambiens

90°

65°

45°

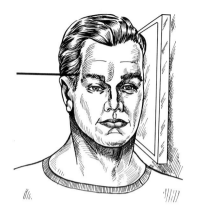
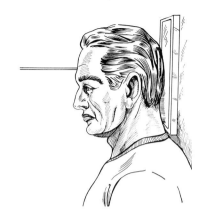

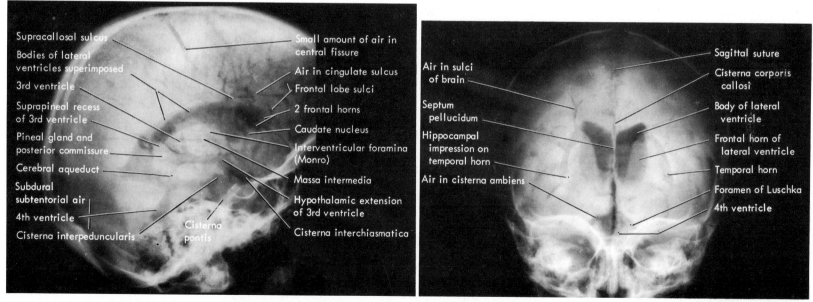

Supracallosal sulcus

Bodies of lateral
ventricles superimposed

3rd ventricle

Suprapineal recess
of 3rd ventricle

Pineal gland and
posterior commissure

Cerebral aqueduct

Subdural
subtentorial air

4th ventricle

Cisterna interpeduncularis

Cisterna
pontis

Small amount of air in
central fissure

Air in cingulate sulcus

Frontal lobe sulci

2 frontal horns

Caudate nucleus

Interventricular foramina
(Monro)

Massa intermedia

Hypothalamic extension
of 3rd ventricle

Cisterna interchiasmatica

Air in sulci
of brain

Septum
pellucidum

Hippocampal
impression on
temporal horn

Air in cisterna ambiens

Sagittal suture

Cisterna corporis
callosi

Body of lateral
ventricle

Frontal horn of
lateral ventricle

Temporal horn

Foramen of Luschka

4th ventricle

FIGURE 5-12. Positioning for and radiographs (intensified) obtained during pneumoencephalography with patient erect and beam horizontal, A-P and lateral projections.

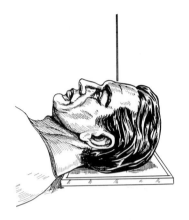

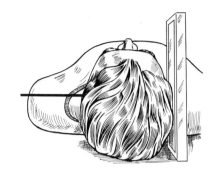

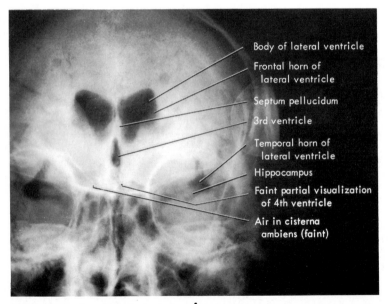

Body of lateral ventricle

Frontal horn of
lateral ventricle

Septum pellucidum

3rd ventricle

Temporal horn of
lateral ventricle

Hippocampus

Faint partial visualization
of 4th ventricle

Air in cisterna
ambiens (faint)

A

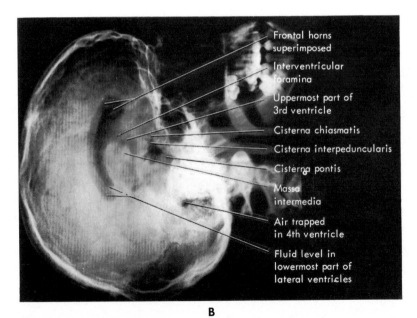

Frontal horns
superimposed

Interventricular
foramina

Uppermost part of
3rd ventricle

Cisterna chiasmatis

Cisterna interpeduncularis

Cisterna pontis

Massa
intermedia

Air trapped
in 4th ventricle

Fluid level in
lowermost part of
lateral ventricles

B

FIGURE 5-13. Positioning for and radiographs (intensified) obtained during pneumoencephalography with patient recumbent, supine. **A,** Vertical beam, A-P; **B,** horizontal beam, lateral (both laterals may be taken).

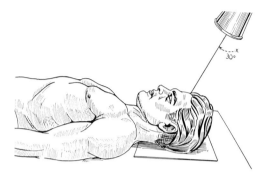

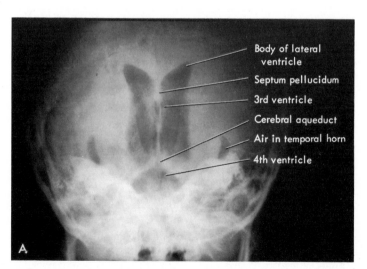

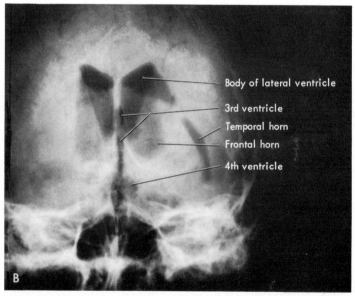

FIGURE 5-14. Positioning for and radiographs (intensified) obtained during pneumoencephalography with patient supine in Towne's projections. **A,** 30 degree angulation of central ray caudad; **B,** 15 degree angulation of central ray caudad.

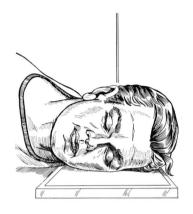
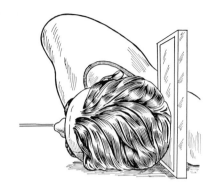

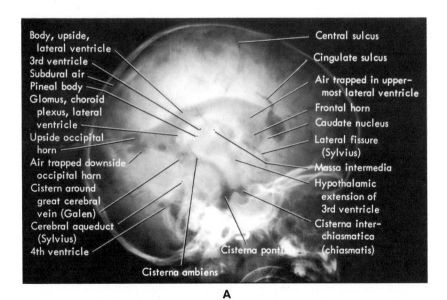

Body, upside,
  lateral ventricle
3rd ventricle
Subdural air
Pineal body
Glomus, choroid
  plexus, lateral
  ventricle
Upside occipital
  horn
Air trapped downside
  occipital horn
Cistern around
  great cerebral
  vein (Galen)
Cerebral aqueduct
  (Sylvius)
4th ventricle

Cisterna ambiens

Central sulcus
Cingulate sulcus
Air trapped in upper-
  most lateral ventricle
Frontal horn
Caudate nucleus
Lateral fissure
  (Sylvius)
Massa intermedia
Hypothalamic
  extension of
  3rd ventricle
Cisterna inter-
  chiasmatica
  (chiasmatis)

Cisterna pontis

A

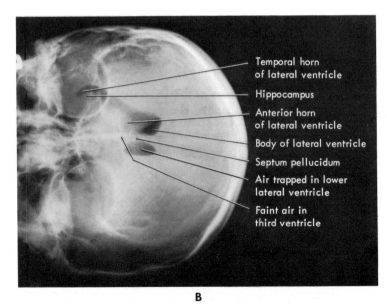

Temporal horn
of lateral ventricle
Hippocampus
Anterior horn
of lateral ventricle
Body of lateral ventricle
Septum pellucidum
Air trapped in lower
lateral ventricle
Faint air in
third ventricle

B

FIGURE 5-15. Positioning for and radiographs (intensified) obtained during pneumoencephalography with patient lying down, right side of head uppermost. **A,** Vertical beam; **B,** horizontal beam. A similar set of two films is obtained with the left side of the head uppermost.

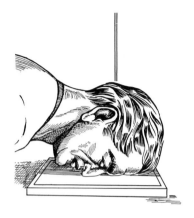
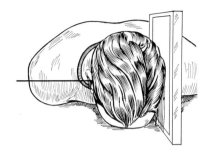

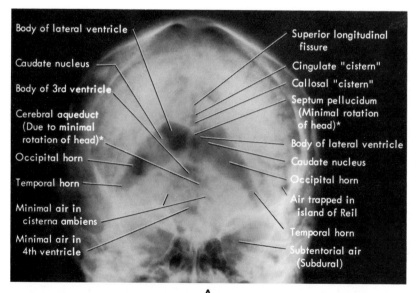

Body of lateral ventricle
Caudate nucleus
Body of 3rd ventricle
Cerebral aqueduct (Due to minimal rotation of head)*
Occipital horn
Temporal horn
Minimal air in cisterna ambiens
Minimal air in 4th ventricle

Superior longitudinal fissure
Cingulate "cistern"
Callosal "cistern"
Septum pellucidum (Minimal rotation of head)*
Body of lateral ventricle
Caudate nucleus
Occipital horn
Air trapped in island of Reil
Temporal horn
Subtentorial air (Subdural)

A

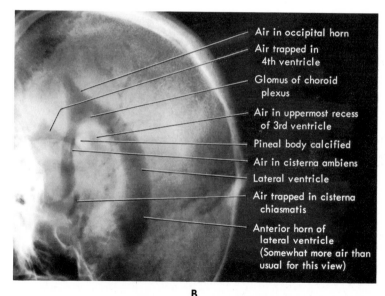

Air in occipital horn
Air trapped in 4th ventricle
Glomus of choroid plexus
Air in uppermost recess of 3rd ventricle
Pineal body calcified
Air in cisterna ambiens
Lateral ventricle
Air trapped in cisterna chiasmatis
Anterior horn of lateral ventricle (Somewhat more air than usual for this view)

B

FIGURE 5-16. Positioning for and radiographs (intensified) obtained during pneumoencephalography with patient prone, brow down. **A,** Vertical beam; **B,** horizontal beam. *Note that minimal rotation of head as indicated by relationship of mastoid processes with condyloid processes (mandible) may distort the septum pellucidum and third ventricle, as well as make the lateral ventricles appear slightly asymmetrical.

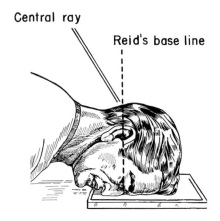

Central ray

Reid's base line

POINTS OF PRACTICAL INTEREST ABOUT FIGURE 5-17

1. Since the air rises to the uppermost portions of the ventricular system, this view has its chief application in visualization of the occipital horns, the posterior portions of the lateral ventricles, the posterior part of the third ventricle, and the fourth ventricle.

2. The true Towne position, with the patient supine and the central ray angled 35 degrees toward the feet, is most applicable to visualization of the temporal horns and the anterior sectors of the lateral ventricles.

3. The term "Reid's base line" as used in this text is actually the canthomeatal line—from the outer canthus of the eye to the external auditory meatus. Originally, Reid's base line was described as a line drawn from the infraorbital rim to the external auditory meatus. We seldom use the latter reference line, since the canthomeatal line is more clearly defined on the patient.

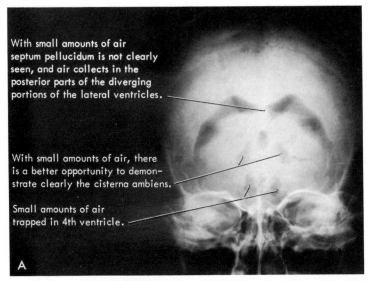

With small amounts of air septum pellucidum is not clearly seen, and air collects in the posterior parts of the diverging portions of the lateral ventricles.

With small amounts of air, there is a better opportunity to demonstrate clearly the cisterna ambiens.

Small amounts of air trapped in 4th ventricle.

A

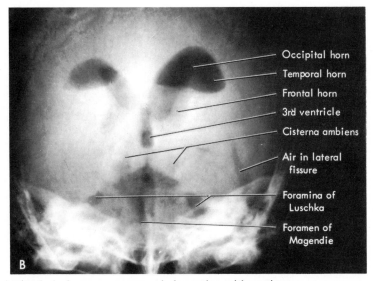

Occipital horn

Temporal horn

Frontal horn

3rd ventricle

Cisterna ambiens

Air in lateral fissure

Foramina of Luschka

Foramen of Magendie

B

FIGURE 5-17. Positioning for and radiographs (intensified) obtained during pneumoencephalography with patient prone, reverse Towne's projection. **A,** Central ray angled 12 degrees to Reid's baseline; **B,** central ray angled 25 degrees to Reid's baseline. (Foramina of Luschka label probable, not certain).

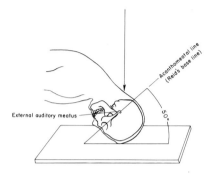

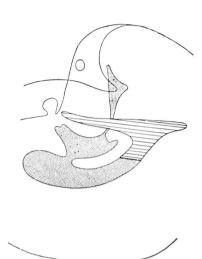

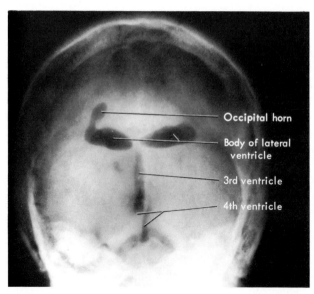

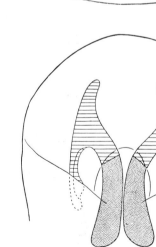

FIGURE 5-18. Positioning for radiograph (intensified) and tracings of basovertical view; patient prone, beam vertical. A horizontal beam lateral view (diagram, upper right) is also obtained with the patient in this position. (Tracings from Robertson, E. G.: *Pneumoencephalography*. Charles C Thomas.)

VENTRICULOGRAPHY

If increased intracranial pressure is present, herniation of brain substance through the foramen magnum (and death) may occur at the time lumbar puncture is performed and cerebrospinal fluid is removed. To prevent this, when air studies of the ventricles are necessary, cerebral puncture is accomplished through the parietal lobes, and cerebrospinal fluid is removed and replaced by air. The same series of films is obtained. The subarachnoid space outside the ventricular system is ordinarily not well demonstrated by this technique.

On occasion, for better visualization of the cerebral aqueduct, 1 to 2 ml. of Pantopaque may be injected into the lateral ventricle. When the patient's head is moved appropriately, the oil, which is heavier than cerebrospinal fluid, will move downward by gravity toward the cerebral aqueduct and fourth ventricle, and films may be taken to demonstrate the adjoining anatomy.

This method of positive contrast ventriculography is utilized particularly when other techniques have failed to reveal sufficient detail for an accurate diagnosis.

CEREBRAL ANGIOGRAPHY

Comment on Examination Technique

Basically, this method of examination involves the direct or indirect introduction of a suitable contrast agent into the major blood vessels of the brain. This may be accomplished by needle puncture of the carotid arteries or the vertebral artery, by threading a catheter via the brachial or femoral artery to an appropriate position for injection, or by the retrograde injection of the contrast agent into the brachial or subclavian artery directly.

If the injection is made directly into the carotid or vertebral artery, usually 6 to 8 ml. will suffice if injected rapidly; if it is made into the arch of the aorta or more peripherally, a greater volume such as 30 to 40 ml. may be necessary (see Chapter 10).

Serial exposures are routinely made in anteroposterior half axial (Fig. 5-19) lateral projections (horizontal beam), simultaneously, at two per second for three seconds, and one per second for four seconds. The half axial angulation is 15 to 20 degrees for carotid angiography and 30 degrees for vertebral. Occasionally, 30 degree oblique or basilar views are also obtained.

If the injection is made below the bifurcation of the common carotid artery, a visualization of the external carotid artery is also obtained, although its circulation is a few seconds slower than the internal carotid. (This technique is especially helpful in meningiomas.) If it is made into the subclavian artery, the vertebral artery of that side is visualized simultaneously, along with its flow pattern with respect to the basilar artery and its major ramifications.

The ideal frontal perspective in most instances is one in which the supraorbital ridge is directly superimposed over the petrous ridge. The condyloid processes of the mandible must be absolutely symmetrical with respect to the mastoid processes. In the lateral views, there must be a perfect superimposition of the rami of the mandible and the temporomandibular joints.

It will be noted that if emphasis on the vertebral circulation is required, the horizontal x-ray beam is centered 3 cm. below the external auditory meatus for the lateral views. In carotid angiography, the horizontal beam is centered 3 cm. above and 1 cm. anterior to the meatus (Fig. 5-19).

The exposures are begun near the end of the injection period. Injections may be repeated with somewhat different timing after the initial films are seen. In general, the arterial phase occurs within the first two seconds; the capillary phase, two seconds thereafter; and the venous phase in the final two to three seconds. These sequences may have to be varied depending upon individual requirements.

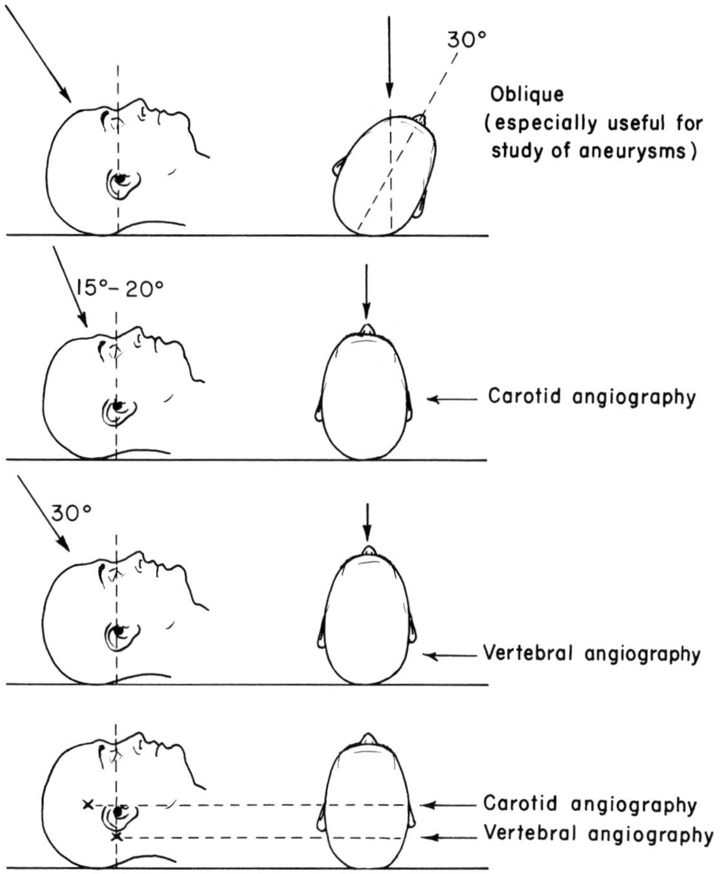

Anatomy

FIGURE 5-19. Positioning for carotid and vertebral angiography. The axial view (Figure 4-16) may also be used on occasion to demonstrate the basilar artery and its branches.

External Carotid Artery. Radiologically, the important branches for identification are: (1) the occipital; (2) the superficial temporal; and (3) the internal maxillary, which in turn gives rise to the middle meningeal and small orbital branches that communicate with the ophthalmic branch of the internal carotid.

Internal Carotid Artery. The important parts and branches for radiologic identification are (1) the carotid sinus and (2) the ophthalmic, (3) the posterior communicating (joining the posterior cerebral), (4) the anterior choroidal and (5) and (6), terminally, the anterior and middle cerebral arteries.

The important branches of the anterior cerebral for identification on both frontal and lateral perspectives are: (1) the frontopolar; (2) the pericallosal; and (3) the callosomarginal. The anterior communicating is usually too small to identify.

The important branches of the middle cerebral for identification are: (1) the lenticulostriate arterial twigs, (2) the ascending frontoparietal, (3) the posterior parietal, (4) the angular and (5) the posterior temporal.

A few of the important relationships of these main branches are indicated in Figures 5-21 and 5-23.

Vertebral Artery. The vertebral arteries ordinarily arise from the subclavian on either side (Fig. 5-25). They enter the foramen transversarium on each side at the level of the sixth cervical vertebra and ascend in the foramen transversarium of each successive cervical vertebra (see Chapter 6) to the C 2 level, where each vertebral swings laterally for about 1 cm. It then traverses the foramen transversarium of C 1 and enters the cranial cavity at the lateral border of the foramen magnum. Its important branches, apart from small muscular branches in the neck, are the following: (1) the posterior meningeal, (2) the anterior and posterior spinal and (3) the posterior inferior cerebellar. This latter branch is of great

(Text continues on Page 164.)

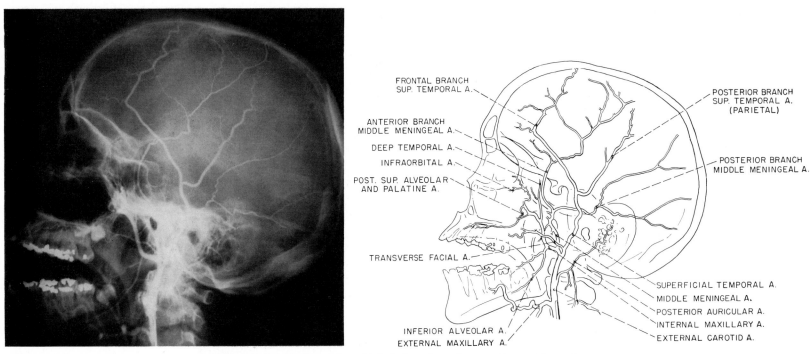

FIGURE 5-20. Radiograph and labeled tracing of external carotid arteriogram.

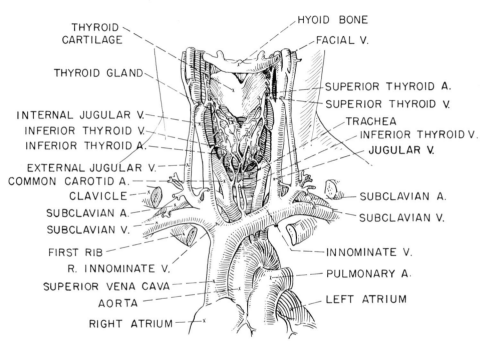

FIGURE 5-21. Diagram of major circulation in the neck.

Labels on figure:
THYROID CARTILAGE
THYROID GLAND
INTERNAL JUGULAR V.
INFERIOR THYROID V.
INFERIOR THYROID A.
EXTERNAL JUGULAR V.
COMMON CAROTID A.
CLAVICLE
SUBCLAVIAN A.
SUBCLAVIAN V.
FIRST RIB
R. INNOMINATE V.
SUPERIOR VENA CAVA
AORTA
RIGHT ATRIUM
HYOID BONE
FACIAL V.
SUPERIOR THYROID A.
SUPERIOR THYROID V.
TRACHEA
INFERIOR THYROID V.
JUGULAR V.
SUBCLAVIAN A.
SUBCLAVIAN V.
INNOMINATE V.
PULMONARY A.
LEFT ATRIUM

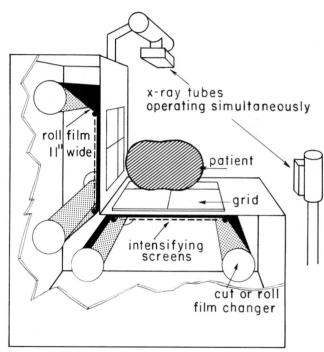

Labels on figure:
x-ray tubes operating simultaneously
roll film 11" wide
patient
grid
intensifying screens
cut or roll film changer

FIGURE 5-22. Diagram of a type of roll film changer in considerable use for obtaining rapid serial films of an anatomic part such as the head or the heart in two perpendicular planes simultaneously. Body may be rotated to any position. (Modified from Clark, K. C.: *Positioning in Radiography*. William Heinemann Medical Books, Ltd., 1964.)

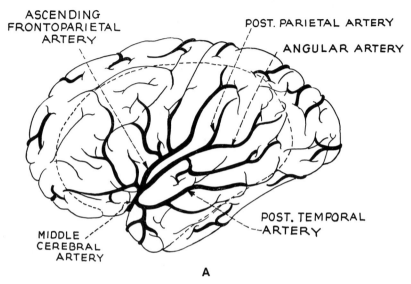

ASCENDING
FRONTOPARIETAL
ARTERY

POST. PARIETAL ARTERY

ANGULAR ARTERY

POST. TEMPORAL
ARTERY

MIDDLE
CEREBRAL
ARTERY

A

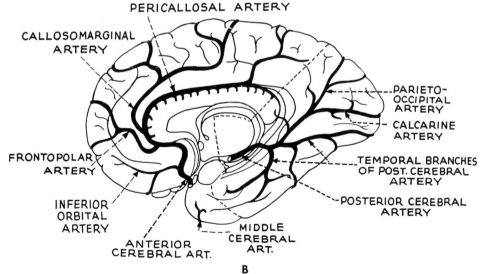

PERICALLOSAL ARTERY

CALLOSOMARGINAL
ARTERY

PARIETO-
OCCIPITAL
ARTERY

CALCARINE
ARTERY

FRONTOPOLAR
ARTERY

TEMPORAL BRANCHES
OF POST. CEREBRAL
ARTERY

POSTERIOR CEREBRAL
ARTERY

INFERIOR
ORBITAL
ARTERY

ANTERIOR
CEREBRAL ART.

MIDDLE
CEREBRAL
ART.

B

FIGURE 5-23.   Chief divisions of the internal carotid artery. **A,** Lateral aspect; **B,** median sagittal aspect.

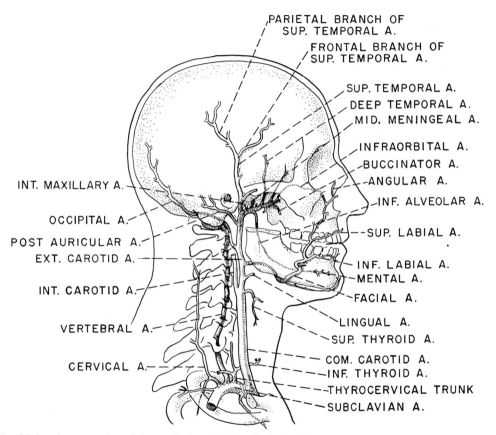

PARIETAL BRANCH OF
SUP. TEMPORAL A.

FRONTAL BRANCH OF
SUP. TEMPORAL A.

SUP. TEMPORAL A.
DEEP TEMPORAL A.
MID. MENINGEAL A.

INFRAORBITAL A.
BUCCINATOR A.
ANGULAR A.
INF. ALVEOLAR A.

INT. MAXILLARY A.

SUP. LABIAL A.

OCCIPITAL A.

POST AURICULAR A.
EXT. CAROTID A.

INF. LABIAL A.
MENTAL A.
FACIAL A.

INT. CAROTID A.

LINGUAL A.
SUP. THYROID A.

VERTEBRAL A.

COM. CAROTID A.
INF. THYROID A.
THYROCERVICAL TRUNK
SUBCLAVIAN A.

CERVICAL A.

FIGURE 5-24. Major deep arteries of the neck, lateral view. Relationship to temporal and meningeal branches is shown.

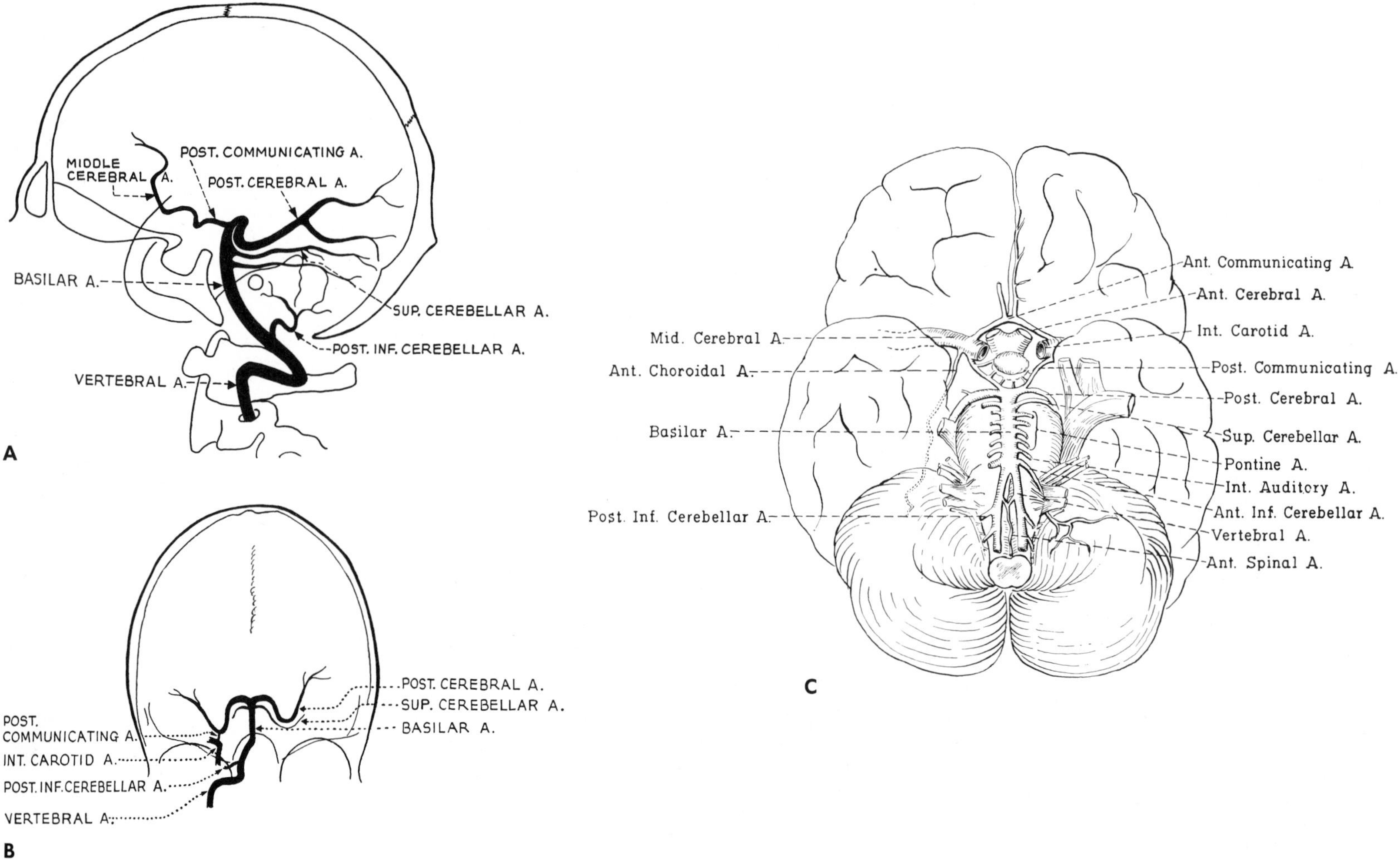

A

MIDDLE CEREBRAL A.

POST. COMMUNICATING A.

POST. CEREBRAL A.

BASILAR A.

SUP. CEREBELLAR A.

POST. INF. CEREBELLAR A.

VERTEBRAL A.

B

POST. CEREBRAL A.

SUP. CEREBELLAR A.

BASILAR A.

POST. COMMUNICATING A.

INT. CAROTID A.

POST. INF. CEREBELLAR A.

VERTEBRAL A.

C

Mid. Cerebral A.

Ant. Choroidal A.

Basilar A.

Post. Inf. Cerebellar A.

Ant. Communicating A.

Ant. Cerebral A.

Int. Carotid A.

Post. Communicating A.

Post. Cerebral A.

Sup. Cerebellar A.

Pontine A.

Int. Auditory A.

Ant. Inf. Cerebellar A.

Vertebral A.

Ant. Spinal A.

FIGURE 5-25. **A,** Diagram of vertebral angiogram, lateral projection; **B,** Towne's projection. **C,** Anatomy of the vertebral artery and branches in relationship with the base of the brain.

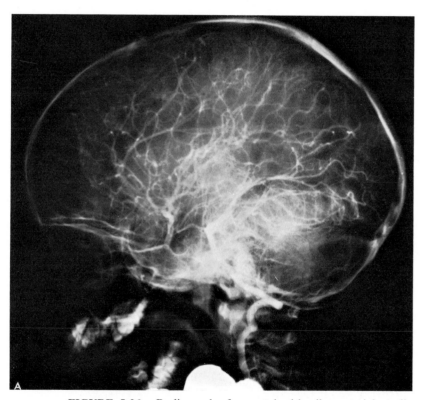
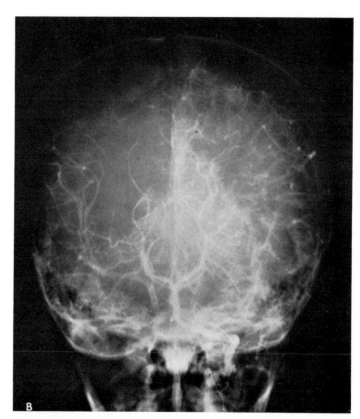

FIGURE 5-26. Radiographs for vertebral-basilar arterial studies. **A,** Lateral projection; **B,** Towne's anteroposterior projection.

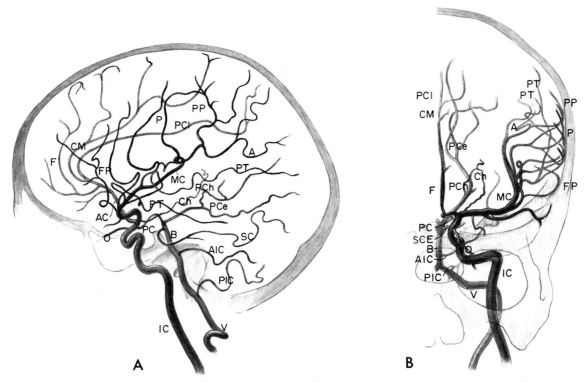

FIGURE 5-27.   Internal carotid and basilar arteriograms. **A,** Diagram of lateral view; **B,** diagram of A-P view. A, angular; AC, anterior cerebral; AIC, anterior inferior cerebellar; B, basilar; Ch, choroidal; CM, callosomarginal; F, frontopolar; FP, frontoparietal; IC, internal carotid; MC, middle cerebral; O, ophthalmic; P, parietal; PC, posterior communicating; PCe, posterior cerebral; PCh, posterior choroidal; PCl, pericollosal; PIC, posterior inferior cerebellar; PP, posterior parietal; PT, posterior temporal; SC, superior cerebellar; SCE, superior cerebellar; V, vertebral.

    C, Lateral radiograph, arterial phase; **D,** anteroposterior radiograph, arterial phase; **E,** geometric relationships on anteroposterior view.

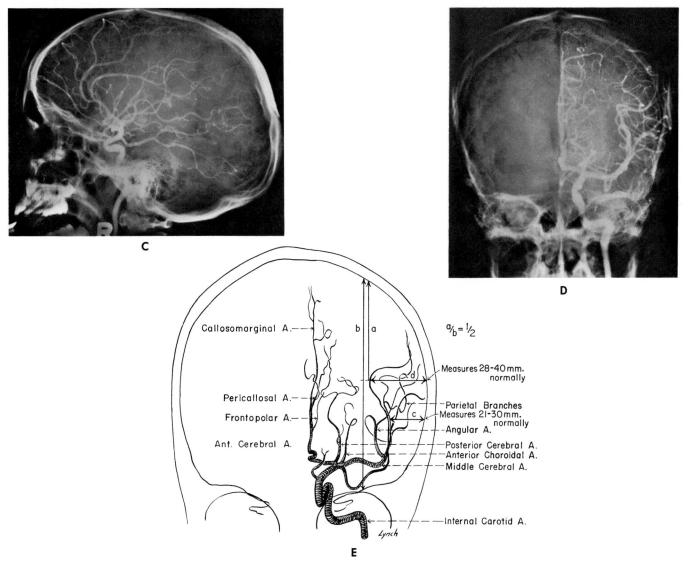

C

D

Callosomarginal A.

b | a   a/b = 1/2

Measures 28-40 mm.
normally

Pericallosal A.

Parietal Branches
Measures 21-30 mm.
normally

Frontopolar A.

Angular A.

Ant. Cerebral A.

Posterior Cerebral A.
Anterior Choroidal A.
Middle Cerebral A.

Internal Carotid A.

Lynch

E

FIGURE 5-27. *(Continued).* See legend on preceding page.

importance, since it lies, in its first part, close to the medial part of the cerebellar tonsil, and more distally, close to the floor of the fourth ventricle and its choroid plexus. If it can be identified 5 mm. or more below the level of the foramen magnum, it is virtually certain that there is a downward herniation of the cerebellar tonsil through the foramen magnum. Near the upper medulla, the two vertebral arteries merge medially to form the basilar artery.

Basilar Artery. This artery runs between the clivus and the pons, in the cisterna pontis (Fig. 5-25). In the interpeduncular cistern, it divides into the two posterior cerebral arteries. The main branches to be identified are: (1) the pontine twigs and (2) the internal auditory, (3) the anterior inferior cerebellar and (4) the superior cerebellar arteries. The last-mentioned encircles the brain stem in the cisterna ambiens, but unlike the posterior cerebral, it finally ramifies beneath the tentorium cerebelli over the upper part of the cerebellum.

Unfortunately for our diagnostic accuracy, the appearance of the basilar artery varies considerably, as it wanders from one side to the other of the brain stem.

Posterior Cerebral Artery. Beyond the posterior communicating artery, it is important to identify the following branches: (1) the thalamostriate; (2) the posterior choroidal, three on each side; (3) the anterior and posterior temporal; (4) the posterior occipital; and (5) the calcarine arteries, terminally ramifying over the temporal and occipital lobes. The posterior cerebral follows the midbrain in the cisterna ambiens, near the edge, but above the tentorial notch. Herniation downward may be detected with protrusion of the brain stem through this notch.

Circle of Willis. This anastomotic arterial circle consists of: (1) the two anterior cerebrals connected by the anterior communicating and (2) the internal carotids connected with the posterior cerebrals by the two posterior communicating arteries. The basilar artery forms the common linkage posteriorly.

Deep Cerebral Veins. The important deep veins to identify are: (1) the septal; (2) the anterior caudate or terminal; (3) the striothalamic; (4) the internal cerebral, which courses medially along the roof of the third ventricle to fuse posteriorly to form (5) the great cerebral vein of Galen, the midline vein that courses slightly upward and posteriorly to empty into the straight venous sinus; and (6) the basal vein of Rosenthal, which winds its way around the midbrain near the brain stem to empty into the great cerebral vein of Galen.

The Venous Sinuses. As previously indicated, the venous sinuses are contained within the dura mater (Fig. 5-2A and B). Those that are important to identify are: (1) the superior longitudinal sinus, (2) the inferior longitudinal sinus, (3) the straight sinus, (4) the lateral sinus; (5) the superior petrosal sinus, (6) the inferior petrosal sinus, (7) the sphenoparietal sinus and (8) the cavernous sinus.

The Superficial Cerebral Veins. These drain into the dural venous sinuses and consist of the following main groups: (1) the anastomotic veins of Trolard, superiorly; (2) the anastomotic vein of Labbe, inferiorly; (3) the middle cerebral vein in the lateral (Sylvian) fissure, emptying into the sphenoparietal and cavernous sinuses, and (4) the superior cerebral veins, which are superficial and empty into the superior longitudinal sinus.

The Venous Angle. It will be noted that this represents the confluent point of the striothalamic vein, and the septal vein, and the origin of the internal cerebral vein (Fig. 5-28). Anatomically, the angle is usually situated at the interventricular foramen on each side of the midline. These veins are of considerable importance, since they serve to delineate much of the body and anterior horn of the lateral ventricle and the roof of the third ventricle. The basal vein of Rosenthal, which together with the internal cerebral vein empties into the great cerebral vein of Galen, winds its way around the midbrain in close approximation to the posterior cerebral artery.

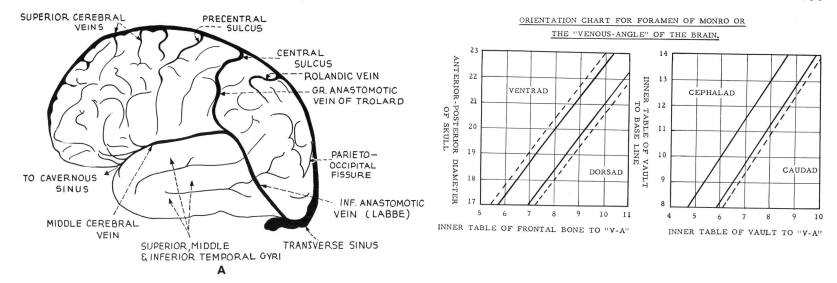

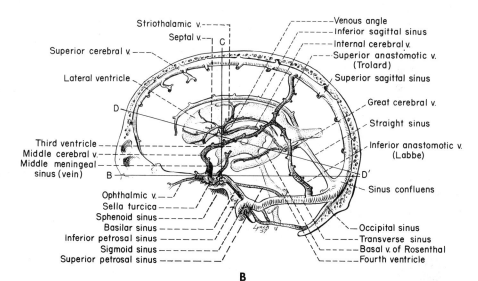

FIGURE 5-28. **A,** Venous drainage of the brain, superolateral aspect. **B,** Diagram of inner aspect, lateral view of venous drainage of the brain. The lines shown are drawn for orientation of the venous angle and foramen of Monro in accordance with the orientation charts of Mokrohisky et al.: The base line *BD'* passes from the nasion through the tuberculum sellae to the occiput; *A* represents the anterior vertex of the venous angle, and *CA* is the perpendicular drawn through *A* to base line *BD'*; *DD'* is the longest anteroposterior diameter of the skull through *A*. On the orientation charts shown, *DD'* is related to *DA* on the graph at left; and the distance of point *C* to line *BD'* is related to *CA* on the graph at right.

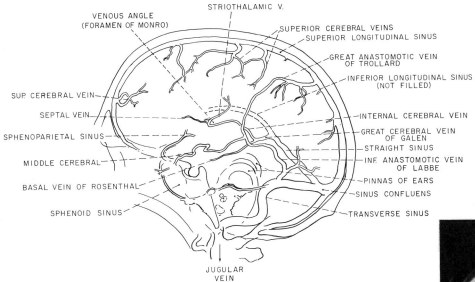

VENOUS ANGLE
(FORAMEN OF MONRO)

STRIOTHALAMIC V.

SUPERIOR CEREBRAL VEINS
SUPERIOR LONGITUDINAL SINUS

GREAT ANASTOMOTIC VEIN
OF TROLLARD

INFERIOR LONGITUDINAL SINUS
(NOT FILLED)

SUP CEREBRAL VEIN

SEPTAL VEIN

SPHENOPARIETAL SINUS

MIDDLE CEREBRAL

BASAL VEIN OF ROSENTHAL

SPHENOID SINUS

INTERNAL CEREBRAL VEIN

GREAT CEREBRAL VEIN
OF GALEN

STRAIGHT SINUS

INF. ANASTOMOTIC VEIN
OF LABBE

PINNAS OF EARS

SINUS CONFLUENS

TRANSVERSE SINUS

JUGULAR
VEIN

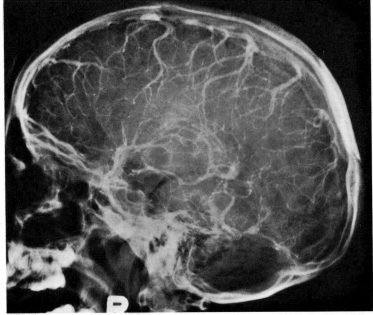

FIGURE 5-29A.   Diagram of venogram and representative radiograph, lateral view.

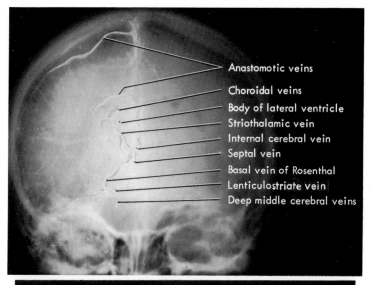

Anastomotic veins

Choroidal veins

Body of lateral ventricle

Striothalamic vein

Internal cerebral vein

Septal vein

Basal vein of Rosenthal

Lenticulostriate vein

Deep middle cerebral veins

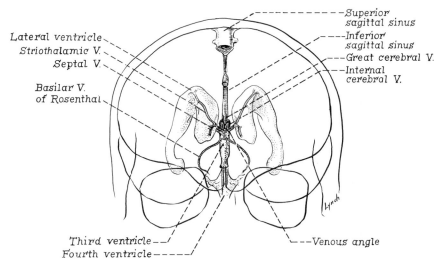

Superior sagittal sinus

Inferior sagittal sinus

Great cerebral V.

Internal cerebral V.

Lateral ventricle
Striothalamic V.
Septal V.

Basilar V. of Rosenthal

Third ventricle
Fourth ventricle

Venous angle

FIGURE 5-29B. Diagram of venogram, A-P view, and representative radiograph (intensified).

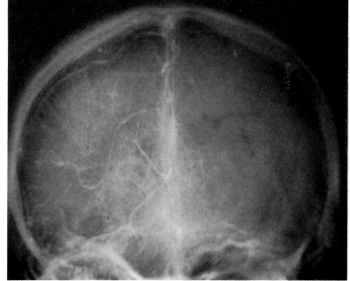

Chapter 6 — The Vertebral Column and Myelography

THE VERTEBRAL COLUMN

The vertebral column is composed of separate articulating segments called vertebrae. These are 33 in number and distributed as follows: 7 cervical, 12 thoracic, 5 lumbar, 5 sacral and 4 coccygeal (Fig. 6-1).

Occasionally there is an extra vertebra in either the thoracic or lumbar spine, or there may be one less vertebra than normal, particularly in the lumbar spine. In the latter case, there may be an extra vertebra fused with the coccyx, either completely or partially.

A vertebra consists of the following parts: (1) the body, (2) the transverse process on each side, (3) the pedicles, (4) the laminae, (5) the superior articular processes, (6) the inferior articular processes, (7) the spinous processes and (8) the partes interarticulares situated between the two articular processes.

In the cervical spine, the transverse and costal processes fuse to form the "lateral mass," with the foramen transversaria between. In the thoracic spine, the costal process remains separate and participates in the formation of the head and neck of the rib with which it articulates. In the lumbar and sacral spine, the costal and transverse processes are completely fused.

The following joints are identified in the spinal column: (1) amphiarthrodial joints between the vertebral bodies (intervertebral disk); (2) synovial joints (diarthrodial joints) between the articular processes on each side of adjoining vertebrae (also called apophyseal joints); (3) costovertebral joints which represent synovial joints at the junction of ribs and vertebrae; and (4) synovial joints between the posterolateral margins of the lower five cervical vertebral bodies (joints of Luschka) (Fig. 6-2A and B).

The intervertebral disk which lies between each two vertebral bodies (from C 2 to S 1) is composed of fibrocartilage, with a gelatinous central matrix known as the nucleus pulposus. It is firmly attached to adjoining vertebral bodies.

The thoracic spine has several distinguishing characteristics.

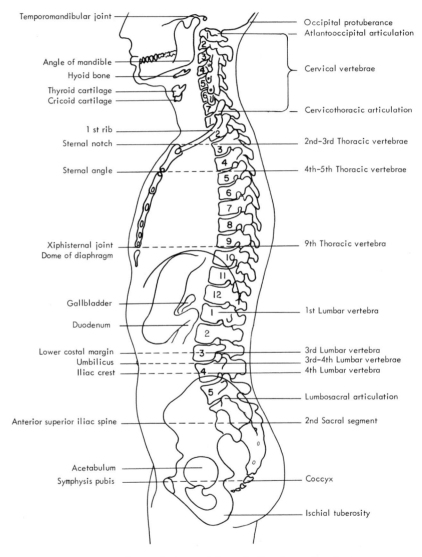

FIGURE 6-1. Lateral view of the spinal column in relation to some anterior structures (Modified from Clark).

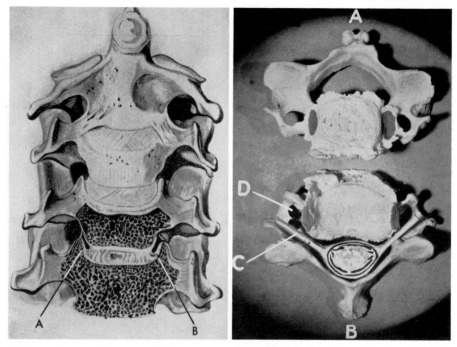

FIGURE 6-2. **A,** Reproduction from Luschka's "Monograph," showing the joints (A and B) between the posterolateral aspects of the sectioned lower cervical vertebral bodies. **B,** Photograph of the fifth (A) and sixth (B) cervical vertebrae showing Luschka joints in relationship to the mixed nerve roots and vertebral foramina. The joints are painted for contrast; the female segment is seen on A and the male part on B. It is apparent that Luschka joints are situated ventromedial to the nerves (C) which emerge through the intervertebral foramina and also medial to the vertebral vessels and sympathetics which pass through the vertebral foramina (D). (From Boreadis, A. G., and Gershon-Cohen, J.: Radiology *66*, 1956.)

The vertebral bodies of the upper eight segments articulate with two ribs on each side, and the lower four articulate only with the one rib with which they are numerically associated. There are also small costal facets on each transverse process of the upper 10 thoracic vertebrae. The two different joints formed are called the costovertebral and costotransverse joints, respectively, with separate synovial cavities and joint capsules in each instance.

The paraspinal line (paravertebral soft tissue shadows, Fig. 6-11), well delineated in frontal radiographs of the thoracic spine, must be differentiated from manifestations of disease. A left paraspinal shadow, delimited by the left pleural reflection, is commonly visualized on films of the thoracic spine. It roughly parallels the left margin of the vertebral column and the aorta and lies between these two structures.

(*Text continues on page 185.*)

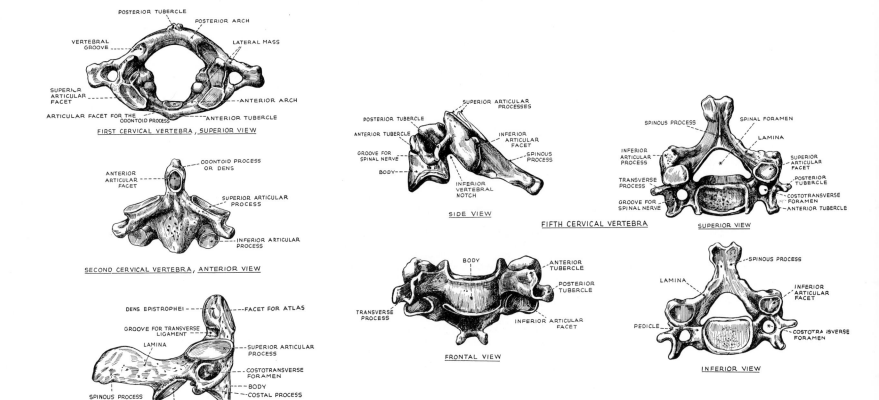

FIGURE 6-3. Distinguishing characteristics of cervical vertebrae.

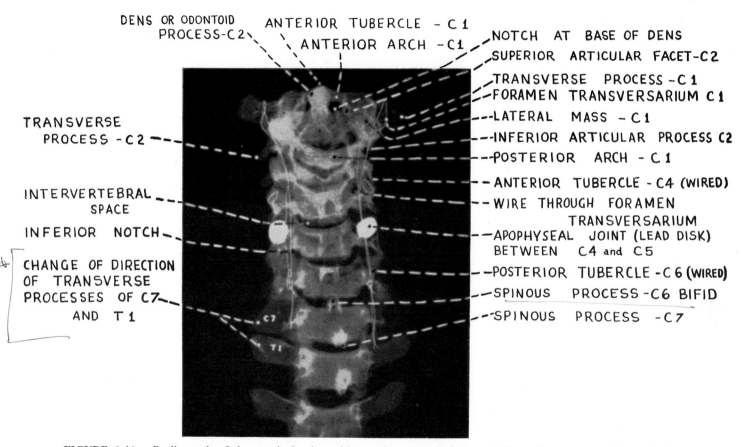

DENS OR ODONTOID
PROCESS-C2

ANTERIOR TUBERCLE - C1
ANTERIOR ARCH - C1

NOTCH AT BASE OF DENS
SUPERIOR ARTICULAR FACET-C2
TRANSVERSE PROCESS - C1
FORAMEN TRANSVERSARIUM C1
LATERAL MASS - C1
INFERIOR ARTICULAR PROCESS C2
POSTERIOR ARCH - C1
ANTERIOR TUBERCLE - C4 (WIRED)
WIRE THROUGH FORAMEN
TRANSVERSARIUM
APOPHYSEAL JOINT (LEAD DISK)
BETWEEN C4 and C5
POSTERIOR TUBERCLE - C6 (WIRED)
SPINOUS PROCESS - C6 BIFID
SPINOUS PROCESS - C7

TRANSVERSE
PROCESS - C2

INTERVERTEBRAL
SPACE
INFERIOR NOTCH

CHANGE OF DIRECTION
OF TRANSVERSE
PROCESSES OF C7
AND T1

FIGURE 6-4A Radiograph of the cervical spine with certain anatomic features indicated, anteroposterior projection.

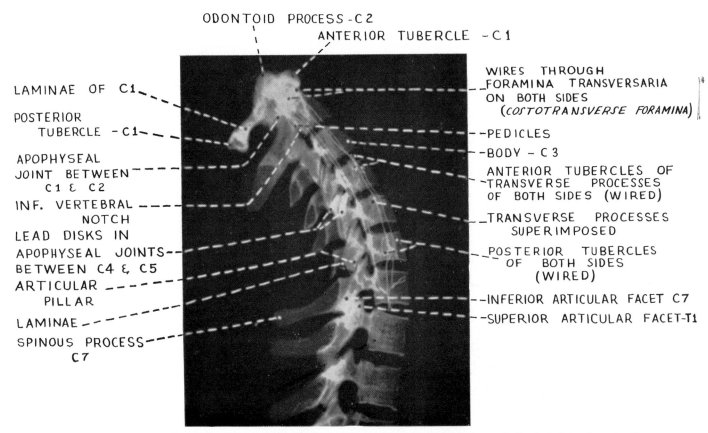

ODONTOID PROCESS - C2

ANTERIOR TUBERCLE - C1

LAMINAE OF C1

POSTERIOR
    TUBERCLE - C1

APOPHYSEAL
JOINT BETWEEN
    C1 & C2

INF. VERTEBRAL
        NOTCH
LEAD DISKS IN
APOPHYSEAL JOINTS
BETWEEN C4 & C5
ARTICULAR
    PILLAR

LAMINAE

SPINOUS PROCESS
        C7

WIRES THROUGH
FORAMINA TRANSVERSARIA
ON BOTH SIDES
    (COSTOTRANSVERSE FORAMINA)

PEDICLES

BODY - C3

ANTERIOR TUBERCLES OF
TRANSVERSE PROCESSES
OF BOTH SIDES (WIRED)

TRANSVERSE PROCESSES
    SUPERIMPOSED

POSTERIOR TUBERCLES
    OF BOTH SIDES
        (WIRED)

INFERIOR ARTICULAR FACET C7

SUPERIOR ARTICULAR FACET - T1

FIGURE 6-4B. Radiograph of the cervical spine with certain anatomic features indicated, lateral projection.

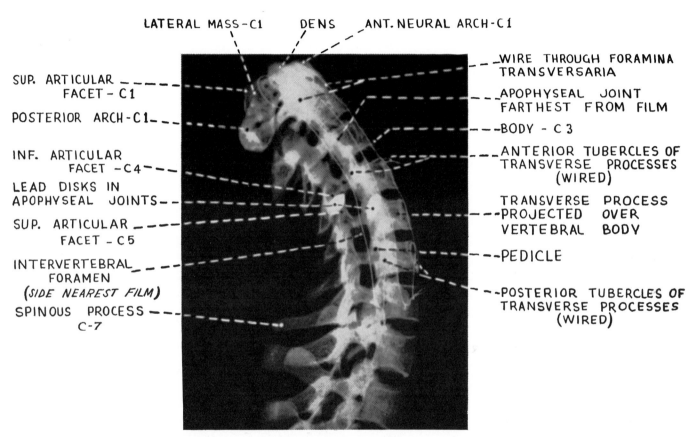

LATERAL MASS – C1   DENS   ANT. NEURAL ARCH – C1

SUP. ARTICULAR
FACET – C1

POSTERIOR ARCH – C1

INF. ARTICULAR
FACET – C4

LEAD DISKS IN
APOPHYSEAL JOINTS

SUP. ARTICULAR
FACET – C5

INTERVERTEBRAL
FORAMEN
(SIDE NEAREST FILM)

SPINOUS PROCESS
C-7

WIRE THROUGH FORAMINA
TRANSVERSARIA

APOPHYSEAL JOINT
FARTHEST FROM FILM

BODY – C3

ANTERIOR TUBERCLES OF
TRANSVERSE PROCESSES
(WIRED)

TRANSVERSE PROCESS
PROJECTED OVER
VERTEBRAL BODY

PEDICLE

POSTERIOR TUBERCLES OF
TRANSVERSE PROCESSES
(WIRED)

FIGURE 6-4C. Radiograph of the cervical spine with certain anatomic features indicated, oblique projection.

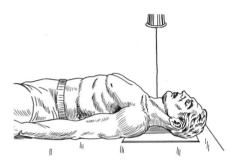

POINTS OF PRACTICAL INTEREST ABOUT FIGURE 6-5

1. The sagittal plane of the head is centered to the longitudinal axis of the table and the patient's chin is extended sufficiently so that the lower edge of his anterior teeth is in the same perpendicular line as the tip of the mastoid processes.

2. The head should be immobilized by means of either sandbags or head clamps. These have been omitted in the drawings for the sake of clarity.

3. The central ray passes through the most prominent point of the thyroid cartilage. This ordinarily lies anterior to the fourth cervical segment.

4. Alternately, the central ray may be angled 15 or 20 degrees toward the head, which gives one a somewhat clearer concept of the lower intervertebral spaces and a better view for demonstration of possible cervical ribs.

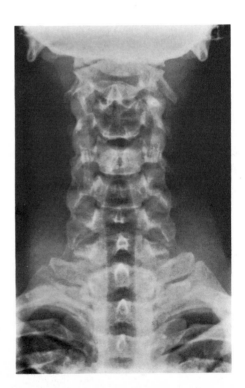

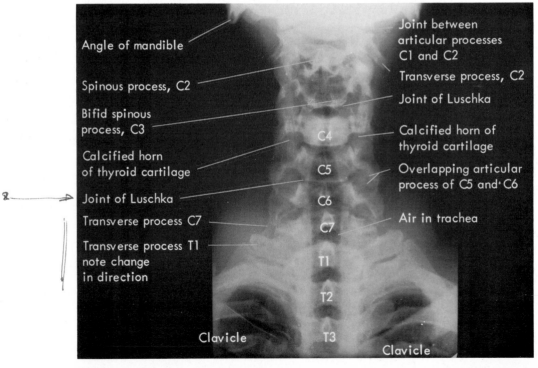

Angle of mandible

Joint between articular processes C1 and C2

Spinous process, C2

Transverse process, C2

Bifid spinous process, C3

Joint of Luschka

Calcified horn of thyroid cartilage

C4

Calcified horn of thyroid cartilage

C5

Overlapping articular process of C5 and C6

Joint of Luschka

C6

Transverse process C7

C7

Air in trachea

Transverse process T1 note change in direction

T1

T2

Clavicle

T3

Clavicle

FIGURE 6-5.   Anteroposterior view of cervical spine.

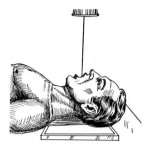

POINTS OF PRACTICAL INTEREST ABOUT FIGURE 6-6

1. The patient's mouth is opened as widely as possible and it may be kept in this position by a large cork or balsa wood block.

2. A line drawn between the lower margin of the anterior upper teeth and the tip of the mastoid process must be perpendicular to the film.

3. If the patient will softly say "Ah" during the exposure, the tongue will be more closely fixed to the floor of the mouth so that its shadow will not be projected over the atlas and axis.

4. Body-section radiographs of the odontoid process and adjoining joints are frequently very helpful (Fig. 6-7).

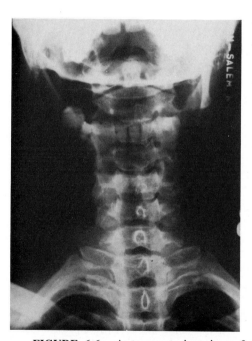

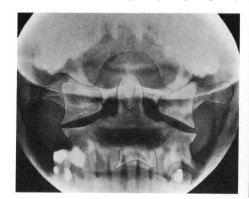

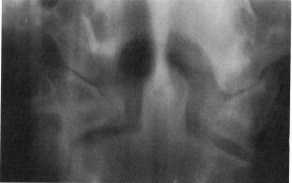

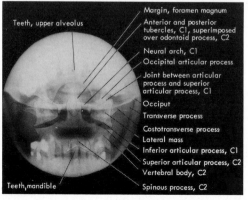

FIGURE 6-6. Anteroposterior view of the cervical spine obtained with a rhythmic motion of the lower jaw during the exposure. The head, of course, is rigidly immobilized to prevent movement of the cervical spine. When a view is obtained in this manner a concept of the upper two cervical segments may be obtained which otherwise is not possible in this projection, since these segments are invariably obscured by the shadow of the mandible (Ottonello method).

FIGURE 6-7. Anteroposterior view of upper cervical spine with mouth open particularly to show odontoid process. (Radiograph intensified.)

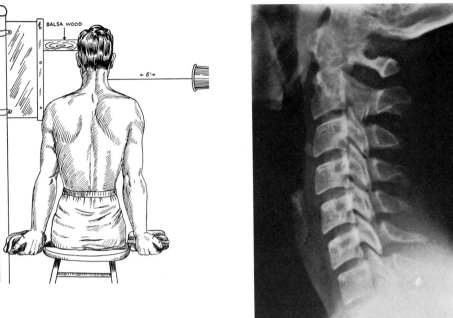

POINTS OF PRACTICAL INTEREST ABOUT FIGURE 6-8A

1. The shoulders should be lowered by weights held in the patient's hands, and all *seven* cervical vertebrae must be clearly seen.

2. The hand is supported in a perfectly vertical position, with the sagittal plane perfectly parallel to the cassette.

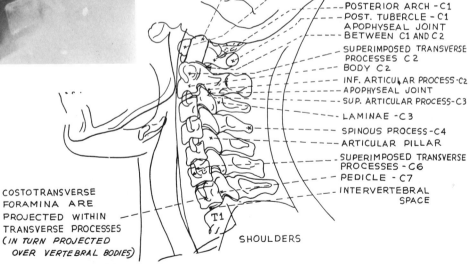

DENS (ODONTOID PROCESS)
ANT. TUBERCLE -C1
POSTERIOR ARCH -C1
POST. TUBERCLE - C1
APOPHYSEAL JOINT BETWEEN C1 AND C2
SUPERIMPOSED TRANSVERSE PROCESSES C2
BODY C2
INF. ARTICULAR PROCESS -C2
APOPHYSEAL JOINT
SUP. ARTICULAR PROCESS -C3
LAMINAE -C3
SPINOUS PROCESS -C4
ARTICULAR PILLAR
SUPERIMPOSED TRANSVERSE PROCESSES -C6
PEDICLE - C7
INTERVERTEBRAL SPACE

COSTOTRANSVERSE FORAMINA ARE PROJECTED WITHIN TRANSVERSE PROCESSES (*IN TURN PROJECTED OVER VERTEBRAL BODIES*)

T1

SHOULDERS

FIGURE 6-8A.   Lateral view of cervical spine and positioning of patient for erect (6 foot film-target distance) and recumbent views. The erect view shown is the Grandy technique, described by C. C. Grandy in 1925 (Radiology 5:128-129, 1925).

Normal Sagittal Measurements*

Region Evaluated	Normal Sagittal Measurements for Children 15 Years and Under (120 cases)		Normal Sagittal Measurements for Adults (480 cases)	
	Average (mm.)	Range (mm.)	Average (mm.)	Range (mm.)
Retropharyngeal space	3.5	2–7	3.4	1–7
Retrotracheal space	7.9	5–14	14.0	9–22
Cervical spinal canal:				
At first cervical vertebra	21.9	18–27	21.4	16–30
At second cervical vertebra	20.9	18–25	19.2	16–28
At third cervical vertebra	17.4	14–21	19.1	14–25
At fifth cervical vertebra	16.5	14–21	18.5	14–25
At seventh cervical vertebra	16.0	15–20	17.5	13–24

*From Whiley, M. H., et al.: Radiology, *71*:350, 1958.

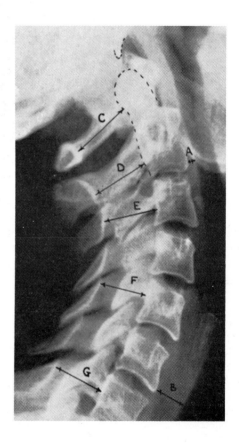

FIGURE 6-8B. Normal lateral view of neck indicating regions evaluated. *A*, Retropharyngeal space, second cervical vertebra; *B*, retrotracheal space, sixth cervical vertebra; *C* to *G*, cervical spinal canal; *C*, first cervical vertebra; *D*, second cervical vertebra; *E*, third cervical vertebra; *F*, fifth cervical vertebra; *G*, seventh cervical vertebra (from Wholey, M. H., Brewer, A. J., and Baker, H. L., Jr.: Radiology *71*:350, 1958).

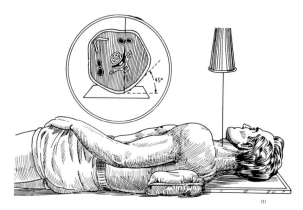

POINTS OF PRACTICAL INTEREST ABOUT FIGURE 6-9

1. This view may be obtained in either the erect or recumbent position.

2. The entire body of the patient is rotated, and if he is supine, sandbags are placed beneath the shoulder and the buttocks to support his position at an angle of 45 degrees with the table top. The sagittal axis of the patient's head is perfectly straight with regard to that of the entire body.

3. The central ray is directed over the cervical spine at the level of the fourth cervical segment (at the level of the most prominent portion of the thyroid cartilage).

4. Alternately an additional angulation of the tube 15 degrees toward the head may be employed, with the patient in the position just described.

5. It is best to employ a focal-film distance of at least 48 inches since the cervical spine is at such a great distance from the film in this projection.

6. Oblique studies of both sides are routinely obtained

7. The intervertebral foramina that are farthest from the film are the ones that are shown most clearly.

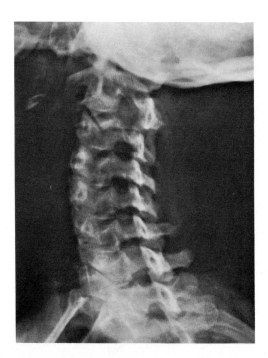

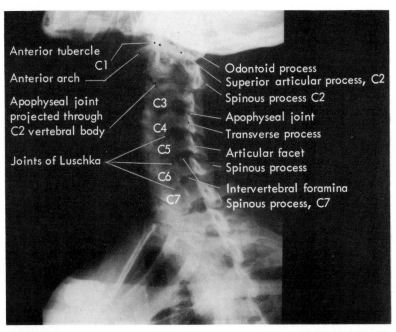

Anterior tubercle
C1
Anterior arch

Apophyseal joint
projected through
C2 vertebral body

C3

C4

Joints of Luschka
C5

C6

C7

Odontoid process
Superior articular process, C2
Spinous process C2
Apophyseal joint
Transverse process
Articular facet
Spinous process
Intervertebral foramina
Spinous process, C7

FIGURE 6-9.   Oblique view of cervical spine.

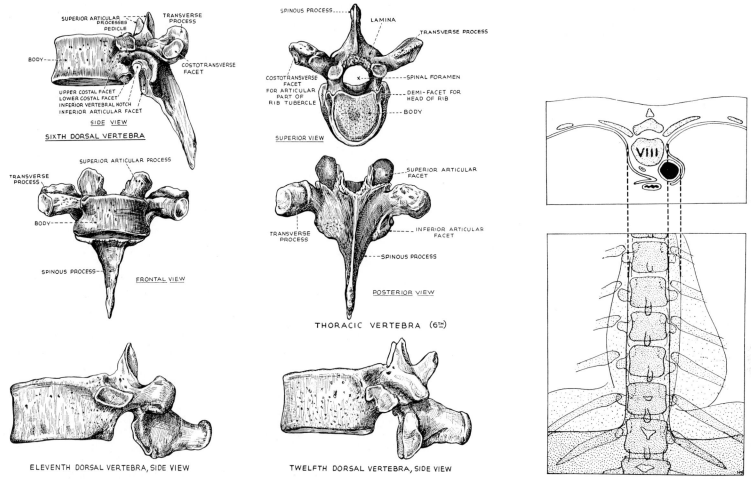

Labels (Figure 6-10):

SIXTH DORSAL VERTEBRA — SIDE VIEW:
SUPERIOR ARTICULAR PROCESSES — PEDICLE — TRANSVERSE PROCESS — BODY — COSTOTRANSVERSE FACET — UPPER COSTAL FACET — LOWER COSTAL FACET — INFERIOR VERTEBRAL NOTCH — INFERIOR ARTICULAR FACET

FRONTAL VIEW:
TRANSVERSE PROCESS — SUPERIOR ARTICULAR PROCESS — BODY — SPINOUS PROCESS

SUPERIOR VIEW:
SPINOUS PROCESS — LAMINA — TRANSVERSE PROCESS — SPINAL FORAMEN — DEMI-FACET FOR HEAD OF RIB — BODY — COSTOTRANSVERSE FACET FOR ARTICULAR PART OF RIB TUBERCLE

THORACIC VERTEBRA (6TH) — POSTERIOR VIEW:
SUPERIOR ARTICULAR FACET — TRANSVERSE PROCESS — INFERIOR ARTICULAR FACET — SPINOUS PROCESS

ELEVENTH DORSAL VERTEBRA, SIDE VIEW

TWELFTH DORSAL VERTEBRA, SIDE VIEW

FIGURE 6-10.   Distinguishing characteristics of dorsal vertebrae.

FIGURE 6-11.   *Upper,* Cross section through the posterior mediastinum at the level of the eighth thoracic vertebra. *Lower,* Diagram taken from a roentgenogram depicting the posterior portions of the visceral and parietal pleura as lines along the vertebral column. Dotted lines indicate anatomical substrates of pleural lines and aortic lines in cross section. (From Lachman, E.: Anat. Rec. *83*, 1942.)

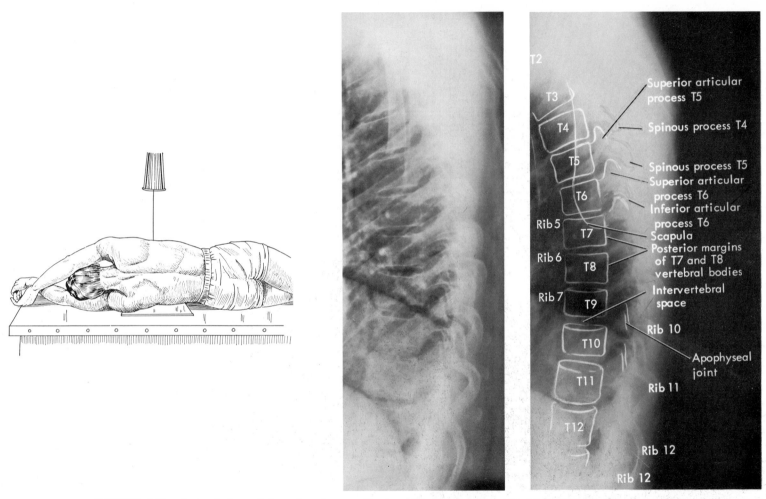

FIGURE 6-12. Lateral view of thoracic spine: positioning of patient, radiograph and labeled tracing.

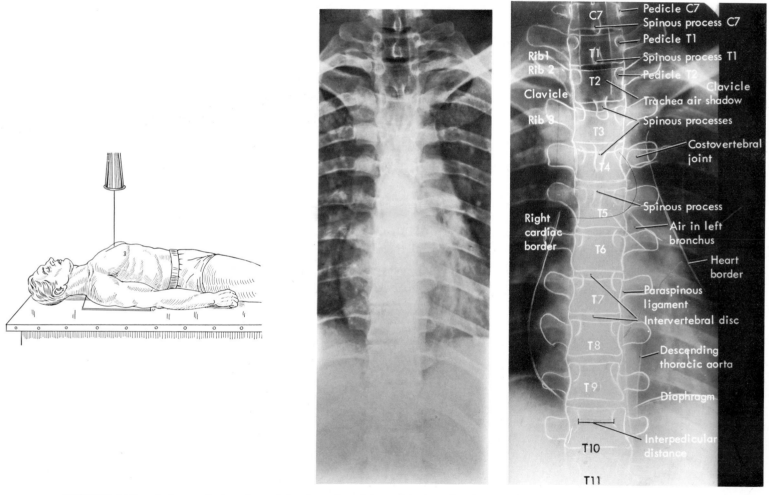

FIGURE 6-13. Anteroposterior view of the thoracic spine: positioning of patient, radiograph and labeled tracing.

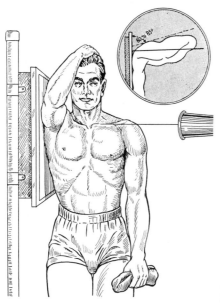

POINTS OF PRACTICAL INTEREST ABOUT FIGURE 6-14

1. The patient's midaxillary plane is placed against the midline of the film. The shoulder that is farthest from the film is depressed as much as possible with a heavy weight in the hand, whereas that which is closest to the film is rotated forward by placing the hand on the head and flexing the elbow. There may be a very slight rotation of the patient's body, 5 to 10 degrees as shown.

2 The patient's axilla closest to the film is centered on the film, and the central ray is directed perpendicular to the film at this central point.

3 The central ray is perpendicular to the film if the remote shoulder can be depressed adequately, but an angle of 15 degrees toward the feet may be employed when the shoulder cannot be well depressed.

4. A view of the uppermost two thoracic segments is not obtained on a routine lateral thoracic spine film, and when these two segments must be visualized some special means such as this must be employed.

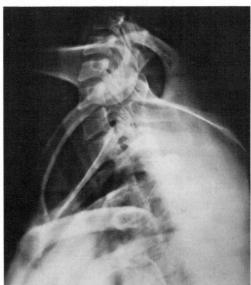
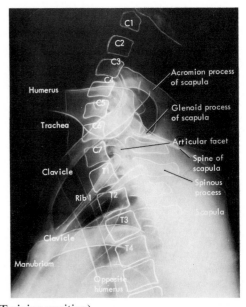

FIGURE 6-14. Lateral (slightly oblique) view of upper two thoracic segments (Twining position).

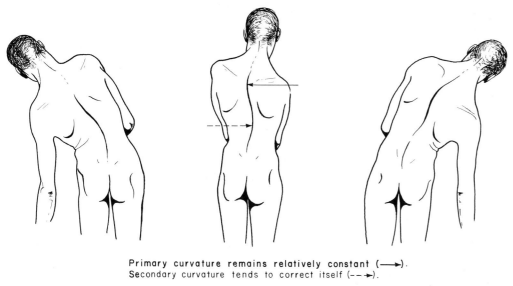

Primary curvature remains relatively constant (——➤).
Secondary curvature tends to correct itself (— —➤).

FIGURE 6-15 Method for positioning patient for study of scoliosis of the spine.

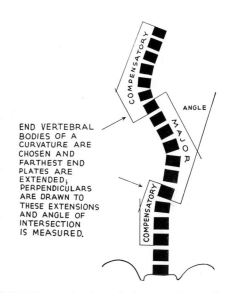

END VERTEBRAL BODIES OF A CURVATURE ARE CHOSEN AND FARTHEST END PLATES ARE EXTENDED; PERPENDICULARS ARE DRAWN TO THESE EXTENSIONS AND ANGLE OF INTERSECTION IS MEASURED.

COMPENSATORY

ANGLE

MAJOR

COMPENSATORY

FIGURE 6-16. Method of measuring scoliosis.

STUDIES FOR ABNORMALITIES IN SPINAL CURVATURE

Definition of Terms

Scoliosis: Rotation or torsion of several vertebrae in their longitudinal axis.

Lordosis: Increased concavity of the spine on its posterior aspect

Kyphosis: Angulation of the spine on its posterior aspect.

Gibbus: Posterior angulation of the spine with no significant disturbance in the line of weight bearing.

Each of these processes has a fulcrum around which the major curvature occurs. A method of measuring scoliosis is indicated in Figure 6-16. One can differentiate a primary scoliosis from the secondary site of curvature by the method shown in Figure 6-15 The primary curvature cannot be significantly changed by bending to one side or the other, or by tilting the pelvis; a secondary curvature will change with tilting the pelvis or bending.

STUDIES FOR STABILITY OF VERTEBRAL SEGMENTS WITH RESPECT TO ONE ANOTHER

Definition of Terms

Subluxations and *dislocations* refer to varying degrees of malalignment of a part with respect to a contiguous part, at the joint site between them.

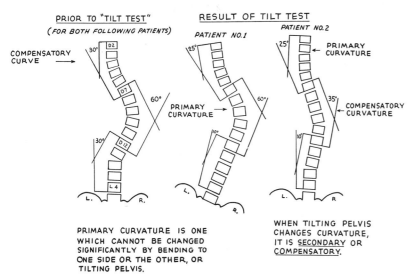

FIGURE 6-17. Determination of primary and secondary curvatures in dorsal scoliosis. (Modified from Ferguson, A. B.: *Roentgen Diagnosis of Extremities and Spine.* New York, Paul B. Hoeber, Inc , 1949.)

Sites of Subluxation or Dislocation in the Spine

Subluxation or dislocation occurs most frequently at the following sites: (1) the first two cervical segments; (2) the levels of C 4, C 5, C 6, and C 7; and (3) the lower lumbar region in relation to a phenomenon known as spondylolisthesis.

Spondylolisthesis refers to the slipping forward of a vertebral body with respect to the adjoining body, usually because of defective ossification, and hence inadequate bony support, at the pars interarticularis.

Films for Demonstration of Instability or Subluxation

Films to test instability of any part of the spine may be obtained under the careful guidance of a physician. Usually they will be sequential films in flexion and extension in the lateral projection centering over the area of suspected abnormality. A method for accomplishing this in the lumbar region is illustrated in Figure 6-18B.

THE VERTEBRAL CANAL AND SPINAL SUBARACHNOID SPACE

The spinal cord lies loosely in its meninges and extends from the foramen magnum to the lower border of the first lumbar vertebra. It has two bulbous enlargements supplying nerves to the upper and lower extremities respectively. From the L 1 level, there is a slender filament that extends downward to the first coccygeal segment

As in the case of the brain, the spinal subarachnoid space contains fluid in direct communication with the ventricles and subarachnoid space surrounding the brain.

The spinal nerves arise at considerably higher levels than their corresponding intervertebral foramina. The cauda equina is formed by the spinal nerves that extend below the termination of the cord at the L 1 level. As these nerves leave the spinal canal, there is a sleeve of meninges, called the nerve sheath, which is carried with them. A small pouch on the inferior aspect of the sleeve is called the axillary pouch. In the lumbar region, the nerve sheath curves under the vertebral pedicle and below the inferior margin of the intervertebral disk—a point of considerable practical clinical importance. Here it is vulnerable to pressure from extruded elements of the intervertebral disk itself

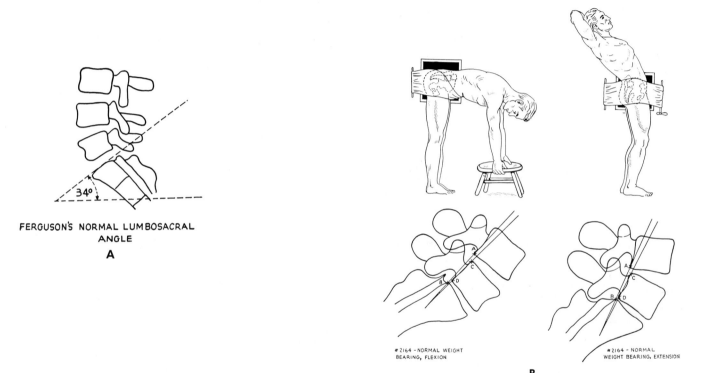

FERGUSON'S NORMAL LUMBOSACRAL
ANGLE

A

#2164 – NORMAL WEIGHT
BEARING, FLEXION

#2164 – NORMAL
WEIGHT BEARING, EXTENSION

B

FIGURE 6-18. Measurement of the lumbosacral angle. **A,** Ferguson's method of determining the normal lumbosacral angle in the lateral projection. **B,** Method of measuring stability at the lumbosacral angle by obtaining films showing weight bearing in flexion and extension, and of measuring the alignment of the fifth lumbar vertebra with respect to the fourth lumbar vertebra and the sacrum.

RELATIONSHIP OF CERVICAL VERTEBRAL BODIES IN
FLEXION, NEUTRAL, AND EXTENSION POSITIONS

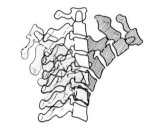

A

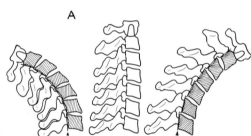

-NOTE STEPLIKE RELATIONSHIP OF POSTERIOR MARGINS
OF VERTEBRAL BODIES IN NORMAL ALIGNMENT.

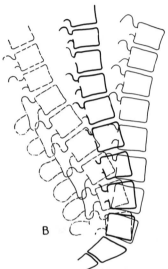

B

SUPERIMPOSED TRACINGS OF LUMBAR SPINE IN FLEXION
AND EXTENSION AS WELL AS NEUTRAL POSITION.
RELATIVE MOVEMENTS OF L3, L4, AND L5 GIVE SOME
INDICATION OF PRESENCE OR ABSENCE OF DISC
ABNORMALITIES, SINCE A RELATIVE IMMOBILITY
IS NOTED UNDER THESE CIRCUMSTANCES.

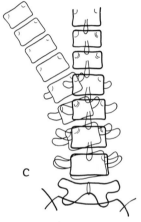

C

RELATIVE MOVEMENT OF L3, L4, and L5
MAY ASSIST IN LOCALIZING INTRASPINAL
DISEASE. NORMAL RELATIONSHIPS ARE
SHOWN IN A. IMMOBILITY MAY ASSIST
IN LOCALIZING DISEASE.

FIGURE 6-19. Flexion, extension and lateral bending studies of the cervical and lumbar spine (tracings only). By superimposition of the several views of a single anatomic part (such as the cervical spine) one can readily visualize the total range of movement, and degrees of movement can be measured and plotted. The plotting of these measurements usually is a smooth curve with gradual increments from one segment to another. Any change in the smoothness of this curve may be of significance in localizing altered mobility from any cause.

When films are obtained for this purpose, movement is permissible only in the anatomic part being studied so that good superimposition is possible. If cineradiographic equipment is available, a similar study may be undertaken and readily visualized.

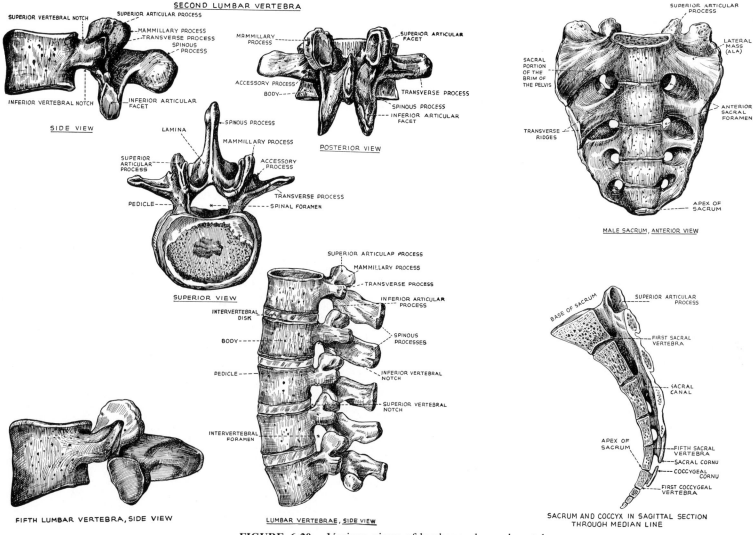

SECOND LUMBAR VERTEBRA

SUPERIOR VERTEBRAL NOTCH
SUPERIOR ARTICULAR PROCESS
MAMMILLARY PROCESS
TRANSVERSE PROCESS
SPINOUS PROCESS

INFERIOR VERTEBRAL NOTCH
INFERIOR ARTICULAR FACET

SIDE VIEW

MAMMILLARY PROCESS
SUPERIOR ARTICULAR FACET
ACCESSORY PROCESS
BODY
TRANSVERSE PROCESS
SPINOUS PROCESS
INFERIOR ARTICULAR FACET

POSTERIOR VIEW

LAMINA
SPINOUS PROCESS
MAMMILLARY PROCESS
SUPERIOR ARTICULAR PROCESS
ACCESSORY PROCESS
PEDICLE
TRANSVERSE PROCESS
SPINAL FORAMEN

SUPERIOR VIEW

SUPERIOR ARTICULAR PROCESS
MAMMILLARY PROCESS
TRANSVERSE PROCESS
INFERIOR ARTICULAR PROCESS
INTERVERTEBRAL DISK
BODY
SPINOUS PROCESSES
PEDICLE
INFERIOR VERTEBRAL NOTCH
SUPERIOR VERTEBRAL NOTCH
INTERVERTEBRAL FORAMEN

FIFTH LUMBAR VERTEBRA, SIDE VIEW

LUMBAR VERTEBRAE, SIDE VIEW

SUPERIOR ARTICULAR PROCESS
LATERAL MASS (ALA)
SACRAL PORTION OF THE BRIM OF THE PELVIS
ANTERIOR SACRAL FORAMEN
TRANSVERSE RIDGES
APEX OF SACRUM

MALE SACRUM, ANTERIOR VIEW

BASE OF SACRUM
SUPERIOR ARTICULAR PROCESS
FIRST SACRAL VERTEBRA
SACRAL CANAL
APEX OF SACRUM
FIFTH SACRAL VERTEBRA
SACRAL CORNU
COCCYGEAL CORNU
FIRST COCCYGEAL VERTEBRA

SACRUM AND COCCYX IN SAGITTAL SECTION THROUGH MEDIAN LINE

FIGURE 6-20. Various views of lumbar and sacral vertebrae.

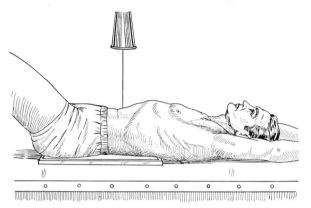

POINTS OF PRACTICAL INTEREST ABOUT FIGURE 6-21

1. The lumbar curvature will impose a degree of distortion and magnification on those lumbar vertebrae which are farthest from the film. To diminish this effect, the knees are flexed as shown in Figure 6-21, which straightens the lumbar spine to some extent.

2 The student should acquire sufficient knowledge of anatomy to visualize the entire vertebral segment from the frontal and lateral perspectives. This can best be accomplished by studying the labeled radiographs with vertebrae in hand

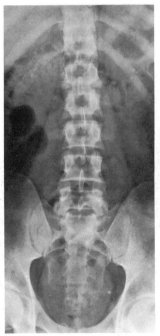

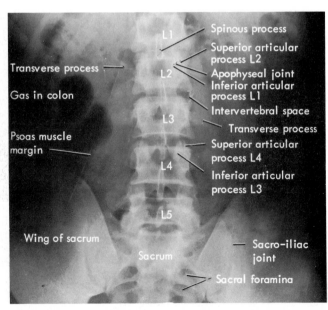

FIGURE 6-21.   Anteroposterior view of lumbosacral spine: positioning of patient, radiograph and labeled tracing.

POINTS OF PRACTICAL INTEREST ABOUT FIGURE 6-22

1. The hips and knees are flexed to a comfortable position, and balsa wood blocks are placed in the depression above the iliac crest so that the thoracic spine, lumbar spine and sacrum are parallel with the table top. A Potter-Bucky diaphragm is always employed.

2. Usually, a separate exposure is required for the fifth lumbar, sacrum and coccyx, since more penetrating x-rays are required. A suitable wedge filter may be employed to combine the two on a single exposure.

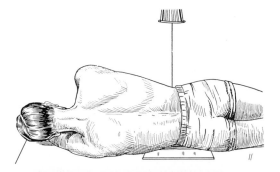

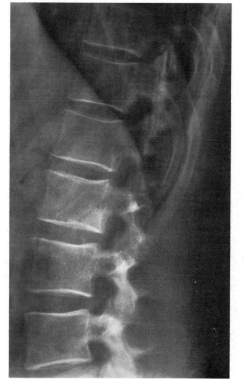

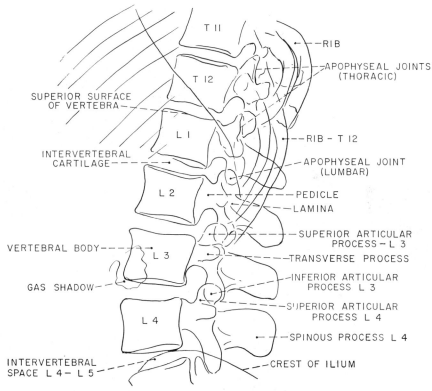

FIGURE 6-22 Lateral view of the lumbosacral spine.

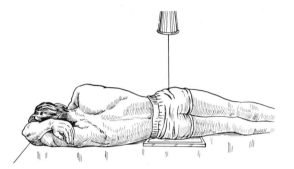

POINTS OF PRACTICAL INTEREST ABOUT FIGURE 6-23

1. To help immobilize the patient, his hips and knees are flexed to a comfortable position.

2. The coronal plane passing 3 inches posterior to the midaxillary line is adjusted to the longitudinal axis of the table.

3. It is usually desirable to place folded sheets or balsa wood blocks in the depression above the iliac crest to maintain the lower thoracic spine in a perfectly parallel relationship with the table top

4. Although the film here is demonstrated immediately beneath the patient, a Potter-Bucky diaphragm is always employed.

5 If it is the coccyx that is the major interest, a somewhat lighter exposure technique must be employed and less detail with regard to the sacrum will then be obtained.

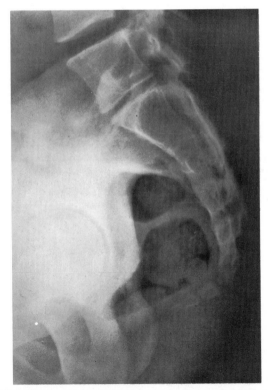

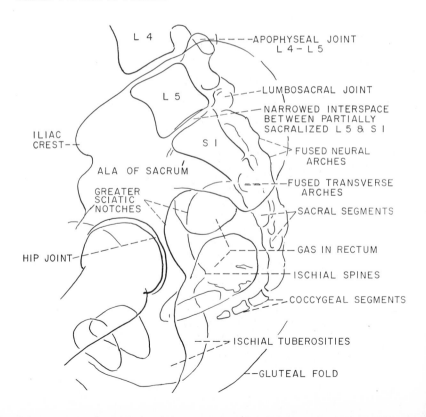

FIGURE 6-23. Special lateral view of sacrum and coccyx.

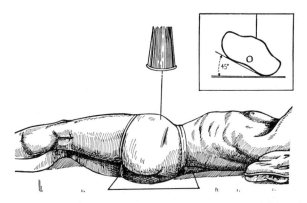

POINTS OF PRACTICAL INTEREST ABOUT FIGURE 6-24

1. The patient's body is placed obliquely with respect to the table top at an angle of 25 to 45 degrees. The coronal plane passing through the spinous processes is centered to the midline of the table.

2. If the lower lumbar apophyseal joints are of greatest interest, the central ray passes through the level of the raised iliac crest. If the upper lumbar apophyseal joints are desired, the central ray passes through a point about 1 inch above the raised iliac crest.

3. The apophyseal joints closest to the film will be shown to best advantage, but occasionally it will require several attempts with varying degrees of angulation to obtain a clear view of all the apophyseal joints. This may be necessary since the plane of the joint varies somewhat as one descends the lumbar spine.

4. The sacroiliac joint that is farthest from the film will be opened up to best advantage. An angle of approximately 25 degrees is usually most satisfactory for the sacroiliac joint depiction.

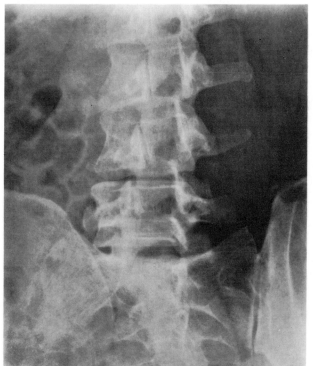

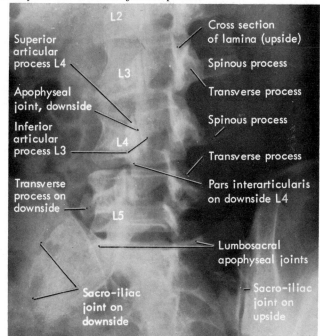

FIGURE 6-24.   Oblique view of lumbosacral spine.

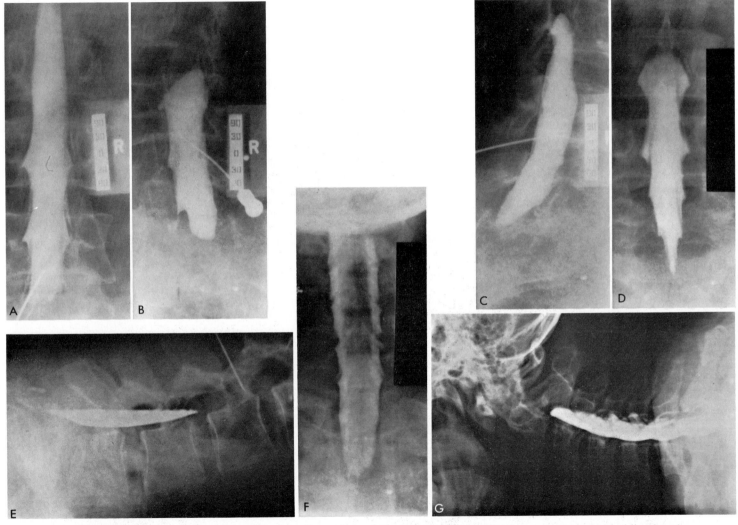

FIGURE 6-25. Example radiographs of lumbar and cervical myelograms. **A** to **D,** Anteroposterior and oblique projections of lumbar myelograms; **E,** lateral horizontal beam study of lumbosacral myelogram; **F,** anteroposterior view of cervical myelogram; **G,** lateral horizontal beam study of cervical myelogram.

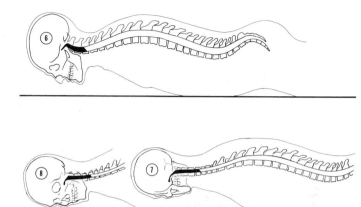

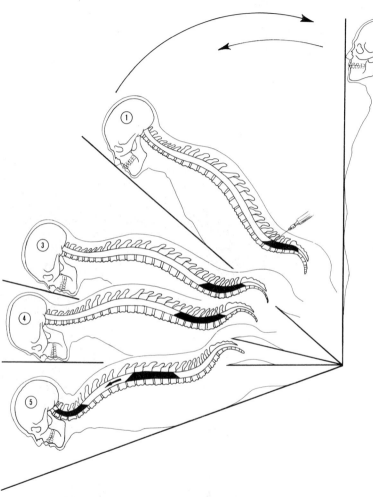

A

B

FIGURE 6-26. Position of patient during myelography: **A,** lumbar and cervical; **B,** for visualization of region of clivus and internal acoustic meati (see text for description).

Contrast Myelography

The two major methods of study involve the introduction of either a positive contrast medium such as Pantopaque or a gaseous medium such as air into the subarachnoid space by lumbar puncture. The Pantopaque technique is by far the most frequently employed.

With the patient prone, 3 to 12 ml. of the iodized oil is introduced at the level of the third or fourth lumbar interspace (Fig. 6-26A). The needle is usually left in place to facilitate removal of the contrast medium after completion of the examination. Because the oil is heavier than spinal fluid, the patient is tilted so that the subarachnoid space can be studied completely. First the patient is almost erect, so that the caudal sac may be studied in posteroanterior oblique and lateral decubitus projections (Fig. 6-26A). Then, under fluoroscopic control, the table is tilted until the medium reaches the thoracic spine. Here, the oil column may break up, but by tilting the table and at the same time hyperextending the patient's head, the oil medium is trapped in the cervical region.

Once the main bulk of medium is in the cervical region, the table may be placed horizontal. By carefully flexing the patient's

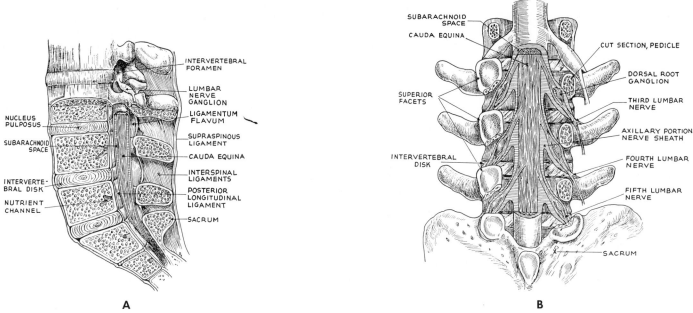

FIGURE 6-27. **A,** Structure of intervertebral disk and its relationship to the subarachnoid space and adjoining ligamentous structures. **B,** Relationship of spinal nerve roots to axillary pouches of the subarachnoid space.

head, and possibly at the same time tilting the table head downward, the entire cervical subarachnoid space can be visualized to the level of the foramen magnum. Again posteroanterior and lateral decubitus films are obtained

If it is desired that the internal acoustic meatus and clivus be delineated, the following procedure is carefully carried out (Fig. 6-26B). After the oil medium is on the clivus, but not in the cranial cavity proper, the person manipulating the patient's head carefully rotates it with the chin toward the right, lowering it just enough to trap a droplet of oil in the internal acoustic meatus. When this has been accomplished, appropriate films are immediately obtained, and the oil is once again returned to its position on the clivus. In similar fashion, the head is then rotated to the opposite side, and a similar

film and fluoroscopic study of the opposite meatus is obtained. It is best to place an opaque object such as a lead number in each external auditory meatus to facilitate orientation during fluoroscopy. It is imperative that during this procedure there be careful cooperation between the fluoroscopist and the person holding the patient's head Moreover, image amplification and closed circuit television fluoroscopy are deemed most desirable if the best results are to be achieved

Although intracranial Pantopaque is undesirable, it is probable that no serious sequelae would result if this should occur. With proper expertise and cooperation of patient and examining team, usually all of the Pantopaque can be recovered through the lumbar needle.

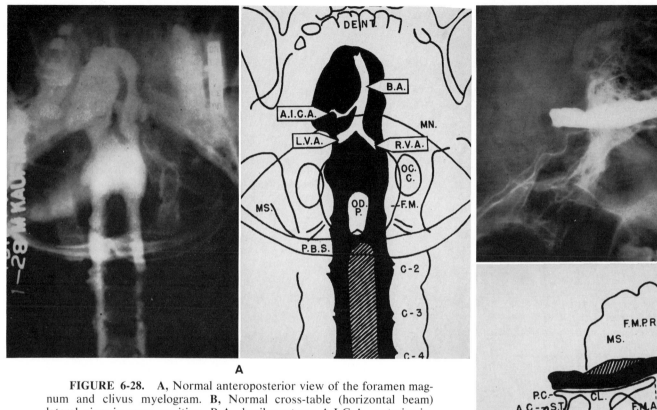

A

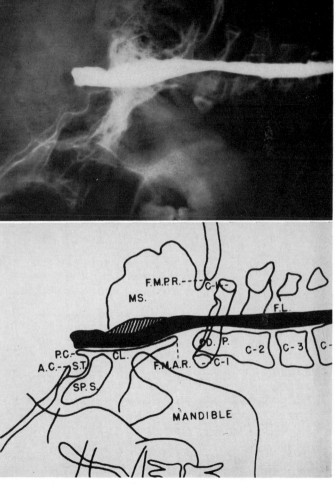

B

FIGURE 6-28. **A,** Normal anteroposterior view of the foramen magnum and clivus myelogram. **B,** Normal cross-table (horizontal beam) lateral view in same position. B.A., basilar artery; A.I.C.A., anterior inferior cerebellar artery; L.V.A., left vertebral artery; R.V.A., right vertebral artery; OC. C., occipital condyle; OD. P., odontoid process; MS., mastoids; F.M., foramen magnum; P.B.S., posterior base of skull; F.M.P.R., foramen magnum posterior rim; F.M.A.R., foramen magnum anterior rim; CL, clivus; A.C., anterior clinoids; P.C., posterior clinoids; S.T., sella turcica; SP.S., sphenoid sinus; F.L., fluid level of Pantopaque. (From Malis, L. I.: Radiology 76, 1958.)

Chapter 7 — The Upper Respiratory Passages and the Chest

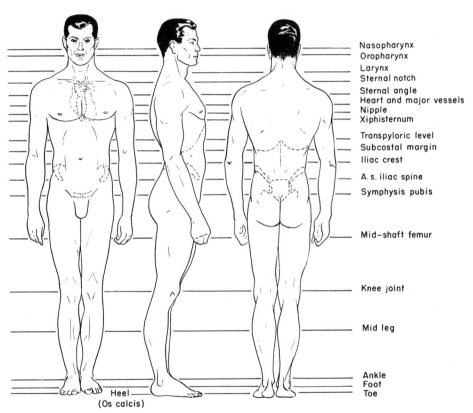

Nasopharynx
Oropharynx
Larynx
Sternal notch
Sternal angle
Heart and major vessels
Nipple
Xiphisternum

Transpyloric level
Subcostal margin
Iliac crest

A. s. iliac spine

Symphysis pubis

Mid–shaft femur

Knee joint

Mid leg

Ankle
Foot
Toe

Heel
(Os calcis)

FIGURE 7-1.   Important body surface reference points.

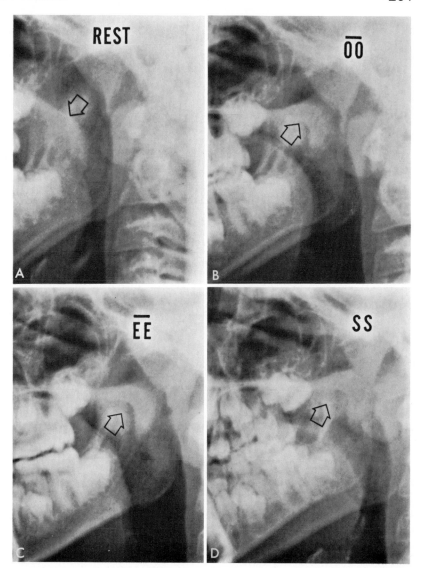

FIGURE 7-2. Phonation studies showing good mobility of the soft palate: **A,** resting state; **B,** o͞o; **C,** e͞e, **D,** ss. Note the complete approximation of the soft palate with the posterior nasopharyngeal wall in **D.**

These studies may be supplemented by cineradiographic examination and by an associated study of the swallowing function.

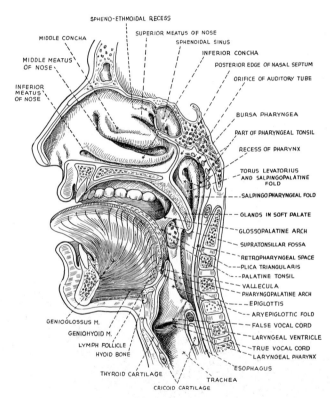

FIGURE 7-3. Sagittal section of the head and neck to demonstrate the structure of the nasopharynx and larynx.

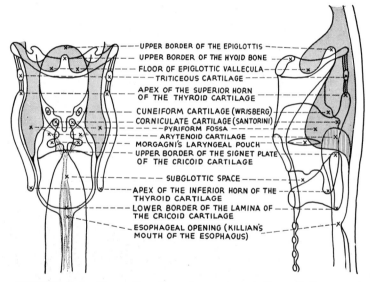

FIGURE 7-4. General schematic representation of the roentgen anatomy of the larynx and pharynx.

THE UPPER RESPIRATORY PASSAGES

From the radiographic standpoint, the neck is studied in many different ways, depending upon the organ system of interest in a particular clinical problem. The major radiographic techniques for the neck, apart from the muscles and nerves, involve angiology of the major arteries and veins (Chapter 5) and studies of the cervical spine and spinal cord (Chapter 6), of the upper respiratory passages (considered here) and of the upper alimentary tract (Chapter 8).

The upper air passages include the nasal air passages (see Chapter 5); the nasopharynx, which extends from the nasal cavity and base of the skull to the uvula and margin of the soft palate; the oropharynx, which extends from the soft palate to the epiglottis and its pharyngo-epiglottic folds, opposite the hyoid bone; and the laryngeal pharynx, which extends from the hyoid bone above to the upper boundary of the esophagus below, opposite the sixth cervical vertebra (Fig. 7-1).

The pharynx not only communicates with the nasal and oral cavities, but also with the middle ear via the auditory (eustachian) tube, the esophagus and the trachea (Fig. 7-3).

The Nasopharynx

The air passages allow ready identification of the nasal turbinates, the orifice of the auditory tube and the soft palate (see Fig. 7-3). The width of the posterior wall of the nasopharynx can be readily measured and adenoid hypertrophy identified. Soft palate movements with phonation can also be studied in considerable detail to assist in analysis of speech defects. In its simplest form, the latter is accomplished by obtaining four views, all in the lateral projection centering over the soft palate: (1) the resting state with normal breathing and no phonation; (2) the patient saying the sound "SSSS"; (3) the patient speaking the long vowel "EEEEEE" and (4) the patient saying the long vowel "AAAAAA" (Fig. 7-2). This can of course be coupled with cineradiographic studies and special film examinations of the swallowing function.

The Oropharynx

As indicated in Chapter 5, the mouth may be studied in relation to teeth, salivary glands, tongue and posterior oropharyngeal wall thickness (Fig. 7-4). The width of this last soft tissue space is important in certain clinical conditions, those of infectious or neoplastic origin particularly (Fig. 7-6).

The Laryngeal Pharynx

The larynx is encased in a cartilaginous framework, which sometimes undergoes partial calcification (Fig. 7-5). The epiglottic cartilage lies in front of and above the superior opening of the larynx and acts to deflect the swallowed bolus of food to either side into the pyriform fossae. The aryepiglottic folds act as a sphincter, preventing the food bolus from entering the larynx and trachea.

The false and true vocal cords, as well as the ventricle between them, are readily detected on good radiographs. Body-section radiography is particularly useful for demonstrating movement of the vocal cords with phonation (Fig. 7-8).

Laryngograms may also be obtained with opaque media, with and without phonation. In this procedure, a topical anesthetic (0.5 per cent Dyclone) is sprayed onto and in the pharynx and larynx, and 10 to 20 ml. of Dionosil oily is dropped slowly over the tongue during quiet inspiration. Frontal and lateral spot film radiographs (Fig. 7-7) are made during nasal inspiration, phonation, straining down against the closed glottis, and breathing in against the closed glottis.

(Text continues on page 208.)

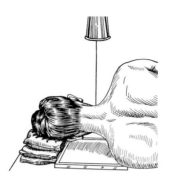

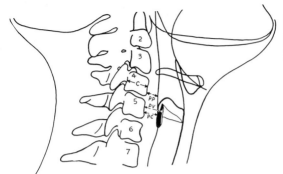

UPPER NORMAL LIMITS OF SOFT TISSUE SPACES OF NECK				
AGE	POSTPHARYNGEAL SOFT TISSUE		POSTLARYNGEAL SOFT TISSUE	
0-1	1.5 c		2.c	
1-2	.5 c		1.5 c	
2-3	.5 c		1.2 c	POSTVENTRICULAR
3-6	.4 c		1.2 c	
6-14	.3 c		1.2 c	
ADULT	MALE .3c	FEMALE .3c	MALE .7c	FEMALE .6c	POSTCRICOID

PV = POSTVENTRICULAR SOFT TISSUE
PP = POSTPHARYNGEAL SOFT TISSUE   PC = POSTCRICOID SOFT TISSUE
C = ANTERO-POSTERIOR DIMENSION OF C-4 VERTEBRAL BODY AT ITS MIDDLE

FIGURE 7-6. Relative widths of the posterior oropharynx and the soft tissues of the neck posterior to the larynx. (After Hay, P. D.: Ann. Roentgenol. *9*, 1930.)

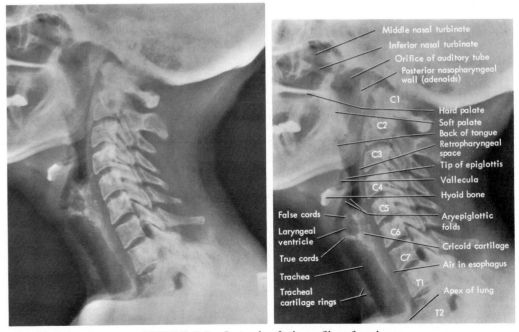

FIGURE 7-5. Lateral soft tissue film of neck.

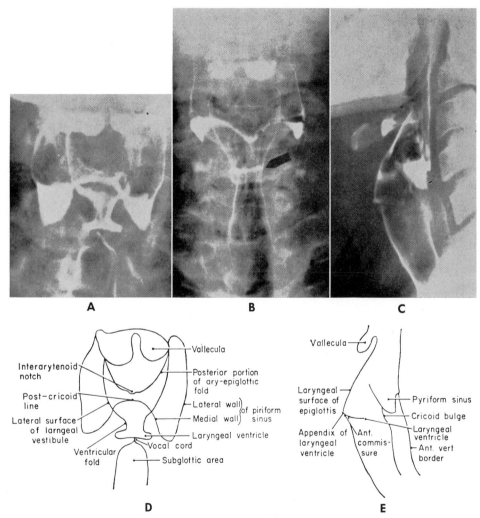

FIGURE 7-7. Laryngograms of a normal larynx employing Dionosil oily after local anesthesia of the pharynx and larynx. **A,** Phonation. The vocal cords meet in the midline. **B,** Quiet respiration. The cords are not now visualized. **C,** Lateral view during quiet respiration. Since the cords are abducted, the laryngeal ventricle is not clearly delineated. However, the line of the epiglottis and anterior wall of the trachea is almost continuous, being broken only by the anterior commissure of the larynx. **D,** Line diagram of **A. E,** Line diagram of **C.** (From Medina, J., Seaman, W., Carbajal, P., and Baker, D. C.: Radiology 77:533, 1961.)

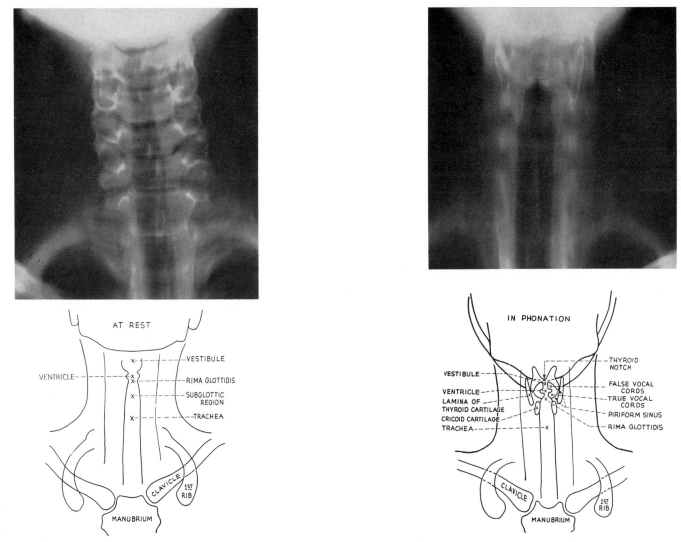

FIGURE 7-8.   Anteroposterior body-section radiograph of larynx at rest and during phonation.

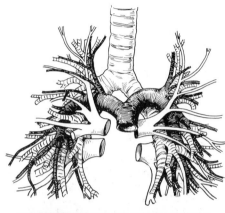

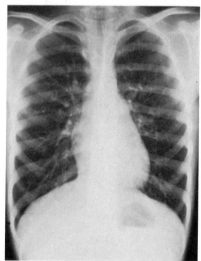

FIGURE 7-9. Pulmonary arteries (black) and pulmonary veins (unshaded) shown in relation to the tracheobronchial tree (transversely striped).

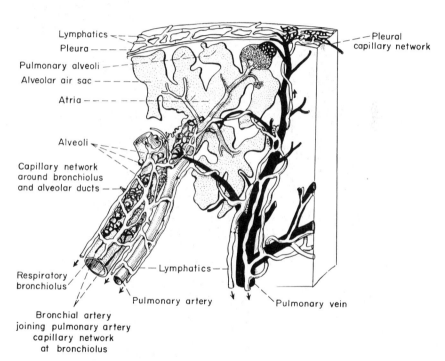

FIGURE 7-10. Primary lobule of the lung (Modified from Miller, W. S.: *The Lung.* Charles C Thomas.)

THE CHEST

No effort will be made to describe in detail the anatomy of the chest; for this information, the student is referred to the authors' companion volume, *An Atlas of Normal Radiographic Anatomy,* 2nd edition. The illustrations dealing with the anatomy of this region will be self-sufficient from a practical point of view.

The Trachea, Bronchi and Primary Lung Lobule

The trachea is a partially cartilaginous midline structure that extends the air passage from the larynx to the bronchi, which, in turn, furnish air access to the lungs. In the region of the lung hili, or roots, there is a complex interrelationship of the tracheobronchial tree and the pulmonary arteries and veins (Fig. 7-9A). In radiographs of excellent quality, these relationships can usually be fairly well defined (Fig. 7-9).

The bronchi are readily studied by the technique of bronchography. Here, the usual method involves the passage of a catheter into the trachea after good local anesthesia of the pharynx and tracheobronchial tree (with 0.5 per cent Dyclone). Dionosil (oily contrast) is the medium usually employed. This is introduced through the intratracheal catheter in small quantities as shown in Figure 7-12, while the patient is carefully positioned to attain optimum distribution of the contrast agent. Films are thereafter obtained as shown in Figure 7-13. It is important in this technique to identify every major bronchus and subdivision thereof.

The bronchi continue to ramify until, at a point where the walls no longer contain cartilage, they form the tubular bronchioli. These, in turn, lead into the *primary lobule of the lung,* where all of the main respiratory exchange occurs (Fig. 7-10). In so far as possible, every effort is made to obtain sufficient detail in chest radiography to allow interpretation of this gaseous exchange.

The primary lung lobules are grouped into pulmonary segments by their blood supply, and these segments ultimately are grouped together to form lobes of the lung. The right lung is subdivided into three lobes, and the left into two; the lobes are separated from one another by fissures, which represent extensions of the visceral pleura into the lung area (Fig. 7-11). Visualization of the fissures, if it can be accomplished, is very helpful from the standpoint of detecting disease, localizing it or determining its nature.

(*Text continues on page 213.*)

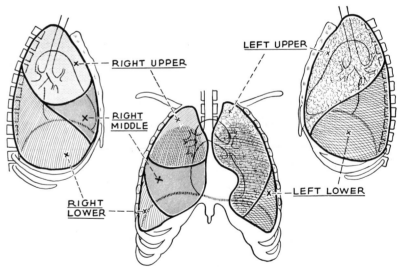

FIGURE 7-11. The lung: lobes and fissures.

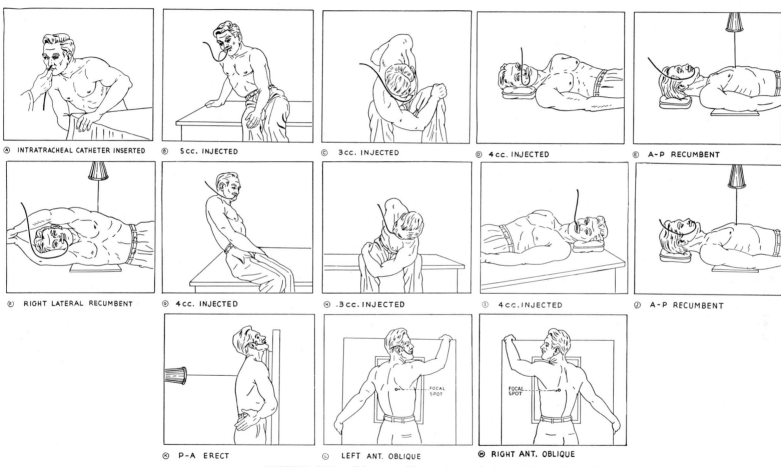

Ⓐ INTRATRACHEAL CATHETER INSERTED   Ⓑ 5 cc. INJECTED   Ⓒ 3 cc. INJECTED   Ⓓ 4 cc. INJECTED   Ⓔ A-P RECUMBENT

Ⓕ RIGHT LATERAL RECUMBENT   Ⓖ 4 cc. INJECTED   Ⓗ .3 cc. INJECTED   Ⓘ 4 cc. INJECTED   Ⓙ A-P RECUMBENT

Ⓚ P-A ERECT   Ⓛ LEFT ANT. OBLIQUE   FOCAL SPOT   FOCAL SPOT   Ⓜ RIGHT ANT. OBLIQUE

FIGURE 7-12. Diagrams illustrating technique of bronchography.

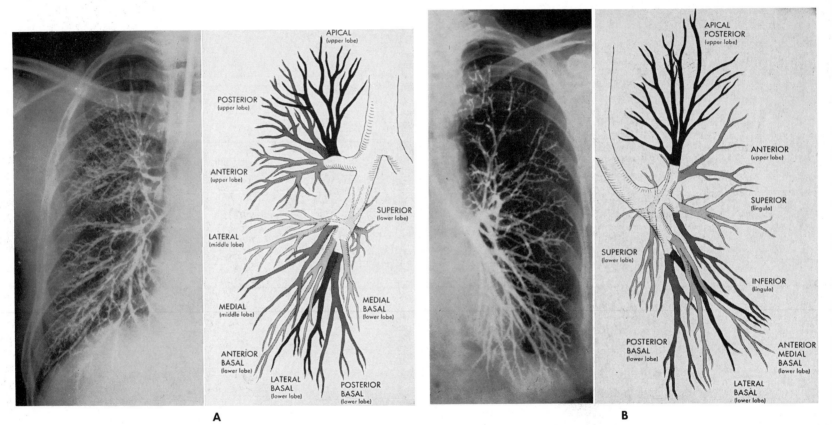

FIGURE 7-13. The normal human bronchial tree: **A,** right posteroanterior projection; **B,** left posteroanterior projection. (From Lehman, J. S., and Crellin, J. A.: Medical Radiography and Photography *31,* 1955.)

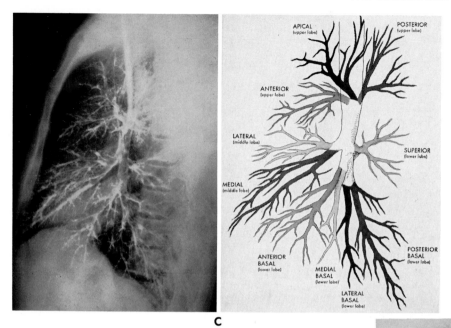

C

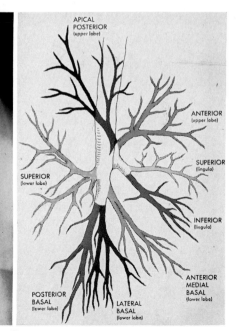

D

FIGURE 7-13. The normal human bronchial tree: **C,** right lateral projection; **D,** left lateral projection. (From Lehman, J. S., and Crellin, J. A.: Medical Radiography and Photography *31,* 1955.)

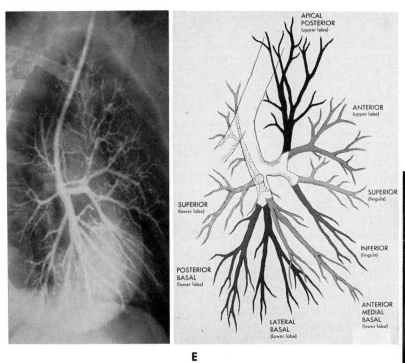

E

F

FIGURE 7-13. The normal human bronchial tree: **E,** right anterior oblique projection; **F,** left anterior oblique projection. (From Lehman, J. S., and Crellin, J. A.: Medical Radiography and Photography *31,* 1955.)

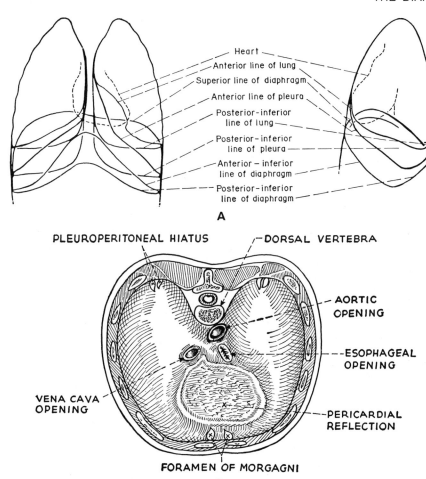

A

PLEUROPERITONEAL HIATUS — DORSAL VERTEBRA

AORTIC OPENING

VENA CAVA OPENING

ESOPHAGEAL OPENING

PERICARDIAL REFLECTION

FORAMEN OF MORGAGNI

B

FIGURE 7-14. A and **B,** Isometric concept of the diaphragm on frontal and lateral views. **C,** Normal openings of the diaphragm.

Labels in Figure A:
Heart
Anterior line of lung
Superior line of diaphragm
Anterior line of pleura
Posterior-inferior line of lung
Posterior-inferior line of pleura
Anterior-inferior line of diaphragm
Posterior-inferior line of diaphragm

The Lung Hili

There are a number of vital structures which enter and leave the lung at its mediastinal surface; these are called the 'root of the lung,' and by common usage comprise the lung hili. The large structures included are: (1) the pulmonary artery; (2) the bronchus; (3) two pulmonary veins; (4) the bronchial arteries and veins; (5) the pulmonary nerves and (6) lymph vessels and lymph nodes.

The Thoracic Cage

The thoracic cage may be literally defined as the entire wall structure which contains the lungs and mediastinum. Each of its elements can be visualized, at least to some extent, radiographically. They are: (1) The soft tissue structures of the thoracic wall, such as the skin, muscles, breasts and nipples; (2) the bony structures consisting of ribs, costal cartilage, sternum and thoracic spine; (3) the pleura and (4) the diaphragm.

There are special radiographic techniques applicable to study of the breasts (soft tissue mammography), the ribs, the sternum, the pleura and the diaphragm.

Ordinarily, the pleura does not cast a significant shadow unless it is infiltrated by disease, has produced a transudate or exudate with fluid accumulation in the pleural space, or has become hemorrhagic, or unless its layers have become separated by air in the pleural space. The latter is sometimes used as a diagnostic procedure, but need not be considered further in this text.

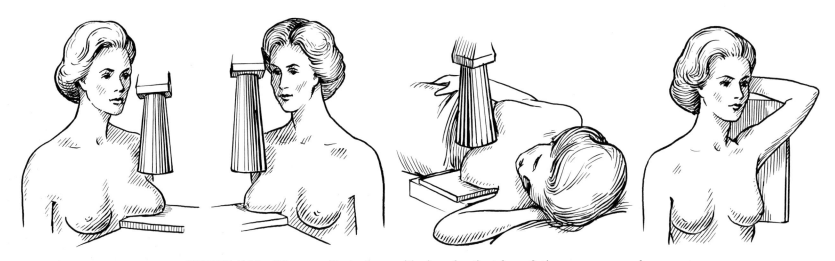

FIGURE 7-15. Diagrams illustrating positioning of patient for soft tissue mammography.

Mammography

General Principles of Technique. The principal factors in mammography are: (1) proper coning, (2) minimal kilovoltage adequate for penetration, (3) increased milliamperage seconds to give adequate exposure, (4) no intensifying screens, (5) minimal filtration of the x-ray beam combined with the kilovoltage used and (6) short object-to-film distance. A fine grain emulsion with the necessary contrast range, comparable to the double emulsion Kodak Industrial Type "M" film must be used (Egan). Developing time is 5 to 8 minutes at 68° F., and 10 minutes' fixation. It is important that the *nipple be in profile* if at all possible.

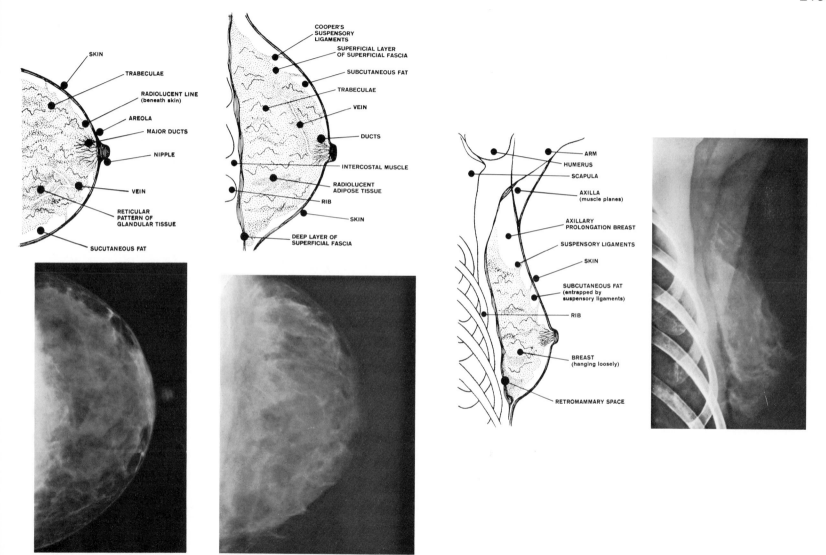

FIGURE 7-16. Representative mammograms in the craniocaudad, mediolateral, and axillary projections and labeled line drawings of each. (From Egan, R. L.: *Mammography*. Charles C Thomas, 1964.)

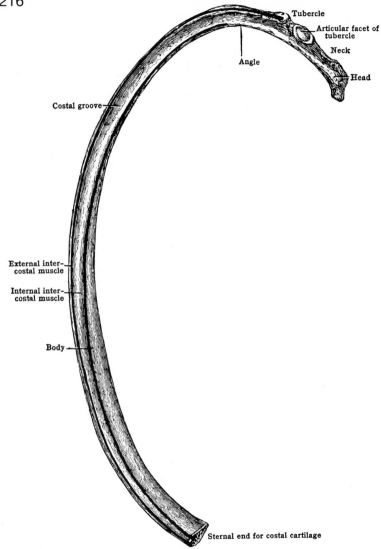

FIGURE 7-17. Anatomic drawing of a typical rib. (From Terry, R. J., in Morris, H.: *Morris' Human Anatomy,* edited by B. J. Anson, The Blakiston Div., McGraw-Hill Book Co., 1966.)

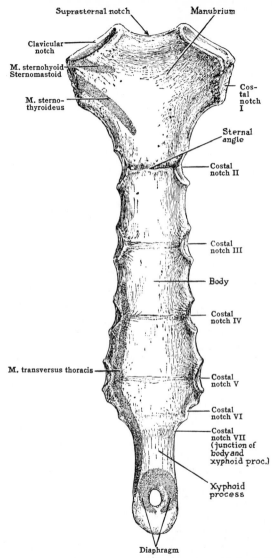

FIGURE 7-18. Gross anatomy of the sternum. (Adapted from Terry, R. J., in Morris, H.: *Morris' Human Anatomy,* edited by B. J. Anson, The Blakiston Div., McGraw-Hill Co., 1966.)

POINTS OF PRACTICAL INTEREST ABOUT FIGURE 7-19

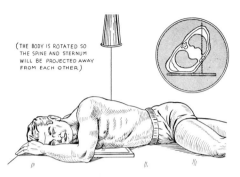

(THE BODY IS ROTATED SO THE SPINE AND STERNUM WILL BE PROJECTED AWAY FROM EACH OTHER)

1. At best, it is sometimes difficult to visualize the sternum with sufficient clarity in this view. Under these circumstances, body-section radiography is recommended. The best technique for this is as follows:

(a) A mobile cart is placed at right angles to the x-ray table, and the patient lies prone on the cart, with his chest overlapping the table, so that he is as nearly as possible *perpendicular to the x-ray table.*

(b) The long axis of the sternum is therefore in contact with the surface of the x-ray table but at right angles to the long axis of this table.

(c) The cassette is placed in the tray so that its long axis corresponds to that of the sternum.

(d) The body-section study is then made in the usual manner, and two or three "cuts" may be made.

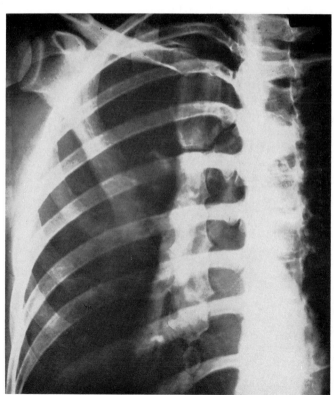

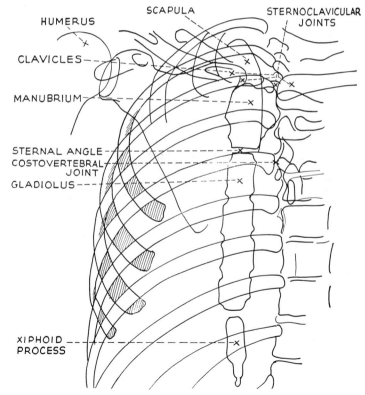

FIGURE 7-19.   Oblique view of sternum and sternoclavicular joints (also ribs).

Sternoclavicular Joints *(Figure 7-20)*

The sternoclavicular joint is a two-chambered synovial or diarthrodial joint with an articular disk between the two chambers. Each chamber is usually distinct and separate from the other, unless the articular disk happens to be unusually thin (as in the case of the temporomandibular joint).

These joints are usually demonstrated on oblique projections such as are employed for the sternum proper, except that the tube is centered over the joint. *A comparison film of the opposite side is always obtained so that the two sternoclavicular joints can be compared in the same patient.*

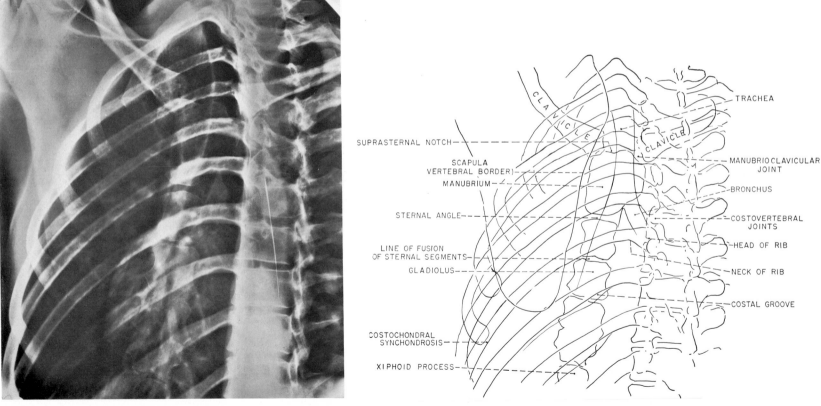

FIGURE 7-20. Oblique view of sternum and sternoclavicular joints (also ribs).

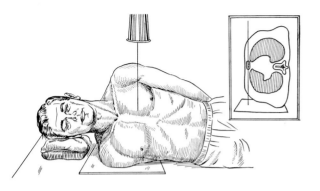

POINTS OF PRACTICAL INTEREST ABOUT FIGURE 7-21

1. This view gives us maximum clarity of the sternum, but unfortunately has the following disadvantages:

(a) When the sternum is depressed at all, it is concealed behind the costal cartilages and some lung in this projection. This is especially true of the condition called "pectus excavatum."

(b) Abnormalities which do not affect the entire width of the sternum may be obscured by the unaffected portion. Body-section radiographs are helpful when this is suspected.

(c) The various segments of the sternum must be recognized, and differentiated from other abnormalities which may be simulated at the costosternal junctions.

2. The retrosternal mediastinal and pleural shadows should always be examined very carefully. This is also true of the shadows which are superficial to the sternum. The clue to abnormality is often found here where it may escape detection by inspection of the sternal shadow only.

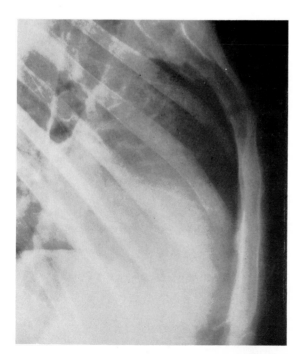
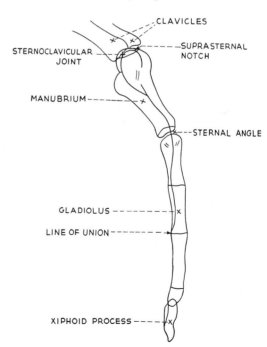

FIGURE 7-21. Lateral view of sternum.

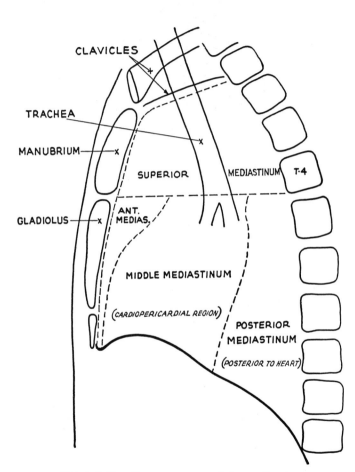

FIGURE 7-22.   Compartments of the mediastinum.

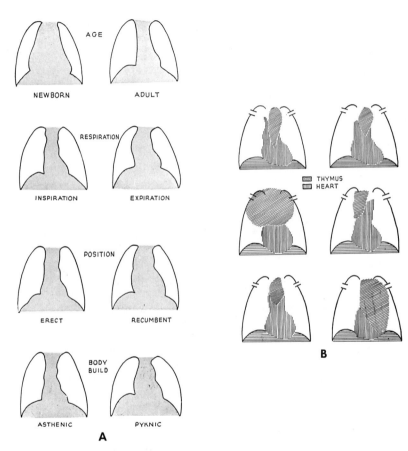

FIGURE 7-23.   A, Normal factors causing variation in the supracardiac shadow and cardiac contour. **B,** Variations in size and position of supracardiac thymic shadow in the infant.

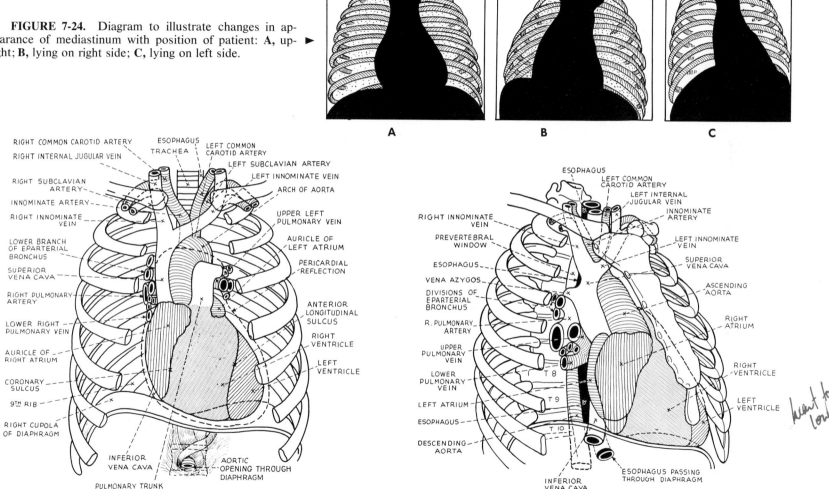

FIGURE 7-24. Diagram to illustrate changes in appearance of mediastinum with position of patient: **A,** upright; **B,** lying on right side; **C,** lying on left side.

A   B   C

FIGURE 7-25. Frontal projection of the heart in the thoracic cage with lung and rib structures removed.

FIGURE 7-26. Right anterior oblique projection of the heart in the thoracic cage with lung and rib structures removed.

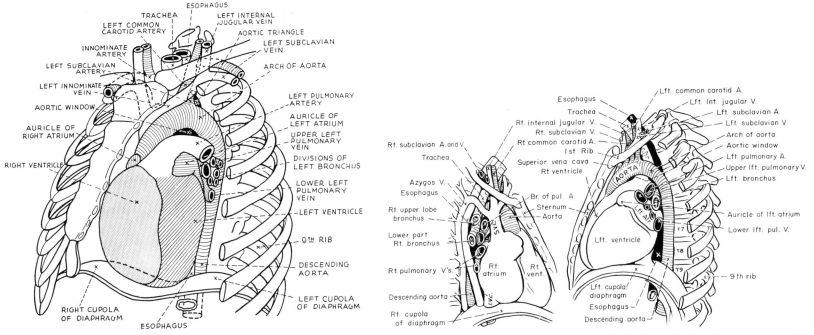

FIGURE 7-27. Left anterior oblique projection of the heart in the thoracic cage with lung and rib structures removed.

FIGURE 7-28. Lateral view of the heart in the thoracic cage with rib structures, pleura and lung removed, as seen from the left side in the larger diagram, and the right side in the smaller.

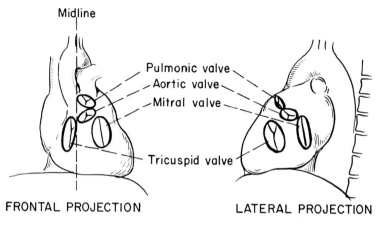

Midline

Pulmonic valve
Aortic valve
Mitral valve

Tricuspid valve

FRONTAL PROJECTION   LATERAL PROJECTION

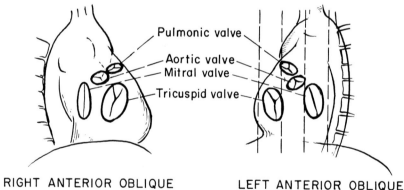

Pulmonic valve
Aortic valve
Mitral valve
Tricuspid valve

RIGHT ANTERIOR OBLIQUE   LEFT ANTERIOR OBLIQUE

FIGURE 7-29. Projections of cardiac valves in routine positions in radiography.

RADIOLOGY OF THE HEART AND MEDIASTINUM

The mediastinum is divided into three anatomical areas: anterior, middle and posterior. The anterior is that radiolucent space which lies anterior to the heart and major blood vessels. The middle mediastinum contains the heart and the major blood vessels leading to and from it. The posterior mediastinum contains those structures which lie posterior to the heart.

The three fundamental principles which especially apply to the radiographic examination of the mediastinum are as follows: Esophagrams (barium in the esophagus) should be employed in every instance; when these are contraindicated by the clinical condition of the patient, the examination is regarded as limited. A somewhat heavier exposure technique than is applicable for lung study is usually necessary for the mediastinum. This may be accomplished by employing a moving grid or an air-gap technique. In the latter, a 6 to 10 inch air gap is allowed between patient and film, and an 8 foot target-to-film distance is employed to diminish distortion and magnification. To obtain the greatest advantage from this method, high kilovoltage and milliamperage (with shortest time possible) is optimum; a three phase, 1000 Ma., 150 kvp generator is best employed for this. Finally, fluoroscopy is highly desirable, to study cardiac and major blood vessel pulsations, swallowing, sniffing, coughing, diaphragmatic excursion, and shifts with inspiration and expiration.

POINTS OF PRACTICAL INTEREST ABOUT FIGURE 7-30

1. The exact course of the esophagus in this projection is noteworthy. At the base of the neck there is a slight deflection toward the left so that the esophageal projection falls behind the left sternoclavicular joint in a perfectly centered film. Thereafter it courses to the right at the level of the transverse portion of the arch of the aorta. From this position, there is a slight gradual deflection toward the left so that the diaphragm is penetrated to the left of the midline. An enlargement in any of the contiguous structures will alter this course perceptibly.

2. It is also important to trace the aortic shadow as it courses to the left of the middle, with its left margin ordinarily separate and distinct from the paraspinous shadow. This is a straight line normally below the level of the arch of the aorta; abnormally, it becomes convex, or S-shaped with elongation of the aorta.

3. The position of the "left" ventricular apex with reference to the left hemidiaphragm is important. This portion of the cardiac silhouette is not always due to the left ventricle, but may be related to the right ventricle, particularly in congenital heart disease.

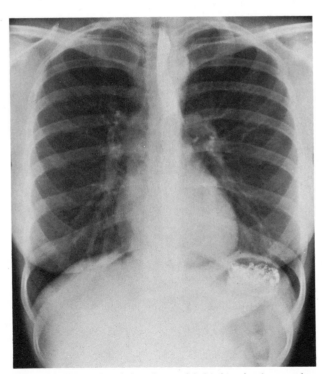

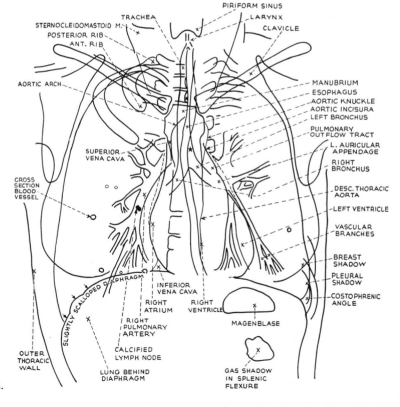

FIGURE 7-30.   Posteroanterior view of the chest with barium in the esophagus.

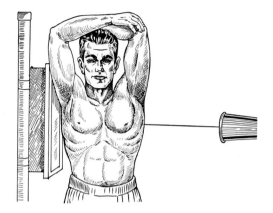

POINTS OF PRACTICAL INTEREST ABOUT FIGURE 7-31

1. Of particular interest and value for identification are:

(a) The relationship of the right ventricle to the posterior margin of the sternum. With enlargement of the right ventricle, its shadow "rises" higher on the sternum.

(b) The degree of clarity of the anterior mediastinal clear space.

(c) The relationship of the left ventricle posteriorly to the shadow of the inferior vena cava. This will allow early and accurate detection of enlargement of the left ventricle.

(d) The relationship of the esophagus to the left atrium.

(e) The relative prominence of the pulmonary arteries. This requires considerable experience, but is very valuable from the standpoint of detecting abnormalities of lymph node origin, or tumor masses.

2. For a clearer demonstration of the trachea and retrosternal structures, the patient's hands are placed behind him on his hips, and his shoulders are rotated backward.

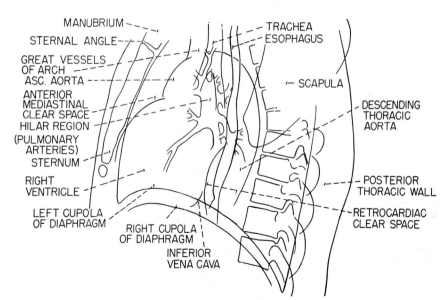

FIGURE 7-31. The lateral view of the chest with barium in the esophagus.

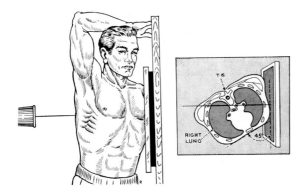

POINTS OF PRACTICAL INTEREST ABOUT FIGURE 7-32

1. The 45 degree obliquity may be increased to 50 or 55 degrees on occasion, to obtain maximum clearance of the spine.

2. Ordinarily the left ventricle clears the spine, and the right ventricle forms a smooth uninterrupted convexity with the ascending portion of the arch of the aorta.

3. This view gives maximum clarity of the bifurcation of the trachea, the arch of the aorta and the posterior basilar portion of the left ventricle. Pulsations are ordinarily of maximum amplitude in this portion of the cardiac silhouette.

4. Although the right ventricle is usually seen very adequately in this view, the straight lateral is preferable, since the relationship of the right ventricle to the retrosternal space is more informative. Likewise, the left ventricle is more accurately evaluated in the straight lateral view by noting its relationship to the shadow of the inferior vena cava. It should not normally project more than 18 mm. beyond this shadow in the lateral projection.

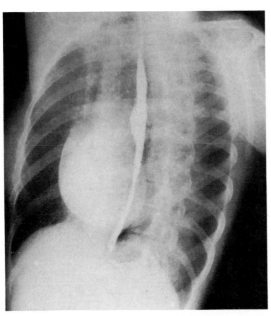

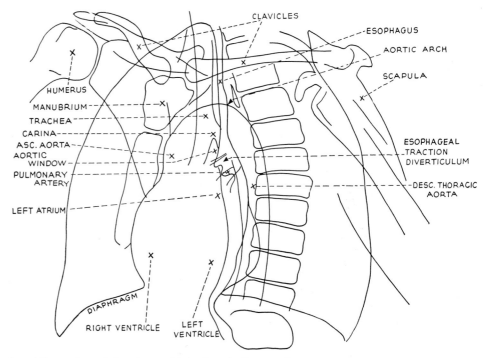

FIGURE 7-32. Left posteroanterior oblique view of the chest with barium in the esophagus.

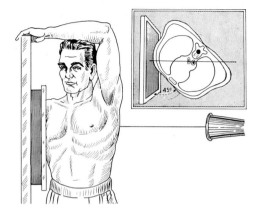

POINTS OF PRACTICAL INTEREST ABOUT FIGURE 7-33

1. The patient's right shoulder is placed against the film and the body turned approximately 45 degrees from the film, resting the left arm in a convenient position, away from the body.

2. The central ray is directed just medial to the scapula nearest the x-ray tube at approximately the level of the sixth or seventh thoracic vertebra.

3. The patient is placed in proper position and then barium paste is administered. He is instructed to swallow and then take a deep breath and hold it while the x-ray exposure is made.

4. The maximum area of the right lung field is demonstrated in this view, but it is partially obscured by the shadow of the spinal column.

5. This view is most advantageous for demonstration of the left atrium and its possible enlargement, since any slight enlargement will cause a significant impression upon the esophagus as indicated.

6. This view is also of value for demonstrating the anterior apical portion of the left ventricle which is most significantly involved in anterior apical myocardial infarction, a rather common disease entity.

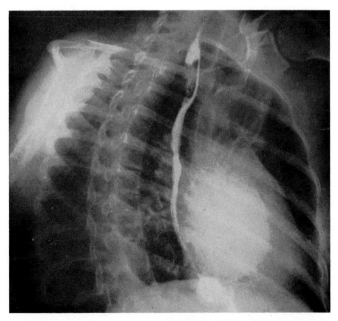

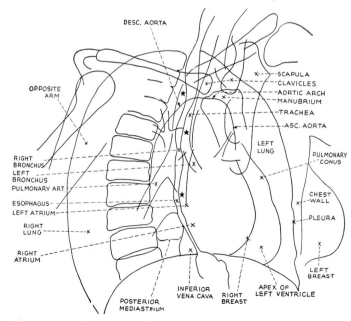

FIGURE 7-33.   Right posteroanterior oblique view of the chest with barium in the esophagus.

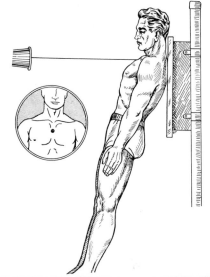

POINTS OF PRACTICAL INTEREST ABOUT FIGURE 7-34

1. By standing the patient approximately 1 foot in front of the vertical cassette stand and then having him lean directly backward, a proper obliquity of the chest is obtained.

2. The top of the cassette is adjusted so that the upper border of the film is about 1 inch above the shoulders.

3. The central ray passes through the region of the manubrium. Occasionally a slight angle of 5 degrees toward the head may prove advantageous in demonstrating the apices more clearly.

4. This view gives one a very distorted view of the lung fields and mediastinum, but is of particular value in showing: (1) the apices more clearly, (2) the interlobar areas of the lungs and (3) the region of the pulmonary sector of the cardiac shadow more clearly.

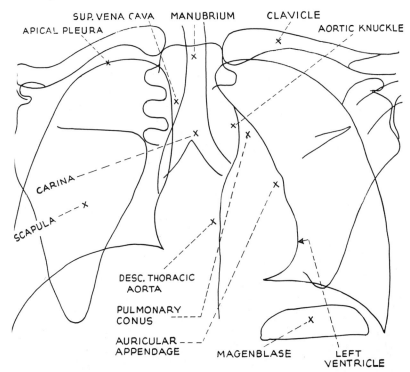

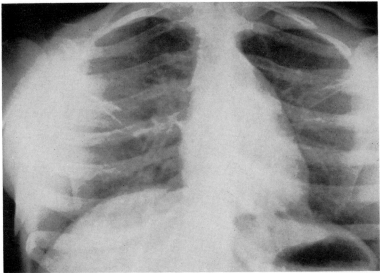

FIGURE 7-34. Apical lordotic view of chest.

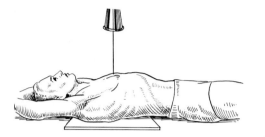

POINTS OF PRACTICAL INTEREST ABOUT FIGURE 7-35

1. Although it is difficult to obtain a view of the upper lung fields in this projection because of the shadows of the scapulae, considerable improvement will result if the patient crosses his arms above his head, thus rotating the scapulae outward.

2. The clavicles, on the other hand, are projected above the lung apices sufficiently so that this area of the lungs may be more clearly shown.

3. Analysis of the cardiac silhouette is not as favorable in this projection in the adult, because of the straightening of the left margin and broadening of the base.

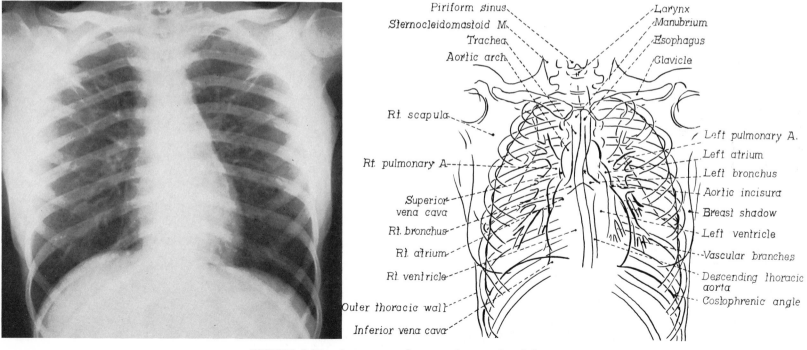

FIGURE 7-35.   Anteroposterior recumbent study of chest.

ADDITIONAL VIEWS OCCASIONALLY EMPLOYED FOR SPECIFIC PURPOSES

Anterior View for the Pulmonary Apices (Patient Supine). The patient is supine with his shoulders elevated on an angle board 20 to 25 degrees. The central ray and film are centered over the suprasternal notch. The film obtained and the anatomy are very similar to that depicted in the apical lordotic view.

The Posteroanterior Lordotic Projection. The patient is in the posteroanterior position, his body bent backward at the waist. The lower chest touches the lower margin of the film, while the upper chest is 4 to 6 inches away from the cassette holder. The thorax may be inclined backward as much as 45 degrees. The central ray is directed at about the fourth thoracic vertebra.

The Posteroanterior Projection with the Patient Lying on His Side (Lateral Decubitus Position), Employing a Horizontal Beam. The patient lies on either the affected or unaffected side, and the thorax is raised above the lower margin of the cassette by a platform or sheets. The central ray is directed through approximately the fourth thoracic vertebra. This position is particularly useful for demonstration of small quantities of free flowing pleural fluid or small degrees of pneumothorax.

The Lateral Projection with the Patient Supine (Dorsal Decubitus Position), Employing a Horizontal Beam. The patient is in the supine position with the thorax elevated several inches above the lower margin of the cassette by means of a platform or folded sheets. The central ray is directed through approximately the fourth thoracic vertebra. A similar view may be obtained with the patient prone (ventral decubitus position). As with the other decubitus views, this one also is useful for demonstration of free flowing pleural fluid.

Chapter 8 — The Abdomen and Genitourinary Systems

RADIOGRAPHIC STUDY OF THE ABDOMEN

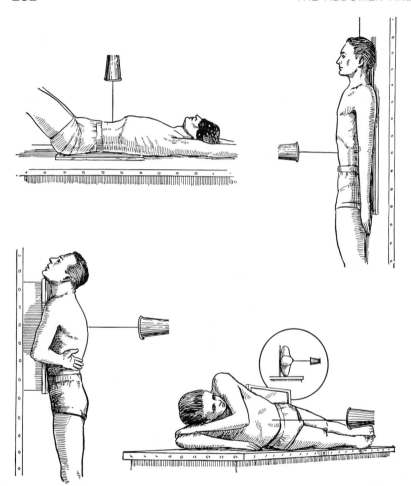

FIGURE 8-1. Routine film studies obtained for plain film survey of abdominal disease. Note that a P-A chest film is part of this routine. (Decubitus left lateral may be preferable.)

The basic positions for study of the abdomen are (Fig. 8-1):

1. Anteroposterior film of the abdomen, recumbent (also called KUB film, the letters standing for kidney, ureter and bladder areas).
2. Anteroposterior film of the abdomen, erect.
3. Patient supine; horizontal x-ray beam.
4. Patient on one side or other; horizontal x-ray beam.
5. Posteroanterior film of chest, including upper abdomen for areas just beneath the diaphragm.

It is best, if time permits, to prepare patients for this examination by thorough cleansing of the gastrointestinal tract, best accomplished by prescribing a cathartic such as 2 ounces of castor oil (or X-Prep Liquid) on the evening prior to the examination and allowing approximately 10 or 12 hours for action. On the morning of the examination, this may be supplemented by enemas until returns are clear.

Air which has escaped from the gastrointestinal tract into the peritoneal space as the result of rupture of a portion of the gut, will rise to the uppermost part of the abdomen—usually beneath the diaphragm. It is absolutely important that the diaphragm be motionless when this film is taken; hence a very rapid exposure technique is essential.

In general, since most of the organs gravitate to the lower abdomen in the erect position, this film is not as good as the recumbent one for best anatomic detail. It is essential, however, that fluid levels, bowel wall thickness, properitoneal fat lines, and fascial planes around kidneys and psoas muscles be clearly shown (Fig. 8-2).

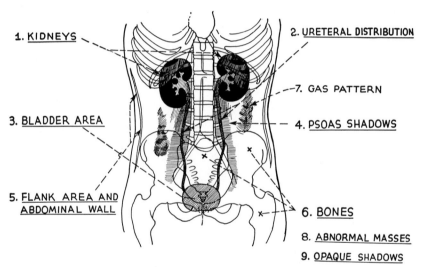

1. KIDNEYS
2. URETERAL DISTRIBUTION
3. BLADDER AREA
7. GAS PATTERN
4. PSOAS SHADOWS
5. FLANK AREA AND ABDOMINAL WALL
6. BONES
8. ABNORMAL MASSES
9. OPAQUE SHADOWS

FIGURE 8-2A. Routine for examination of the recumbent film of the abdomen.

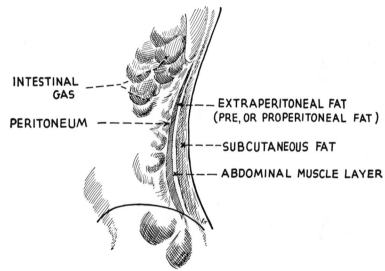

INTESTINAL GAS
PERITONEUM
EXTRAPERITONEAL FAT (PRE, OR PROPERITONEAL FAT)
SUBCUTANEOUS FAT
ABDOMINAL MUSCLE LAYER

FIGURE 8-2B. Diagram of flank anatomy, showing the relationship of the properitoneal fat layer to the rest of the abdominal wall.

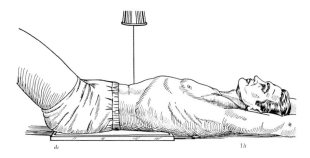

POINTS OF PRACTICAL INTEREST ABOUT FIGURE 8-3

1. The exposure should be made about 2 seconds after suspension of respiration (to avoid motion).

2. The patient's knees should be flexed to a comfortable position with folded sheets or sandbags under them.

3. Respiration is suspended at the end of exhalation.

4. Gonadal shielding should be used whenever possible.

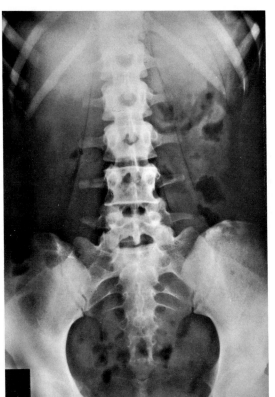

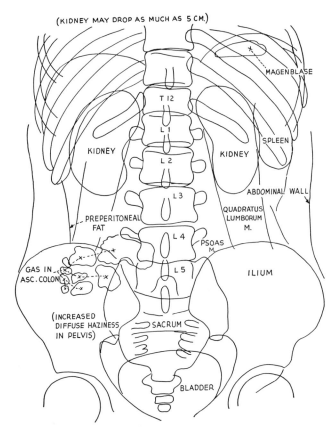

FIGURE 8-3. Anteroposterior view of abdomen (KUB film).

THE SUPRARENAL GLAND

Each suprarenal (adrenal) gland overlies the superior pole of the respective kidney, and lies within Gerota's fascia. The right adrenal gland is conical in shape with concave sides and the appearance of a cocked hat. The left adrenal gland tends to be rather crescentic or semilunar in shape with, occasionally, a convex medial margin. Retroperitoneal pneumography affords the best method for visualization of the suprarenal gland. This examination is best coupled with body-section radiography.

The two main techniques for injecting the gaseous medium are shown in Figure 8-4. The injection may be made directly into the flank above the iliac crest, or a presacral retrorectal route may be used.

The patient is in a prone, semi-upright, or sitting position during the administration of the gaseous injection. If carbon dioxide is used, the films must be obtained very promptly in view of the rapid absorption of the carbon dioxide.

The films obtained are: (1) both supine posterior obliques; (2) an anteroposterior erect; (3) body-section radiography at cuts 6 to 12 cm., 1 cm. intervals from the posterior. If oxygen or air is used, since rapid absorption of the gas does not occur, one may additionally obtain: (4) excretory urograms simultaneously and (5) a 24 hour KUB film.

If air is used, the usual optimum time for radiography is the 2 hour interval following the injection; if the 2 hour study is not optimum, hourly films may be taken thereafter until maximum visualization is obtained.

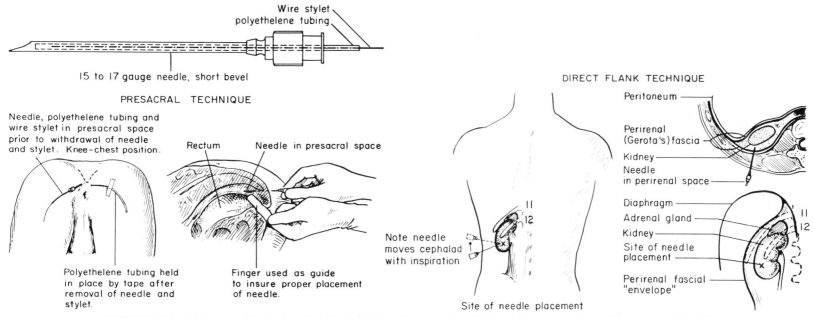

FIGURE 8-4. Diagrams illustrating the direct flank and presacral techniques for retroperitoneal pneumography. (From McLelland, R., Landes, R. R., and Ransom, C. L.: Radiol. Clin. N. A. *3*:116, 117, 120, 1965.)

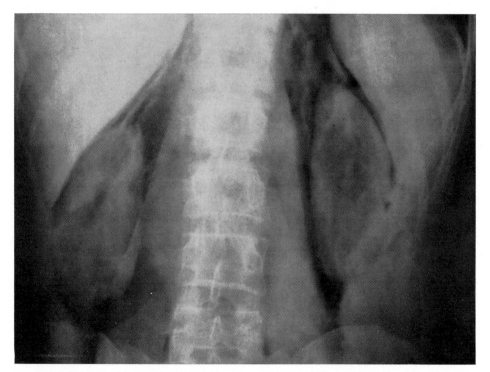

FIGURE 8-5. Normal retroperitoneal pneumogram. (From McLelland, R., Landes, R. R., and Ransom, C. L.: Radiol. Clin. N. A. *3*:115, 1965.)

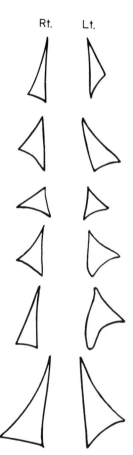

FIGURE 8-6. Tracings of six normal retroperitoneal pneumograms. (From McLelland, R., Landes, R. R., and Ransom, C. L.: Radiol. Clin. N. A. *3*:120, 1965.)

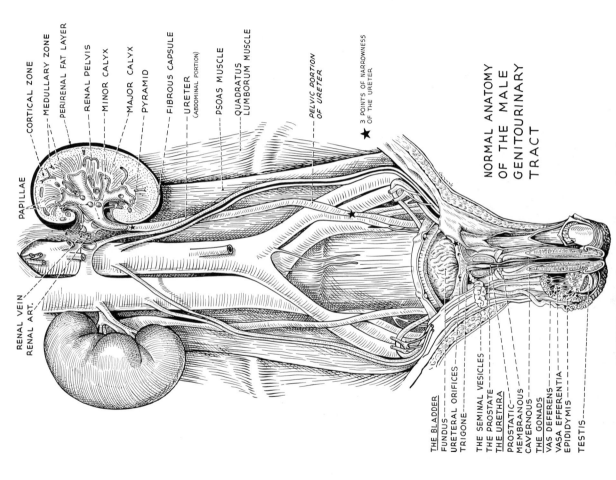

CORTICAL ZONE
MEDULLARY ZONE
PERIRENAL FAT LAYER
RENAL PELVIS
MINOR CALYX
MAJOR CALYX
PYRAMID
FIBROUS CAPSULE
URETER (ABDOMINAL PORTION)
PSOAS MUSCLE
QUADRATUS LUMBORUM MUSCLE

PAPILLAE

PELVIC PORTION OF URETER

3 POINTS OF NARROWNESS OF THE URETER

RENAL VEIN
RENAL ART.

NORMAL ANATOMY OF THE MALE GENITOURINARY TRACT

THE BLADDER
FUNDUS
URETERAL ORIFICES
TRIGONE

THE SEMINAL VESICLES
THE PROSTATE
THE URETHRA
PROSTATIC
MEMBRANOUS
CAVERNOUS
THE GONADS
VAS DEFERENS
VASA EFFERENTIA
EPIDIDYMIS
TESTIS

FIGURE 8-7. Gross anatomy of the urinary tract.

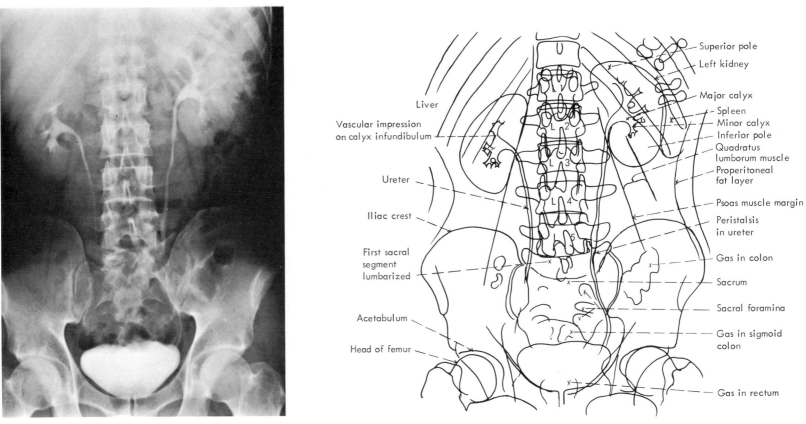

FIGURE 8-8. Representative excretory urogram (also called intravenous pyelogram) obtained 15 minutes after the intravenous injection of a suitable contrast agent (25 ml. 50 per cent Hypaque).

If gas embolism is at all suspected, the patient must be placed in the left lateral decubitus position.

THE URINARY TRACT

Intravenous Pyelography (Excretory Urography)

A KUB (abbreviation for kidney, ureter, bladder) film is obtained prior to the intravenous injection of a suitable contrast agent, followed by serial film studies of the kidneys, ureter and bladder at selected intervals. The intervals will depend upon the anatomic and physiologic information desired. Routine intervals are: 3 minutes, 5 minutes, 10 minutes, and 20 minutes.

Oblique films or prone films (for better demonstration of the ureters) are obtained as occasion demands.

Rapid Sequence Pyelography and "Washout" Pyelography for Study of Hypertension. In this technique, 20 to 30 ml. of the contrast agent is injected rapidly (in 30 seconds or less), and films are obtained every minute thereafter for 5 minutes; next film at 8 minutes, at which time an infusion of 500 ml. of a diuretic solution is begun to be delivered in about 5 minutes. This solution contains 100 ml. of 25 per cent mannitol in 400 ml. isotonic glucose. Films are obtained at 5 minute intervals following the beginning of the infusion for a total of 20 minutes thereafter.

Infusion Pyelography. A constant infusion of a large volume of the contrast agent with an equal volume of isotonic glucose is administered. Usually the contrast agent is employed in a dose of 1 ml. per pound of body weight up to 120 ml., and this total infusion may be given in a period of approximately 3 to 5 minutes. Films are obtained at 3 minutes, 5 minutes, 10 minutes and 20 minutes. Nephrotomograms may be obtained at about the 10 minute interval, or when visualization is optimum for either the nephrogram phase (kidney cortex) or the pyelogram phase (kidney calyces and pelvis).

Contrast Agents. The most commonly employed contrast agents are: 50 per cent Hypaque; 60 per cent Renografin; 50 per cent Miokon; Renovist; 35 to 70 per cent Diodrast; Neo-Iopax; Perabrodil (see Table 8-1).

Special Expedient in Infants. During the examination, a carbonated drink is administered to distend the stomach and thus portray the kidney areas more clearly (Fig. 8-9). Use the dose indicated by the manufacturer of the contrast agent.

Delayed Excretion and Concentration. Delayed film studies are obtained at hourly intervals for as long as eight hours in some instances. Usually, however, the urinary bladder even in these cases is seen to contain most of the administered contrast agent in about two hours.

Voiding Cystourethrograms. Oblique study of the bladder and urethra are obtained while the patient is voiding in a suitable receptacle. It is usually more satisfactory to obtain urethrograms following the instillation of the medium directly into the bladder or while the contrast agent is being injected into the urethra (contrast agent, Thixocon).

The Retrograde Pyelogram

This method requires that catheters be introduced into the ureters by cystoscopic manipulation.

Usually a plain film of the abdomen is obtained after the introduction of these opaque catheters and prior to the injection of the contrast medium. Oblique studies are taken as necessary to determine whether or not a pathologic condition projected in the ureter remains in constant relationship with the ureter with change of projection. An opaque agent is then injected through the ureteral catheters. Organic iodide media are preferred, and 20 to 30 per cent solutions of these are quite satisfactory. Too great an opacity is undesirable since calculi may be obscured. Ordinarily 5 to 10 ml. will suffice. Films are processed immediately to assure optimum visualization, and special films may be obtained thereafter during withdrawal of the catheter (while continuing to inject contrast agent).

When obstruction is suspected, a delayed pyelogram is some-

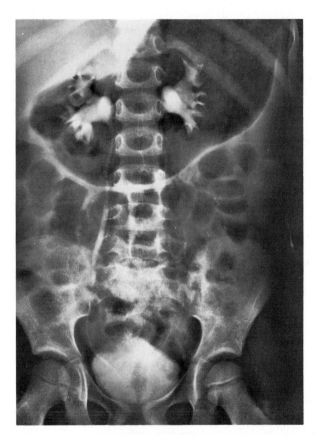

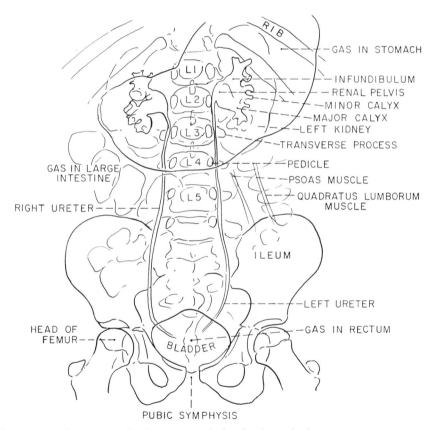

FIGURE 8-9. Intravenous pyelogram on a child. The upper urinary tract is demonstrated clearly through the gas-distended stomach.

TABLE 8-1. Contrast Media Used in Urography and Angiography

Trade Name	Organic Compound	Per Cent Iodine W/V	Concentration of Drug in Commercially Available Solution	Manufacturer's Suggested Dosage			
				Adult Dose	Children's Dose	Subcutaneous Administration	Intramuscular Administration
Neo-Iopax	Sodium iodometha-mate	25.8 38.6	50% 75%	20 cc. of 50% 30 cc. of 50% 20 cc. of 75%	10 cc. of 50%	10% solution (dilute 14 cc. of 75% solution to 100 cc. with normal saline)*	Not recommended
Diodrast	Iodopyracet, U.S.P.	17.5 (35% in 70% solution)	35% (70% also available)	20–30 cc. of 35%	0– 6 mo.: 5 cc. 7–12 mo.: 6– 7 cc. 1– 3 yr.: 7–10 cc. 4– 6 yr.: 10–16 cc. 7– 8 yr.: 16–20 cc.	7% solution (dilute 20 cc. of 35% solution to 100 cc. with normal saline)*	35% solution Children: 10– 20 cc. Adults: 20–30 cc.
Hippuran	Sodium iodohippu-rate	7 (in 20% solution)	Powder only available. Mix 12 gm. with 60 cc. of distilled water to make 20% solution	60 cc. of 20%	0–12 mo.: 6 gm. + 9.55 cc. water 1– 4 yr.: 8 gm. + 12.5 cc. water 4– 8 yr.:10 gm. + 21 cc. water	Not recommended	Not recommended
Urokon	Sodium acetrizoate, U.S.P.	19.74 (46.06% in 70% solution)	30% 70% for difficult cases only or aortography or nephrotomography	25 cc. of 30% 25 cc. of 70%	<4 yr.: 0.7 cc. of 30% solution >4 yr.: 25 cc. of 30% solution	Not recommended	Not recommended
Miokon	Sodium diprotrizo-ate, U.S.P.	28.7	50%	20 cc. of 70% 25 cc. of 50% 30 cc. of 50%	<3 mo.: 6 cc. 3– 6 mo.: 6– 8 cc. 6–12 mo.: 8–10 cc. 1– 2 yr.: 10–15 cc. 2– 6 yr.: 15–20 cc. >6 yr.: 20–25 cc.	Not recommended	Not recommended

TABLE 8-1. *(Continued)*

Trade Name	Organic Compound	Per Cent Iodine W/V	Concentration of Drug in Commercially Available Solution	Manufacturer's Suggested Dosage			
				Adult Dose	Children's Dose	Subcutaneous Administration	Intramuscular Administration
Hypaque-50	Sodium diatrizoate, U.S.P.	30	50% for excretory urography	30 cc. of 50%	0– 6 mo.: 5 cc. 6–12 mo.: 6– 8 cc. 1– 2 yr.: 8–10 cc. 2– 5 yr.: 10–12 cc. 5– 7 yr.: 12–15 cc. 7–11 yr.: 15–18 cc. 11–15 yr.: 18–20 cc.	Dilute with equal quantities of distilled water*	Inject undiluted or diluted with equal parts distilled water
Hypaque-75	Sodium diatrizoate, U.S.P.	39.3	75% 90% for nephro-tomography	50 cc. or more	Infants: 5–10 cc. Older children: 15–20 cc.	Not recommended	Not recommended
Hypaque-90	Sodium diatrizoate, U.S.P.	46	75% 90% for nephro-tomography	50 cc. or more	Infants: 5–10 cc. Older children: 15–20 cc.	Not recommended	Not recommended
Renografin-30	Diatrizoate methyl-glucamine, U.S.P.	15	30%	*Retrograde pyelograms:* 15 cc. (unilateral)	Proportionately smaller for children	Not used	Not used
Renografin-60	Methylglucamine diatrizoate, U.S.P.	29	60%	25 cc. of 60% (over 15 yrs.)	Under 6 mo.: 5 cc. 6–12 mo.: 8 cc. 1– 2 yr.: 10 cc. 2– 5 yr.: 12 cc. 5– 7 yr.: 15 cc. 8–10 yr.: 18 cc. 11–15 yr.: 20 cc.	Not used	Not used
Renografin-76	Diatrizoate methyl-glucamine	37	76%	20–40 cc. of 76% (over 15 yrs.)	Under 6 mo.: 4 cc. 6–12 mo.: 6 cc. 1– 2 yr.: 8 cc. 2– 5 yr.: 10 cc. 5– 7 yr.: 12 cc. 8–10 yr.: 14 cc. 11–15 yr.: 16 cc.	Not used	Not used

TABLE 8-1. *(Continued)*

Trade Name	Organic Compound	Per Cent Iodine D/W	Concentration of Drug in Commercially Available Solution	Manufacturer's Suggested Dosage			
				Adult Dose	Children's Dose	Subcutaneous Administration	Intramuscular Administration
Renovist	Sodium and methyl-glucamine diatrizo-ate	37	69%	25 cc. of 37% solution (over 15 yrs.)	Under 6 mo.: 5 cc. 6–12 mo.: 8 cc. 1– 2 yr.: 10 cc. 2– 5 yr.: 12 cc. 5– 7 yr.: 15 cc. 7–10 yr.: 18 cc. 10–15 yr.: 20 cc.	Not used	Not used
Retrografin	Neomycin sulfate solution with methyl-glucamine diatrizo-ate	15	25% neomycin 30% methylgluca-mine diatrizoate	*Retrograde pyelography:* 15 cc. (unilat-eral)	Proportionately smaller for children	Not used	Not used
Ditriokon	Sodium diprotrizo-ate and diatrizoate	40	68.1%	40–50 cc. (over 12 yrs.)	0.5–1 cc./kg. body weight	Not used	Not used
Conray-60	Meglumine iothala-mate	28.2	60%	25–30 cc. (14 yrs. and over)	Under 6 mo.: 5 cc. 6–12 mo.: 8 cc. 1– 2 yr.: 10 cc. 2– 5 yr.: 12 cc. 5– 8 yr.: 15 cc. 8–12 yr.: 18 cc. 12–14 yr.: 20–30 cc.	Not used	Not used
Conray-400	Sodium iothalamate 66.8%	40	66.8%	40–50 cc. (over 14 yrs.)	0.5–1 cc./kg. under 14 yrs.	Not used	Not used

Manufacturers:

Schering: Neo-Iopax

Winthrop Laboratories: Diodrast and Hypaque

Mallinckrodt Pharmaceuticals: Hippuran, Urokon, Miokon, Ditriokon, and Conray

E. R. Squibb and Sons: Renovist and Renografin

* Subcutaneous injections are given in divided doses over each scapula. Intramuscular injections are given in divided doses into each gluteal region. To increase the rate of absorption, the addition of hyaluronidase to the solution is recommended (150–200 turbidity units on each side for children; 500 for adults).

Nephrotomograms

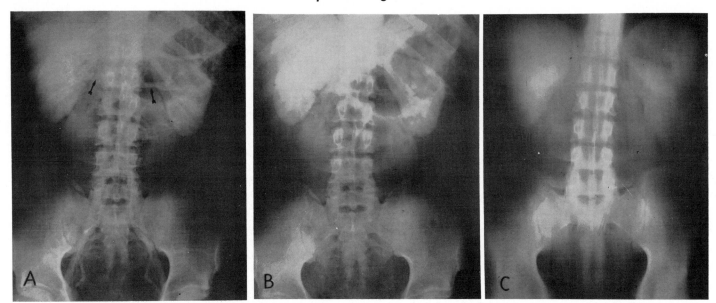

FIGURE 8-10. Twenty-five year old normal male subject. **A,** Plain film taken at predetermined circulation time demonstrates arteriogram phase. Good opacification of abdominal aorta, renal arteries (arrows) and other major arterial trunks. Note beginning opacification of the kidneys. **B,** Plain nephrogram. Film taken immediately after arterial phase. **C,** Nephrotomogram demonstrates clearly opacified kidneys without superimposition of extraneous abdominal shadows. (From Evans, J. A., Dubilier, W., Jr., and Monteith, J.: Am. J. Roentgenol. *71, 1954.*)

times desirable. This may be obtained in the erect position to visualize the point of obstruction to better advantage.

Cystograms

The most commonly used opaque media employed for this purpose are: 5 to 10 per cent sodium iodide; 12 per cent Hippuran; 12 per cent Diodrast, Hypaque, Urokon, Renografin or Neo-Iopax; air; Lipiodol and gum tragacanth mixture; Umbrathor; various mixtures of organic soluble iodides; and sodium iodide. The first two

are the most popular for cystograms; the others are not infrequently employed in urethrography.

The usual film studies obtained are (Fig. 8-13A, C, and D) (1) straight anteroposterior; (2) right posterior oblique (45 degrees); (3) left posterior oblique; (4) Chassard-Lapiné view ("sitting," "squat" or "jackknife view").

Stereoscopic films may be obtained if desired.

If catheterization is not possible, the bladder may be visualized by taking views in similar positions after an intravenous dye has been injected.

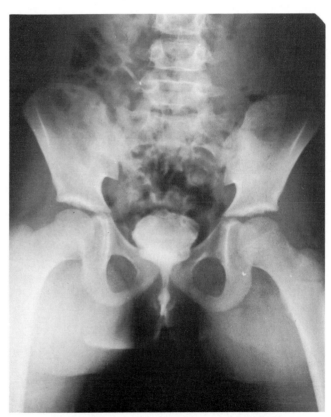

FIGURE 8-11. Normal female urethrogram.

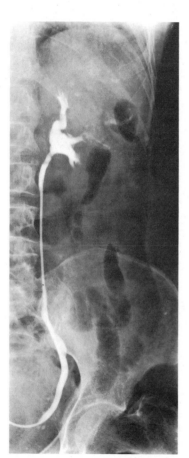

FIGURE 8-12. Representative retrograde pyelogram with ureteral catheter in situ.

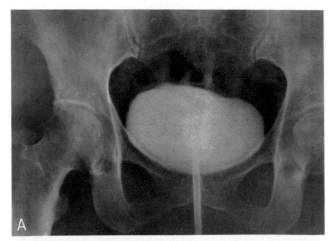

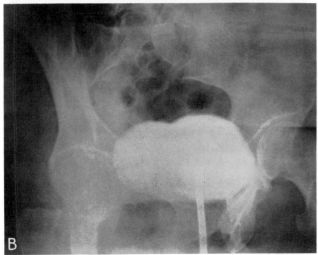

POINTS OF PRACTICAL INTEREST ABOUT FIGURE 8-13

A 5 to 15 degree caudal tilt of the central ray may be used. This will project the pubic symphysis away from the base of the bladder.

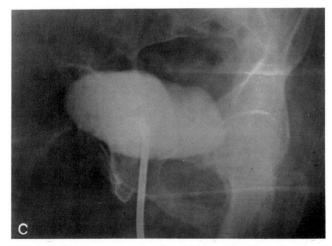

FIGURE 8-13. Representative normal cystograms: **A,** Anteroposterior view; **B,** left posterior oblique view; **C,** right posterior oblique view. A lateral view may also be employed.

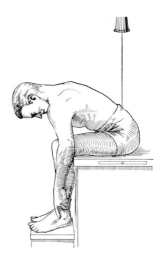

POINTS OF PRACTICAL INTEREST ABOUT FIGURE 8-13 (Continued)

1. The dynamic activity of the urinary bladder may be studied by obtaining films of the bladder area after voiding. This may show a residuum in the bladder (bladder retention) or reflux up the ureters.

2. The thickness of the bladder wall is also important, and may be gauged readily, particularly when the wall is hypertrophied in association with cystitis.

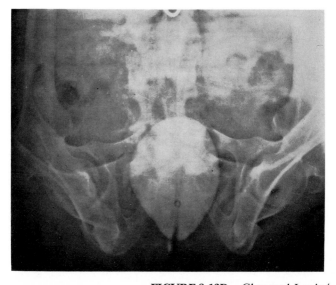

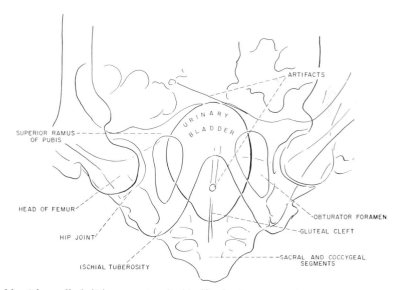

FIGURE 8-13D.   Chassard-Lapiné view of urinary bladder (also called sitting, squat or jackknife view).

Urethrograms *(Figure 8-14)*

This method of examination consists of first obtaining a film of the urethra before the introduction of contrast material into the lumen and thereafter obtaining films of the urethra filled with an opaque medium. Approximately 15 per cent sodium diatrizoate (Hypaque) is usually adequate, although any of the media described under cystograms may be used. This is injected through a urethral nozzle. A resistance to the injection is encountered when the contrast material has reached the external sphincter of the bladder. After this is overcome, the injection must be continued while the radiographs are obtained, since there is a constant leakage of contrast medium into the urinary bladder. Thus not only the anterior urethra but also the membranous and prostatic portions will be visualized.

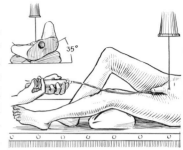
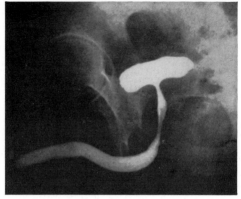

The patient is placed in an oblique position, 35 to 40 degrees, with the lower thigh flexed, and the upper thigh extended. The penis is held parallel with the upper thigh. The central ray is directed at the root of the penis (Fig. 8-14).

The film taken prior to injection of the contrast medium is of value in detecting calculi or foreign bodies that may be present.

A urethrogram in the female is illustrated in Figure 8-11. Whenever possible, anteroposterior and lateral films and cineradiographic studies are made with the patient supine, semierect or standing.

THE MALE GENITAL SYSTEM

Related Gross Anatomy *(Figure 8-15)*

Each testis is formed by numerous lobules, each containing coiled tubules called seminiferous tubules. The spermatozoa are formed in these tubules. These lobules and tubules converge posteriorly toward the rete testis, which consists of a network of tubules that empty by coiled ducts into the head of the epididymis. Here the duct of the epididymis is formed and extends in very tortuous fash-

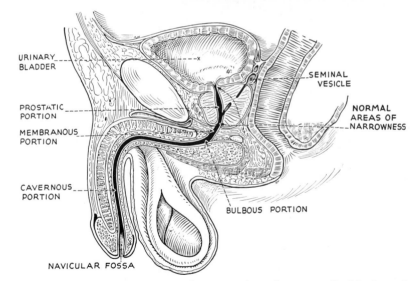

FIGURE 8-14. Representative normal urethrogram: Positioning of patient (lying down or standing), radiograph (reproduced with permission of Goodyear, Beard and Weens and the publishers of Southern Medical Journal) and anatomic sketch of the male urethra and surrounding structures.

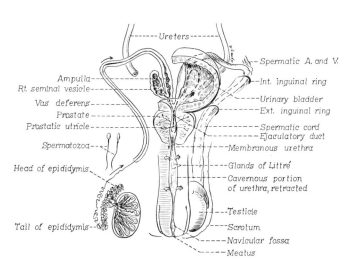

FIGURE 8-15. The male reproductive system. (Modified from Dickinson, R. L.: *Human Sex Anatomy,* Williams and Wilkins Co.)

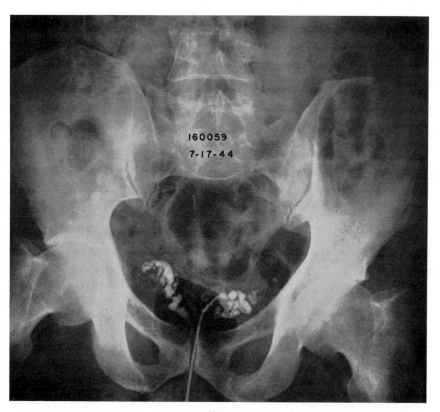

FIGURE 8-16. Representative seminal vesiculogram. (Courtesy of Drs. H. Hauser and C. C. Dundon, Cleveland, Ohio.)

ion to the tail of the epididymis where it becomes the ductus deferns. This latter is a cordlike structure that traverses the posterior aspect of the spermatic cord, and in the vicinity of the trigone of the urinary bladder, undergoes slight bulbous dilatation to form the ampulla of the ductus deferens. Near the lower margin of this ampulla, there is a diverticulum-like structure which extends cephalad and appears racemose in configuration. This is the seminal vesicle. The continuation of the ampulla of the ductus deferens beyond the point of junction with the seminal vesicle is called the ejaculatory duct, and this empties into the lower posterior aspect of the prostatic urethra, one opening on either side of the prostatic utricle. In its course, the ejaculatory duct traverses about two thirds of the length of the prostate.

Technique of Examination

There are only certain portions of the male genital system that can be examined radiographically by presently known methods, and these are not very frequently employed. The examination is confined to a soft tissue study of the prostate, seminal vesicles and scrotal contents, and the direct injection of opaque media into the lumen of the seminal vesicles, vas deferens and ejaculatory duct via the vas deferens.

The usual method employed in the direct injection depends on the exposure of the vas through a small inguinal incision under local anesthesia. This injection is first directed upward to fill the vesicles and then downward to the epididymis to fill the tubules (Fig. 8-16). Either Lipiodol or Renografin may be used. Urethroscopic catheterization has been employed by a few, but ordinarily this procedure is not very feasible in the normal subject. The latter method also does not permit visualization of the vas deferens, and serves only to outline the ejaculatory ducts and seminal vesicles.

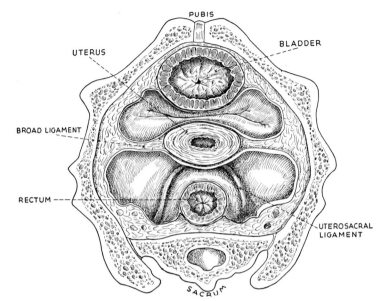

FIGURE 8-17A. Gross anatomy of female reproductive system, frontal view.

THE FEMALE REPRODUCTIVE SYSTEM

The soft tissue structures of this system will be described first and then a brief account will be given of the bony pelvis and its anatomic variations.

Soft Tissues

The organs of the female genital system consist of two ovaries, two oviducts, the uterus, the vagina and the external genitalia. The suspensory and supplementary structures are the broad ligaments

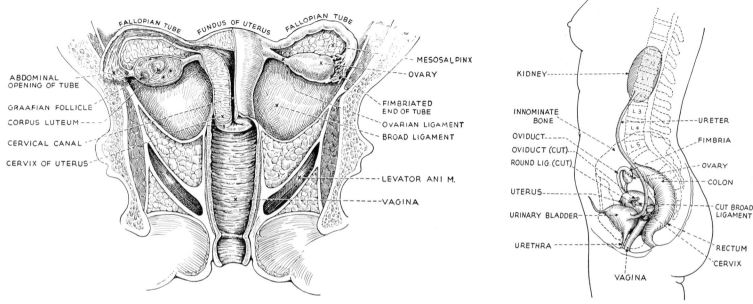

FIGURE 8-17B. Superior cross-sectional diagram of gross anatomy of female reproductive system.

FIGURE 8-17C. Lateral relationships of female genitourinary tract.

(and mesosalpinx) on either side, the round ligament, the mesovarium and mesometrium (Fig. 8-17).

The broad ligament is the transverse fold of peritoneum that extends across the pelvis minor, dividing it into an anterior and a posterior compartment. This has frequently been compared with a "curtain draped over a clothesline." Projecting into the posterior compartment, and attached a little below the upper margin of the broad ligament, is the mesovarium, with the ovary attached to its free edge. That portion of the broad ligament above this is called the mesosalpinx, and that below, the mesometrium.

The ovaries are two almond-shaped organs — one on either side of the pelvis. Their exact position in nulliparous women is somewhat variable, but their long axes are usually vertical in the erect position. The right ovary is usually slightly larger than the left, and the length varies from 2.5 to 5 cm. The width is ordinarily half the length and the thickness half the width.

The oviducts, or uterine tubes, are two trumpet-shaped tubes that run in the superior border of the broad ligament between the uterine horns and the lateral pelvic walls. The dilated end lies over each ovary. Each oviduct is from 7 to 14 cm. in length. Ordinarily, the fimbriated end and mouth of the infundibulum rest upon the medial end of the ovary. The course of the oviducts is rather variable, and may be different on the two sides.

The uterus is a pear-shaped organ with a body or fundus, and a downward extension, the cervix, with supravaginal and vaginal sections. The cavity of the body is flattened transversely and has a triangular shape, being broad above where each cornua communicates with an oviduct and narrow below where it communicates with the canal in the cervix. The direction of the axis of the uterus is quite variable. Ordinarily a moderate degree of anteflexion is considered the normal position, making an angle of 80 to 120 degrees with the horizontal. There may also be a slight list to the right or to the left side.

The vagina extends from the uterus to the external genitalia where it opens to the exterior. Its course roughly parallels the anterior curvature of the sacrum and averages 5 to 7 cm. in length.

Bony Pelvis

In addition to the normal anatomic landmarks of the pelvis (see Chapter 3), certain areas should receive the attention of the radiologist because of their influence on the course of labor. Differences characteristic of male and female types should be borne in mind. These areas are as follows:

The Subpubic Arch (Fig. 8-19).   Note should be made whether the bones of the pubic rami are delicate, average or heavy; whether the pubic angle is wide or curved (female) or narrow and straight (male); and whether the side walls of the forepelvis are divergent, straight or convergent. The configuration of the pelvic arch is a guide to the capacity of the true pelvis.

The Ischial Spines.   These are classified as sharp, average or anthropoid. Sharp spines are definitely a male characteristic and,

when present, direct attention to the necessity for a more detailed examination of the pelvis, as they may be associated with converging side walls of the forepelvis. Anthropod spines are blunt and shallow.

The Sacrosciatic Notch and Sacrum.   The capacity of the posterior pelvic inlet is related to the width of the sacrosciatic notch and the configuration of its apex. The male pelvis shows a long narrow notch with a high rounded apex and the female a wide notch with a blunt apex.

The inclination of the sacrum directly affects the capacity of the birth canal since a forward tilt will offer a barrier to normal delivery. If the forepelvis is wide and divergent, compensation occurs, but if convergent, a funnel pelvis will result. The female sacrum is wide and short compared with that of the male.

The curvature of the sacrum on the lateral projection is also important. Normally the sacrum is concave anteriorly. When this curvature is absent owing to any developmental aberration, the midpelvis is diminished and the progress of labor is impeded. The absence of this curvature will be readily apparent from measurements to be described later.

The Pelvic Inlet.   The pelvic inlet with its variations forms the basis for the classification of all pelves into four major types (Fig. 8-18):

The inlet of the anthropoid pelvis is relatively long in anteroposterior measurements and narrow in transverse diameter. The pelvic arch is usually wider than normal, and the sacrosciatic notch is wide and shallow when seen in the lateral view. The anthropoid type is so called because it closely resembles the pelves found in the higher apes.

The gynecoid pelvis refers to the average type as seen in the human female. The inlet is round or slightly oval, the pubic angle is wide, and the sacrosciatic notch is also wide. The cavity of the pelvis is ample in all directions.

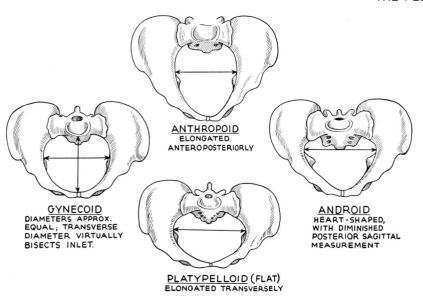

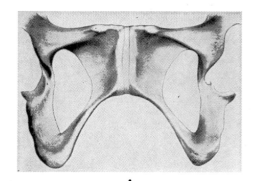

FIGURE 8-18. Different pelvic types (pelvic inlet view).

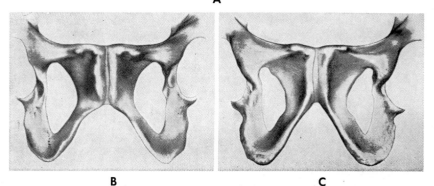

FIGURE 8-19. Variations in size and shape of the subpubic arch: A, delicate bones, wide angle, well-curved female type of pubic rami; B, average bones, moderate angle, average curvature of pubic rami; C, heavy bones, narrow angle, straight masculine type of pubic rami. (Moloy, H.C., and Swenson, P. C.: The use of the roentgen ray in obstetrics. In *Golden's Diagnostic Roentgenology,* vol. 4. edited by L. Robbins, Baltimore, Williams and Wilkins Co., 1967.)

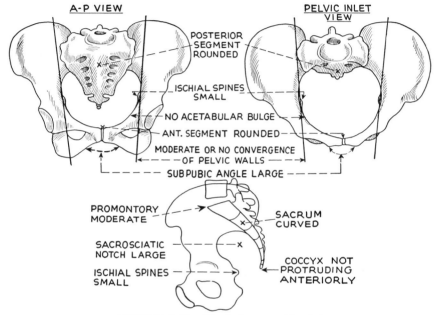

FIGURE 8-20. Typical gynecoid pelvis.

The android pelvis refers to a female pelvis that has marked masculine characteristics. These include what is described as a blunt heart-shaped or wedge-shaped inlet with narrow forepelvis, and the widest diameter is close to the sacral promontory. A narrow masculine type of sciatic notch is present, and the sacrum is set forward in the pelvis. The pubic arch is usually narrow.

The platypelloid or flat pelvis is characterized by an inlet with a transversely oval shape. The anteroposterior diameter is short and the greatest transverse diameter of the pelvis is wide—this diameter occurring well in front of the sacrum. The angle of the forepelvis is wide also, but the sacrosciatic notch and subpubic angle will vary in size.

It should be stated that gradations between all types are seen and individual variations should be described as they appear on the radiograph.

The reader is referred to the work of Caldwell and Moloy on this subject.

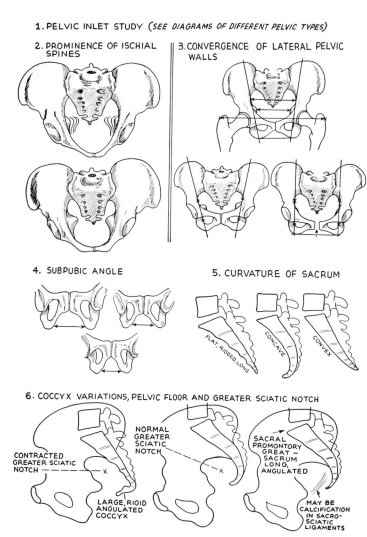

1. PELVIC INLET STUDY (*SEE DIAGRAMS OF DIFFERENT PELVIC TYPES*)

2. PROMINENCE OF ISCHIAL SPINES

3. CONVERGENCE OF LATERAL PELVIC WALLS

4. SUBPUBIC ANGLE

5. CURVATURE OF SACRUM

FLAT, RIDGED, LONG   CONCAVE   CONVEX

6. COCCYX VARIATIONS, PELVIC FLOOR AND GREATER SCIATIC NOTCH

CONTRACTED GREATER SCIATIC NOTCH

NORMAL GREATER SCIATIC NOTCH

SACRAL PROMONTORY GREAT — SACRUM LONG, ANGULATED

LARGE, RIGID ANGULATED COCCYX

MAY BE CALCIFICATION IN SACRO-SCIATIC LIGAMENTS

FIGURE 8-21. Factors studied in pelvic architecture.

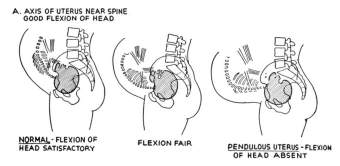

7. UTERINE AXIS FACTOR IN RELATION TO SACRUM AND SACRAL PROMONTORY

A. AXIS OF UTERUS NEAR SPINE GOOD FLEXION OF HEAD

NORMAL - FLEXION OF HEAD SATISFACTORY

FLEXION FAIR

PENDULOUS UTERUS - FLEXION OF HEAD ABSENT

Methods of Study of the Female Genital System

In the entire description that follows of the applications and usefulness of radiographic techniques in investigation of obstetrical and gynecologic problems, the student must bear in mind those aspects of radiologic protection that pertain here (see Chapter 1). The information to be gained must justify the exposure of the patient (and the fetus, if one be present). In any case, radiation exposure of the patient and the fetus in the first trimester of pregnancy is to be avoided unless the problem at hand is critical.

Direct Radiography and Its Applications. Anteroposterior, lateral and oblique views of the pelvis are obtained, and a considerable amount of information is available from these views (Figs. 8-21, 8-22 and 8-23).

1. The configuration of the maternal pelvis can be ascertained as judged by the standard bony types just described. It is important to comment on individual bony differences irrespective of the four major pelvic types.

2. An indication of the age of the fetus is obtained, or a decision as to the maturity of the fetus can be reached. Perhaps, the best index of the former is the fetal length. Haase has suggested that for

clinical purposes the length of the embryo in centimeters may be approximated during the first five months by squaring the number of the month to which the pregnancy has advanced; in the second half of pregnancy by multiplying the month by five.

The radiologist may be called upon to offer an opinion as to the maturity of the fetus. Authorities suggest the following as salient critieria:

An ossification center is present in the distal end of the femur in 90 per cent of term fetuses; ossification of the hyoid bone is complete; and five out of six cases will show ossification in the proximal tibial epiphysis.

Less practical standards are the ossification of the essential parts of vertebrae, the first segments of the coccyx, and the metacarpals and phalanges. It should be remembered that good films are essential to obtain the necessary detail.

3. The presentation and position of the fetus can be determined.

4. The degree of flexion of the fetal head and spine can be noted.

5. The viability of the fetus can be confirmed.

6. The progress of labor can be followed.

7. The diagnosis of multiple pregnancy or fetal abnormality can be made.

8. The detection of the early fetus is possible. Anteroposterior and oblique films of the pelvis are obtained; the position described under the heading of pelvic pneumoperitoneum is also useful. The oblique films are especially helpful as a small fetus may be obscured by the sacrum in the anteroposterior film. Good films will detect the fetal skeleton as early as three and one-half months.

9. The position of the placenta can be ascertained.

Direct anteroposterior and lateral views of the abdomen are usually sufficient in our experience to delineate the placenta as a crescentic shadow lying between the fetus and the boundary of the uterus. A wedge-type barium or plastic filter may be utilized to obtain better detail in placentography.

Combination air rectograms and cystograms are useful in making certain that the placenta is not implanted low in the uterus. When air is injected in the rectum and urinary bladder, and a lateral film of this obtained, a placenta that is implanted low will produce an opacity projected in the air medium and thus may be recognized.

This method is of value in cephalic presentations, and particularly in a central type of placenta praevia in which the placenta intervenes between head and bladder. The erect position must be employed to make sure the fetal head is pressing upon the dome of the urinary bladder, and that gravity and the weight of the fetus are forcing the head downward.

Radiography after the injection of opaque fluid such as Hypaque into the amniotic sac (amniography) has been employed by some.

Amniography. Amniography implies and involves the direct injection into the amniotic fluid of water-soluble iodide compound. The amniotic fluid thereby becomes diffusely opacified, and the placenta is identified as a filling defect encroaching on this space. Anteroposterior and lateral views must be obtained. Ordinarily 40 cc. of 50 per cent Hypaque or its equivalent will suffice. An injection site is chosen in the paraumbilical region within a radius of 5 to 6 cm. from the umbilicus, at a point where the entering needle is least likely to touch the fetus.

Following the injection, the patient is encouraged to walk about for 20 or 30 minutes, if her clinical condition will permit. If not, she is shifted around from position to position so that a good distribution of the contrast agent may be obtained. Films may be obtained at any time between 30 minutes and two hours after the instillation of the medium.

An inherent danger in this procedure is that premature labor may be induced. Films taken after two hours, with a live fetus sometimes show some of the opacified amniotic fluid in the fetal stomach and intestines. In a dead fetus no swallowing will have occurred.

AMNIOGRAPHY AS A GUIDE TO FETOGRAPHY AND INTRAUTERINE FETAL TRANSFUSION. During amniography it has been noted that the fetus swallows the radiopaque medium, with delineation of the gastrointestinal tract of the fetus obtained thereby. This has been advocated as a test for viability of the fetus. Liley, in 1963, demonstrated that he could pass a needle through the maternal abdominal wall, the uterine wall and the abdominal wall of the fetus to instill Rh negative blood into the peritoneal cavity of the fetus. Blood so instilled was absorbed into the fetal peripheral circulation. Others who have repeated this technique have also reported success with it (Queenan and Wyatt; Bowman and Friesen; Duggin and Taylor).

Some of the difficulties of intrauterine transfusion have been described in an editorial in the Journal of the American Medical Association (*191*:138, 1965). It is apparently not unusual to make three or four attempts to enter the peritoneal cavity of a fetus 25 to 26 weeks of age, before a successful intraperitoneal approach is achieved. Considerable x-ray exposure must be involved since films must be obtained after each attempt. Image intensification is of course vital for such a procedure.

Removal of amniotic fluid under fluoroscopic guidance prior to delivery has also been helpful in determining the onset of deterioration from erythroblastosis fetalis in the fetus. Apparently after 29 weeks of gestation, the prognosis of impending fetal death on the basis of the rise in optical density of the amniotic fluid seems to be quite accurate. Prior to this time, the significance of a given rise of optical density of the amniotic fluid is less certain. This has afforded an effective means of selection of fetuses for preterm delivery and postdelivery exchange transfusions. This procedure has been found to be extremely effective in the management of infants with erythroblastosis fetalis (Queenan and Wyatt).

Percutaneous Transfemoral Aortography. Percutaneous transfemoral aortography by the Seldinger technique has opened up a new vista for diagnosis in obstetric and gynecologic conditions. In this technique a needle is first introduced into the artery. Its sharpened inner stylus is withdrawn. A guide spring is slipped through the needle into the arterial lumen. The needle is then removed and the guide remains. Tubing is slipped over the guide into the arterial lumen. (See Chapter 10.)

Fluoroscopy with image amplification is usually employed during manipulation of the guide and tubing thereafter. The tip of the tube is located at the upper abdominal aorta for abdominal aortography and renal arteriography or at the aortic bifurcation for pelvic arteriography. During the injection, blood pressure cuffs are generally used as tourniquets about both thighs to prevent useless run-off of contrast agent into the leg arteries. Benson et al. utilized 20 to 25 cc. of 60 per cent N-methylglucamine or 80 per cent methalamate as the contrast agent. The material was injected rapidly and a series of x-ray films of the desired area obtained. The injection could be made manually, although mechanical pressure injectors are desirable. Ordinarily 12 x-ray exposures were made at one-half second intervals beginning with the injection, but fewer films would have sufficed in most instances. Accurate placental visualization was obtained routinely after a scout film and two exposures made four and six seconds after the start of injection. Thirteen patients with anterpartum hemorrhage were studied and 16 patients with pelvic pain or tumor, exclusive of 17 other patients with carcinoma of the cervix. Twenty-seven additional patients were studied for vascular or renal disease. The details and highly specific anatomy of this specialized procedure are outside the scope of this text, and the reader is referred to Benson et al. for pertinent details.

This procedure was found very useful in a study of the extension of carcinoma of the cervix, uterine tumors, adnexal tumors, problems of pregnancy, and placentography. The placental circulation is usually identified as early as the second month in unruptured extrauterine pregnancy. It appears as a scattered, fine, mottled, or cotton-fluff opacification. There is ordinarily a lingering density in the placenta due to slowing of the circulation in this area.

By means of image amplification and limited fluoroscopy with a limited number of films employed, the extent of exposure of maternal pelvis and fetus should not be inordinate.

Pelvic Mensuration and Fetal Cephalometry. The purpose of this investigation is to determine by the process of measurements made on radiographs whether or not disproportion exists between the fetal head and the maternal pelvis. It should be stated that this examination can only determine the *mathematical* relationship of the two; *no prognostication as to whether or not spontaneous delivery will occur is possible in view of the multitude of other factors that are involved,* such as the extent of molding of the fetal head, or uterine inertia.

These measurements can be made on the routine films described, but the calculations are complicated by the necessity for correction of the magnification present. This problem is overcome by applying a correction factor for magnification, and different methods of pelvimetry differ primarily in their method of correction.

A teleroentgenographic technique may be employed, which minimizes magnification, and the films are usually taken at a distance of 6 feet. This method requires relatively high-powered equipment, but is readily applicable in many hospital laboratories with tall ceilings and floor-to-ceiling tube stands, and we have found it most convenient in our own laboratory. A magnification of approximately 10 per cent is obtained for a part 15 cm. from the film, and this correction is readily applied. A lesser correction is applied for measurement of parts closer to the film. Not only is error in measurement minimized by this method, but better detail is obtained as well as an immediate visual impression of the relative size of the fetal head with respect to the pelvis that has proved very valuable.

In cephalic presentations, the same film may be employed for measurement of both the fetal head and the pelvis. In breech presentations, it is advisable to obtain separate films centered over the fetal head, in addition to the films of the pelvis, to obviate distortion caused by divergence of the x-ray beam.

It should be emphasized that the part to be examined should be parallel with the film surface to eliminate distortion, otherwise distortion must also be taken into consideration (see Chapter 1).

In all these examinations, care must be exercised not to alter the position of the patient in the change from the anteroposterior to lateral projection since the one view is utilized to obtain the measurements used in correction for magnification in the other view. Such care is less important in the teleroentgenographic method since small changes in position do not reflect significant changes in magnification; in all other methods, these changes are especially important, particularly in breech presentations or when the fetal head is not engaged.

Thus, if the patient is supine for the anteroposterior film, she should remain so for the lateral view, and a horizontal x-ray beam should be employed.

The erect position has the advantage of simplifying this procedure, but the greater difficulty of obtaining good films in the erect position on a pregnant woman offsets this advantage.

In all methods other than the teleroentgenographic method a considerable inaccuracy will be introduced if the patient does not remain in the same position for both anteroposterior and lateral views; if it is not possible to do this in any installation, a deficiency in accuracy must be recognized and so stated.

The usual views obtained are as follows: (1) anteroposterior view of the pelvis and fetal head (Fig. 8-22); (2) lateral view of the pelvis and fetal head (Fig. 8-23) and (3) a direct view of the pelvic inlet (Fig. 8-24). The patient sits on the table top, her back making an angle of about 45 degrees with the table. The patient's position is adjusted so that the pelvic inlet will be parallel with the table top. The central ray is directed central to the pelvic inlet. If

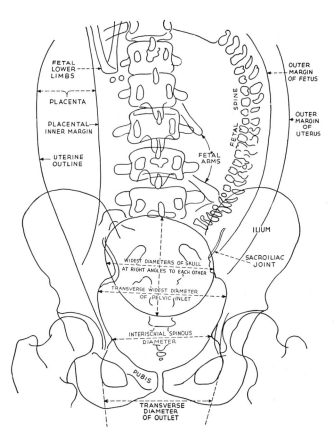

FIGURE 8-22. Tracing of radiograph routinely employed in pelvicephalometry: anteroposterior view (position same as for KUB film).

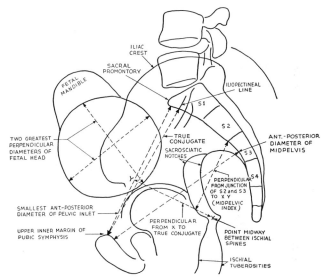

FIGURE 8-23. Tracing of radiograph routinely employed in pelvicephalometry: lateral view (position same as for lateral projection of abdomen or lumbar spine).

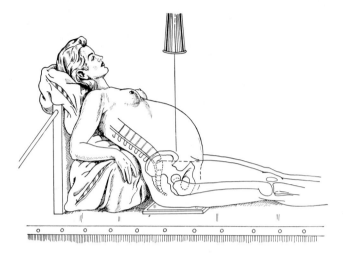

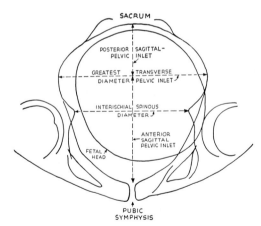

FIGURE 8-24. Positioning of patient for special view of pelvic inlet (note that pelvic inlet is parallel to the table top) and tracing of radiograph so obtained and routinely employed in pelvicephalometry.

possible, a 72 inch film-to-target distance should be employed to produce a minimum magnification. With short film-to-target distances, the pelvic inlet will be considerably magnified and somewhat distorted, in view of the relatively great distance from the pelvic inlet to the film. (4) Occasionally a special view of the pelvic outlet is made with the patient sitting and leaning forward, so that the ischial tuberosites are in contact with the table top, and the remainder of the body does not obscure them.

Whatever method is employed to take these films, it is important to know the film-to-target and film-to-table-top distances accurately to correct for the magnificant present.

If a breech presentation is present, additional anteroposterior and lateral views centering over the fetal head are made.

THE CUSTOMARY MEASUREMENTS MADE ON THE RADIOGRAPHS (Fig. 8-26). It is important to emphasize that we are comparing the measurements of the particular fetus in question with the maternal pelvis and that the data needed are present on the films and are obtained as described. *No average pelvic or fetal measurements are included, as each case has to be judged on its own merits.*

Having obtained satisfactory films, it is necessary to ascertain the following measurements to gauge the size of the inlet.

1. *The greatest transverse diameter of the pelvic inlet* is obtained from the special view of the pelvic inlet and from the anteroposterior view of the pelvis.

2. *The anteroposterior diameter of the pelvic inlet* (true conjugate) is obtained from the lateral projection. The measurement is taken from the posterior margin of the symphysis pubis to the point where the shadow of the iliopectineal line crosses the sacrum, or to the top of the sacral promontory, whichever distance is smaller.

3. *The ratio of the posterior sagittal dimension of the inlet to the total anteroposterior diameter* is obtained. To obtain this measurement, the greatest transverse diameter of the inlet is drawn on the film of the special view of the inlet. Since an accurate measurement for this is available from the anteroposterior view of the pelvis,

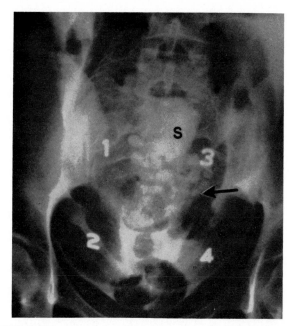

FIGURE 8-25A. Complete breech presentation. Radiopaque material may be seen in the fetal stomach *(S)* and small intestine (arrow). Localizing lead markers surround fetal peritoneal cavity.

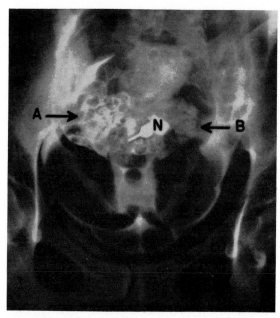

FIGURE 8-25B. Tuohy needle *(N)* in fetal peritoneal cavity. Radiopaque material demonstrated outside fetal small intestine *(A)* and in small intestine *(B)*. (From Queenan, J. T.: J.A.M.A. *191*:944, 1965.)

a magnification correction factor is thus obtained by comparing the latter with the former. On the inlet view a perpendicular is drawn from this greatest dimension to the middle of the sacral promontory and also to the middle of the pubic symphysis. The former measurement is spoken of as the posterior sagittal measurement of the inlet and the latter as the anterior sagittal measurement of the inlet. Accurate correction for these measurements is obtained from the correction factor mentioned earlier. Ideally, the ratio of the anterior to the posterior sagittal diameters of the inlet should approach unity in a gynecoid pelvis.

METHOD FOR CORRECTION OF MAGNIFICATION. The degree of magnification will vary in accordance with the distance between the x-ray tube target and the film, and the distance between the diameter (or distance) to be measured and the film. If the dimension in question is parallel with the film surface, distortion is eliminated. If the target-to-film distance is known and also the object-to-film distance, it is possible to calculate accurately the true measurement of the part. This may be accomplished by graphs or nomograms (Fig. 8-27, 8-28 and 8-29) (Ball, Snow), stereoscopic films. (Caldwell and Moloy), metal notched rules placed next to the part being

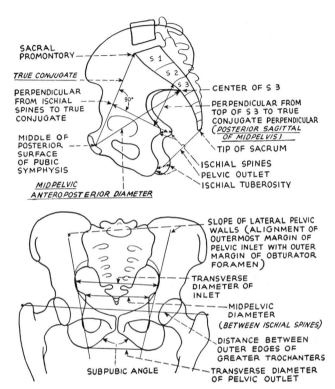

FIGURE 8-26A. Diagrams illustrating the various pelvic measurements which are obtained from routine anteroposterior and lateral teleroentgenograms of the pelvis.

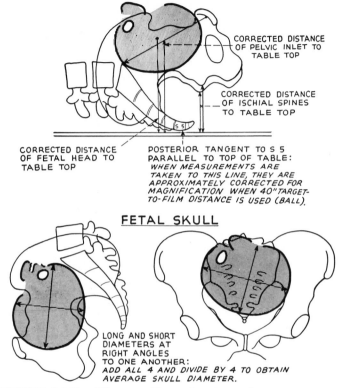

FIGURE 8-26B. Diagrams illustrating the various measurements of the fetal head which are obtained and compared with the pelvic measurements.

radiographed (Colcher-Sussman), or perforated metal plates superimposed on the radiograph (Thoms).

THE INTERPRETATION OF THE MEASUREMENTS. Having obtained the foregoing measurements of the pelvis and the average diameter of the fetal head, each pelvic measurement is compared with the fetal head diameter. Obviously when the average inlet, midpelvic and outlet diameters exceed the average diameter of

the fetal head, no disproportion exists. When the average diameter of the fetal head exceeds the average diameter of any of the pelvic planes, further computation is necessary as follows:

The average pelvic diameter in question is considered the diameter of a sphere and as such the volume of this sphere is calculated or obtained from nomograms (Figs. 8-27 or 8-29). This volume is compared with the fetal head volume as previously com-

FIGURE 8-27. Nomograms for correction of magnification and for conversion of diameters to volumes. With a straight edge, a line is drawn from the object-film distance (1) of a certain dimension through the anode-film distance (2) used when the film was taken to the transfer axis. From this point on the transfer axis, a line is drawn through the dimension as measured on the film (3) which intersects (4) at the true, corrected dimension. With the table at the bottom of the nomogram a circumference or a diameter measurement in centimeters can be transposed directly to volume of a similar sphere in terms of cubic centimeters. (After Holmquest, from *Golden's Diagnostic Roentgenology,* vol. 4, edited by L. Robbins. Baltimore, Williams and Wilkins Co., 1967.)

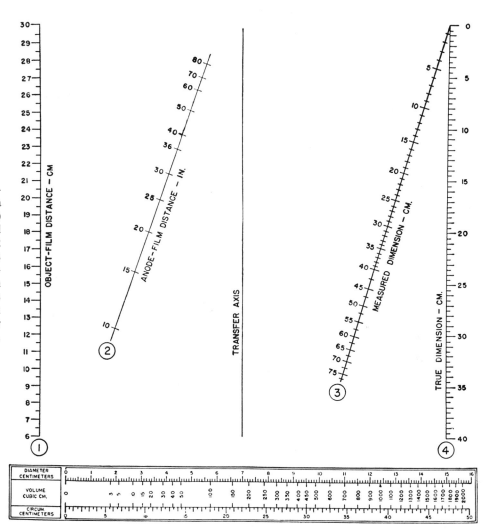

puted. When the fetal head volume exceeds the volume capacity of the inlet by 70 cc. or less, or the volume capacity of the bispinous diameter by 30 to 220 cc., the incidence of cesarean section would be about 33 per cent. Excesses beyond these limits would increase difficult delivery, and cesarean section incidence accordingly, up to 80 to 87 per cent.

In those methods that employ calculation, graphs or nomograms to determine the degree of magnification, the basic procedure is as follows:

1. The desired dimension is measured on the one radiograph, whether it be the anteroposterior or lateral view.

2. The distance that this dimension is placed from the film is determined from the other radiograph. Thus, to determine this object-to-film distance for dimensions measured on the anteroposterior view, the lateral radiograph is employed, and vice versa.

3. There will, however, be an error of magnification on this second radiograph also, which must be corrected before it can be applied as the object-to-table-top distance.

4. In order to obtain object-to-film distance, the object-to-table-top distance is first calculated, and to this figure is added the known table-top-to-film distance (usually 5 cm.).

5. Only those dimensions in the central ray can be measured, unless the teleroentgenographic method is employed in which beam divergence is negligible.

6. The following triangulation laws are applied (Fig. 8-28):

$$\frac{GH \text{ (unknown)}}{DE \text{ (known)}} = \frac{XH}{XE} = \frac{XE - (HB + BE) \text{ (known)}}{XE \qquad \text{(known)}}$$

From this equation, it is obvious that all factors are known except GH, and hence, simple algebraic solution is possible. Snow's special calculator or Ball's nomograms allow one to obtain this algebraic solution directly.

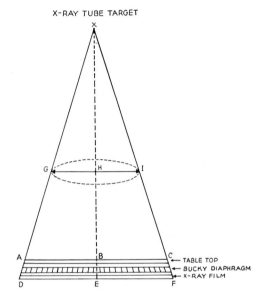

X-RAY TUBE TARGET

XE = TARGET-TO-FILM, DISTANCE (KNOWN)
BE = TABLE TOP-TO-FILM, DISTANCE (KNOWN)
GH = 1/2 THE DIMENSION TO BE MEASURED
DE = THE PROJECTION OF GH ON THE FILM AND HENCE THE MEASUREMENT OBTAINED FROM THE FILM (KNOWN)
HB = THE DISTANCE OF DIMENSION GH FROM THE TABLE TOP (KNOWN FROM FILM IN OPPOSITE VIEW AFTER CORRECTED FOR MAGNIFICATION)

FIGURE 8-28. Triangulation method of determining radiographic magnification (see text for explanation).

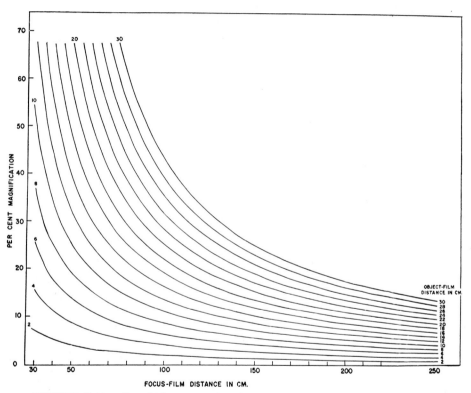

FIGURE 8-29. Graph demonstrating the per cent magnification readily obtained when one knows both the focus-to-film distance and the object-to-film distance in centimeters. (Courtesy of T. H. Oddie, D.Sc.)

EVALUATION OF PELVICEPHALOGRAPHY IN THE LIGHT OF RADIATION HAZARD. Considerable confusion has resulted with respect to the indications and contraindications for the radiologic study of the female pelvis and fetal skull in pregnancy. While radiation is not the only genetic hazard in our environment that can result in increased mutations, every effort should be made to reduce this particular hazard as much as possible. Although it has not been absolutely proved in mammals, it is generally accepted that genetic aberrations from exposure to radiation can occur at virtually any dose level.

The reader is referred to Chapter 1 for a more detailed consideration of the many aspects of radiation protection. From these discussions, however, we may deduce the following conclusions:

1. Roentgen pelvic encephalometry should not be considered a routine procedure. It must be employed only after thorough obstetrical examination and evaluation, and the information to be obtained must be of critical value. Nevertheless, this procedure must be undertaken with the full understanding that the radiologist cannot and should not by himself attempt to predict the outcome of delivery. The data obtained should permit a thorough study of the maternal pelvis in all its aspects and should provide some idea of the relative size, shape, and position of the fetal skull in relation to the maternal pelvis.

2. All precautions should be employed to minimize radiation exposure. These must include high kilovoltage techniques, fast films, fast screens, collimation, additional filtration, increased target-to-film distance and adequate darkroom processing so that repeated exposures are unnecessary.

3. The optimal time for roentgen pelvic encephalometry is during the last two weeks of pregnancy. Under these circumstances, with a cephalic presentation the fetal gonads may actually lie outside the primary beam of radiation if one concentrates on the maternal pelvis.

4. Although information regarding fetal maturity, age and development may be obtained, fetal weight predictions have proved inaccurate and unsatisfactory since no relationship has been established between fetal skull measurements and body weight (Ane).

Pelvic Pneumoperitoneum (Fig. 8-30). A needle is inserted 2 to 3 cm. below and to the left of the umbilicus. Oxygen, carbon dioxide or nitrous oxide is introduced into the peritoneal space with the patient in the Trendelenburg position (hips above the level of the head). Films are thereafter obtained in the posteroanterior position with the patient tilted head downward approximately 50 degrees and the central x-ray beam centered over the rectum, the beam being directed vertically downward.

Pelvic pneumoperitoneum allows visualization of the ovaries, oviducts and uterine fundus. The uterus appears as a dome-shaped structure projection above the pubic symphysis, and measures approximately 3 to 5 cm. on the usual projection. The ovaries are projected on the lateral pelvic walls as ovoid shadows. There is a homogeneous air shadow above.

Hysterosalpingography with Opaque Media (Fig. 8-31). The most common opaque media employed are Lipiodol, Iodochlorol, Lipoiodine, Rayopaque, Skiodan acacia, or Salpix. A suitable cannula, which at the same time obstructs the cervical canal, is inserted into the cervical canal of the uterus. Approximately 6 cc. of the opaque medium is injected and an anteroposterior film is obtained. If there is inadequate filling of any portion another 3 cc. is injected, and stereoscopic films are obtained while injecting an additional 2 to 3 cc. of dye. When iodized oil is used, another film is obtained in 24 hours to detect the extent of overflow into the pelvis through the oviducts. Serial films may be obtained if there is an obvious constriction of one of the tubes, and it is desired to detect the constancy of this finding. When Rayopaque or the other absorbable media are employed, serial films at 15 to 20 minute intervals are obtained. Ordinarily, in 1 to 2 hours all the dye is reabsorbed and appears in the urinary bladder.

Hysterosalpingography is particularly useful in cases of ster-

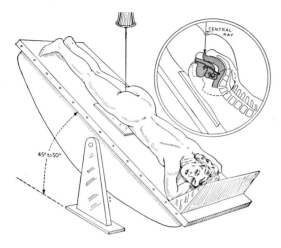

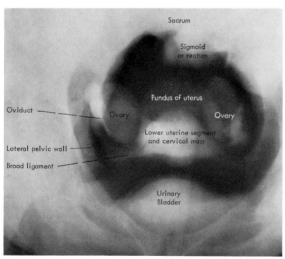

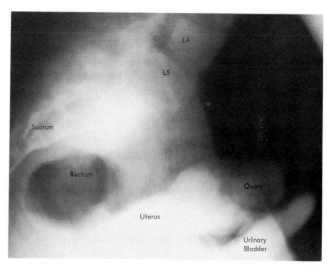

FIGURE 8-30. Pneumoperitoneum of the female pelvis in anteroposterior *(left)* and lateral *(right)* projections. This patient was a 29 year old female with a Stein-Leventhal syndrome proved by surgery, but her ovaries are considered normal in size for a young woman. (Courtesy of Dr. Wilma C. Diner, Department of Radiology, University of Arkansas Medical Center, Little Rock, Arkansas.)

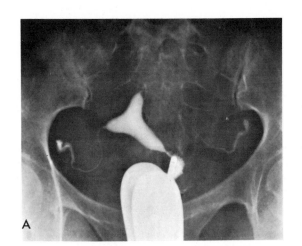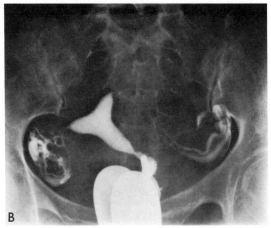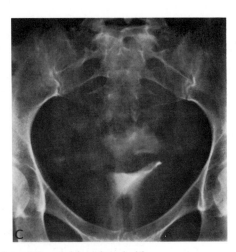

FIGURE 8-31.   Radiographs demonstrating routine films obtained by hysterosalpingography with soluble, absorbable medium. **A,** Film obtained after the insertion of the first 2 cc. fraction. **B,** Radiograph obtained after the fourth insertion of the 2 cc. fraction. This radiograph demonstrates spillage into the pelvic peritoneal space. **C,** Film obtained 20 minutes after the injection, showing the opaque medium still present in the pelvic peritoneal space; but already some of the medium has been absorbed and is appearing in the urinary bladder. Dotted areas indicate the impression of the ovaries upon the contrast medium. A preliminary scout film is also obtained prior to the injection of contrast medium.

ility and to prove or disprove the patency of the tubes. This examination delineates the uterine cavity, shows the length, shape and position of the oviducts, and the patency of one or both tubes. A variable amount of fluid escapes into the pelvis proper.

In recent times, we have found fluoroscopy with image amplification, video tape recording, and cineradiography most helpful.

GENITOGRAPHY IN INTERSEXUAL STATES

The components of sexual differentiation consist of chromosomal, gonadal, internal genital anatomy, external genital anatomy, hormonal aspects, environmental rearing and sexual orientation or gender. The last two elements are largely governed by internal and external genital anatomy; in the case of the male, hormonal activity is required as well.

The clinical studies which are of assistance in the determination of these sexual components are sex chromatin pattern, a study of the external genital anatomy, a knowledge of the internal genital anatomy, urinary hormonal excretion and the nature of the gonads as determined by biopsy.

Genitography is the simplest and best procedure for providing information regarding the internal genital anatomy, particularly prior to the time when knowledge of the nature of the gonads is not essential. Apparently genitography can provide anatomic information not afforded by other means.

The technique of genitography requires the filling of all genital cavities with opaque media. Two methods may be employed: a flushing technique, or a multiple catheter technique. The examination should be performed under fluoroscopy for proper control.

The multiple catheter technique is employed when the flushing technique fails, since in placing a catheter into one cavity, one may miss other passages. The relationship of the urinary bladder may be simultaneously determined by excretory urography. It is suggested that the opaque medium employed be aqueous at first try; if success is not obtained, an oily medium may be thereafter employed.

A simple classification of intersex states is the following: true hermaphroditism, in which both ovaries and testes are present in the same individual; female pseudohermaphrodism, in which ovaries and a masculinized lower genital tract in external genitalia are present; and male pseudohermaphrodism in which the testes are present but female external genitalia are noted. This classification does not include those instances with hypoplastic structures which do not communicate with the exterior of the body.

The basic principle in handling intersex problems is that it is easier to transform a sexually ambiguous person into a female than a male.

There are actually very few circumstances in which the intersex problem can be resolved by masculinization of the external genitalia. Hypospadias is one of these. Shopfner has recommended that genitography be employed particularly in patients with hypospadias in order to detect unsuspected müllerian remnants, which would tend to counteract the benefits derived from correction of the hypospadias. Genitography also affirms the presence or absence of the vagina and shows the relationship of the urethra to it. Such information becomes important in assigning a practical sex to an intersexual patient.

For further detail in regard to this important subject, the reader is referred to Shopfner's comprehensive monograph.

Chapter 9 — The Alimentary and Biliary Tracts

THE ALIMENTARY TRACT

The alimentary tract consists of the mouth and oropharynx, the esophagus, the stomach, the small intestine and the large intestine (colon).

The contrast agent of choice is barium sulfate in water suspension. Colloidal barium sulfate is useful in certain instances, and occasionally, as will be indicated, the barium sulfate may be suspended in isotonic saline. Organic soluble iodides (diatrizoate) are occasionally used also, but offer little advantage ordinarily, and some disadvantage since they are hypertonic.

On certain occasions, advantage is gained by so-called "double contrast" in which, following the introduction of the barium suspension, gas is introduced. In the colon, air is insufflated; in the stomach, the patient is given a carbonated drink such as ginger ale or carbonated water.

The actual radiologic methods include: (1) fluoroscopy; (2) spot film radiography or cineradiography at the time of fluoroscopy and (3) routine radiography in certain positions. Any or all of the usual erect, recumbent, supine, prone, lateral or oblique positions are employed. In our positioning illustrations to follow, only the latter will be considered.

Although our positioning studies are static, it must at all times be recalled that the gastrointestinal tract is a dynamic, moving, functioning system of organs. Their structure must at all times be considered along with their function; the two are inseparable.

We must also always be cognizant of the fact that when we fill the lumen with barium, we are studying the hollow part of the organ and its mucosal lining. The structure of the wall of the organ outside the mucosal layer may not be reflected in the appearance of the rugal pattern, and abnormalities therein may escape detection.

In recent times, angiography has begun to play a part in the examination of the gastrointestinal tract. A percutaneous catheter (Seldinger technique; see Chapter 10) is threaded through the femoral artery (or brachial), up (or down) the aorta to the celiac axis, the superior or inferior mesenteric arteries, and selective injections of a suitable contrast agent are made. A rapid serial filming technique is utilized as described in Chapter 10. Because the procedure is highly specialized, the student is referred to other texts for detailed descriptions of this technique. (Also see Chapter 10.)

It is probable that closed circuit television, with tape recording and possible "kineradiography" thereafter from the television screen, will play an increasing role in examination of the swallowing function and all areas of the gastrointestinal tract. In general, however, a knowledge of the fundamentals elucidated in the following pages will still apply, enhanced by the additional advantages of replay, monitored selection of views for permanent recording, and an understanding of motor physiology unparalleled by our present day, more conventional studies.

RADIOGRAPHY OF THE MOUTH WITH OCCLUSAL TYPE DENTAL FILM

Soft Tissue of the Floor of the Mouth

By placing an occlusal type dental film in the mouth and directing the x-ray beam perpendicular to it, the soft tissues of the submandibular area are penetrated, as well as the mandible (Fig. 9-1). These soft tissues are not visualized in sufficient detail to distinguish such anatomic structures as the salivary glands and ducts, lymph nodes, and tongue, but this method of examination affords a ready means of investigating abnormal calcareous deposits in these structures. Hence an understanding of the normal appearance of this projection is essential.

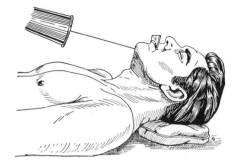

Soft Tissues of the Cheek

This area can be examined in a similar manner by placing an occlusal film on the inside of the cheek. Care must be exercised in placing the film sufficiently posterior to obtain a visualization of as much of Stensen's duct as possible, since occasionally calcareous deposits in this location may lead to obstructive inflammation and symptoms.

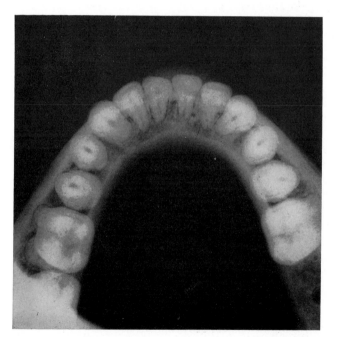

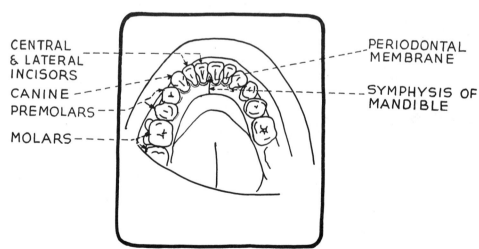

CENTRAL & LATERAL INCISORS

CANINE

PREMOLARS

MOLARS

PERIODONTAL MEMBRANE

SYMPHYSIS OF MANDIBLE

FIGURE 9-1. Occlusal type dental film of floor of mouth.

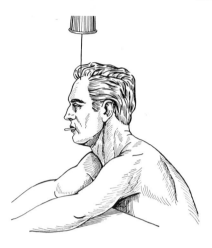

The Hard Palate

Apart from the lateral projection described earlier, a visualization of the hard palate may be obtained by means of an occlusal film in the mouth as illustrated in Figure 9-2. Note that there are considerable differences in density in the various portions of the hard palate, accounted for by the aerated sinuses, the alveolar process, and the bony nasal septum, which overlie the palate. This variation in osseous density is important to consider when one interprets the osseous structure of the hard palate.

The incisive foramen and the major palatine foramen can usually be identified. Frequently, the midline suture as well as the transverse palatine suture can also be noted.

(Text continues on page 284.)

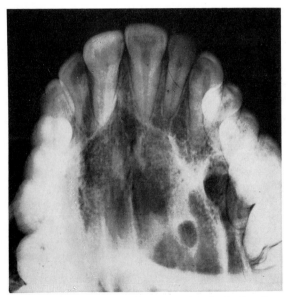

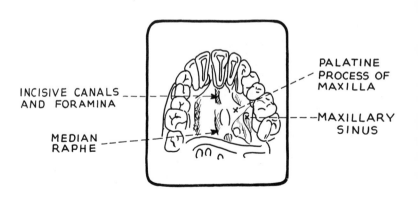

FIGURE 9-2. Method of radiography of hard palate with occlusal type of dental film; showing positioning of patient; radiograph and labeled tracing.

POINTS OF PRACTICAL INTEREST ABOUT FIGURES 9-3, 9-4 AND 9-5

    1. A barium paste is usually employed. This adheres to the wall of the esophagus long enough to allow the technician to obtain good films of the full esophagus. On the other hand, air pockets can occur, and when they are seen, an additional film may be desired to exclude a constant filling defect.

    2. To visualize the mucosal pattern of the esophagus, one may administer a tablespoon of water following the barium paste.

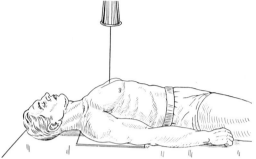

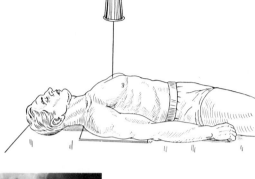

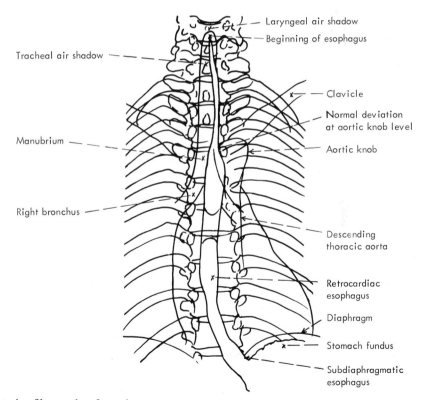

FIGURE 9-3. Anteroposterior film study of esophagus.

POINTS OF PRACTICAL INTEREST ABOUT FIGURES 9-3, 9-4 AND 9-5 *(Continued)*

3. For demonstration of suspected esophageal varices, an effort is made to obtain a clear visualization of the mucosal pattern (as described previously) with the patient performing the Valsalva maneuver (straining down against the closed glottis). Indeed, a film obtained before this maneuver that shows a diminution of the filling defects, followed by a film with the Valsalva maneuver that shows an accentuation of them, is virtually pathognomonic of esophageal varices.

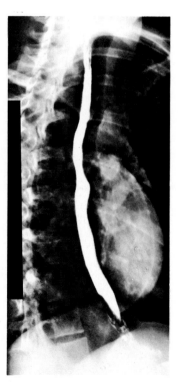

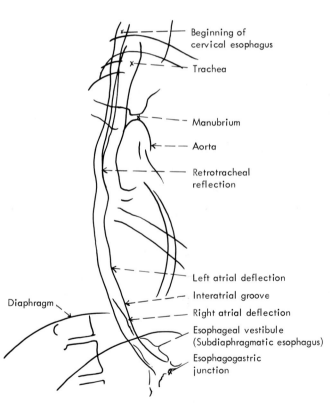

Beginning of cervical esophagus

Trachea

Manubrium

Aorta

Retrotracheal reflection

Left atrial deflection

Interatrial groove

Right atrial deflection

Esophageal vestibule (Subdiaphragmatic esophagus)

Esophagogastric junction

Diaphragm

FIGURE 9-4. Right anterior oblique view of esophagus: positioning of patient, radiograph and labeled tracing. (This same view is frequently taken in the recumbent position as well.)

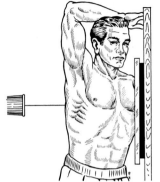

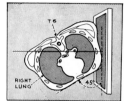

POINTS OF PRACTICAL INTEREST ABOUT FIGURES 9-3, 9-4 AND 9-5
(Continued)

4. In the case involving a search for foreign bodies contained within the esophagus, it is important to obtain the following films before appropriate fluoroscopy: (1) a lateral soft tissue study of the neck, and (2) lateral and/or oblique studies of the esophagus *without* barium. The fluoroscopist then obtains spot films and/or cineradiographs with thick and thin barium, and often with a small cotton ball or capsule made opaque with barium.

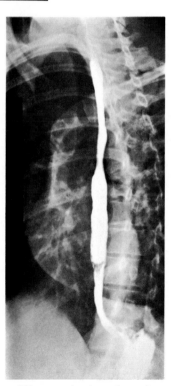

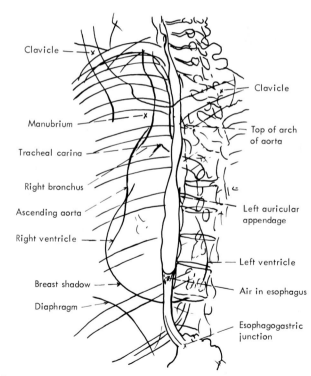

FIGURE 9-5. Left anterior oblique projection of esophagus: positioning of patient (recumbent may also be used), radiograph (intensified) and labeled tracing.

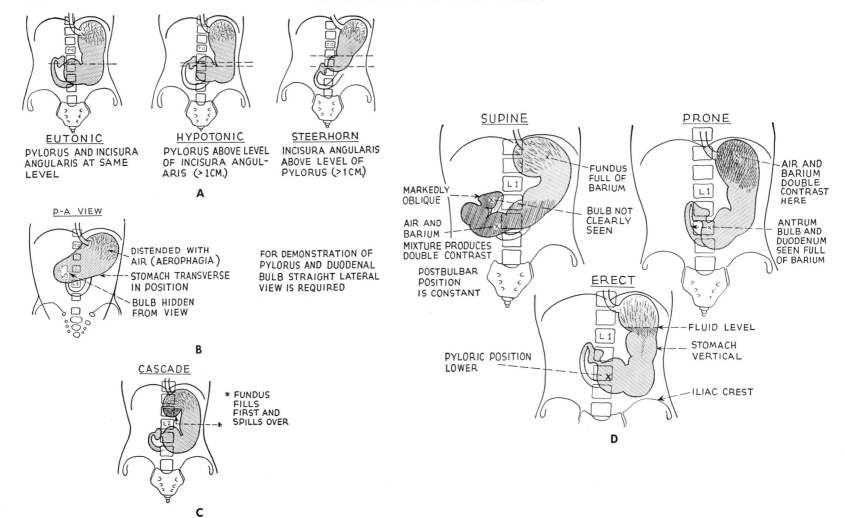

FIGURE 9-6. Variations in stomach contour: **A,** in relation to body build and general stomach type; **B,** the infantile stomach; **C,** the cascade stomach; **D,** in relation to body position.

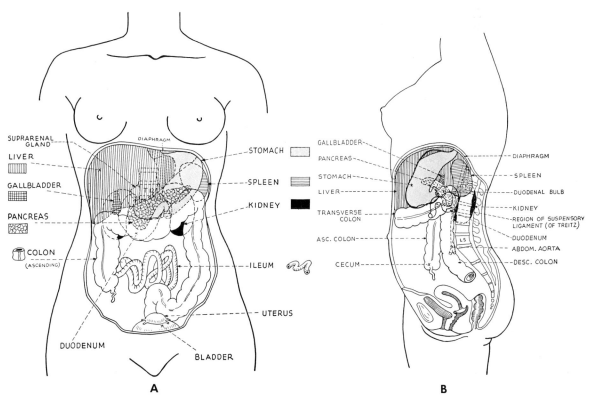

FIGURE 9-7.   Important anatomic relationships of the stomach: **A,** anteroposterior view; **B,** lateral view (right, recumbent).

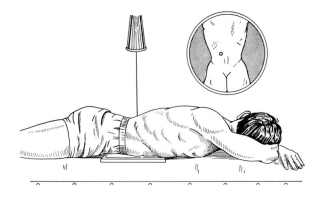

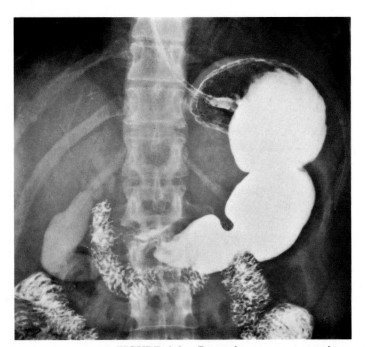

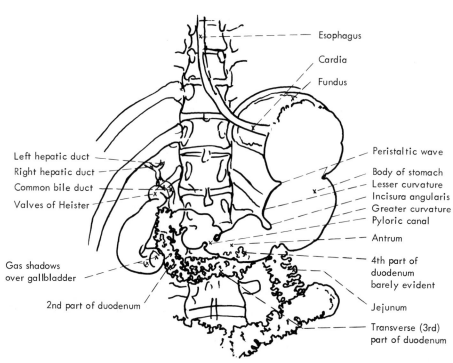

Esophagus

Cardia

Fundus

Peristaltic wave

Left hepatic duct

Right hepatic duct

Common bile duct

Valves of Heister

Body of stomach
Lesser curvature
Incisura angularis
Greater curvature
Pyloric canal

Antrum

4th part of
duodenum
barely evident

Gas shadows
over gallbladder

Jejunum

2nd part of duodenum

Transverse (3rd)
part of duodenum

FIGURE 9-8. Recumbent posteroanterior projection of stomach and duodenum. (An oral cholecystogram was also obtained at this time in the film illustrated.)

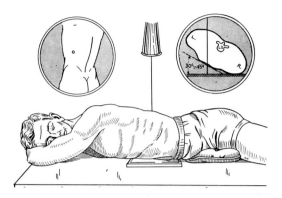

POINTS OF PRACTICAL INTEREST ABOUT FIGURE 9–9:

1. It is often in this position that peristalsis is maximal. Often, when there is an initial delay in gastric evacuation, it is our practice to place the patient in this position for a short while until peristalsis returns and gastric emptying begins.

2. This position is also optimal for passage of a Miller-Abbott or Cantor tube from the stomach into the duodenum, provided the balloon end of the tube is in good relationship with the pyloric antrum. The balloon should not be inflated until this end of the tube reaches the third part of the duodenum.

3. When rigidity of the stomach is suspected, it is well to put the patient in this position and obtain several films in sequence without moving him. The films, which should be taken at the rate of two or three per minute, may thereafter be superimposed to study the extent of change over the intervals of time spanned.

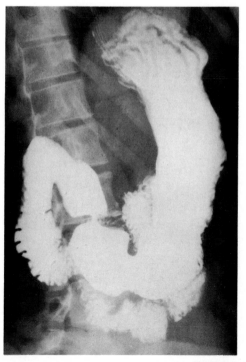

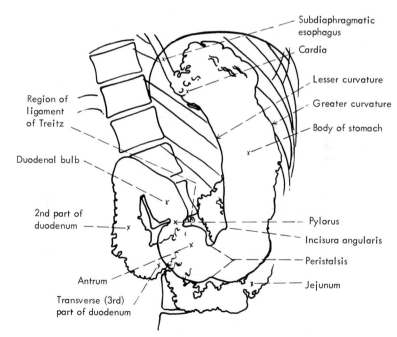

FIGURE 9-9. Right anterior oblique prone projection of stomach and duodenum.

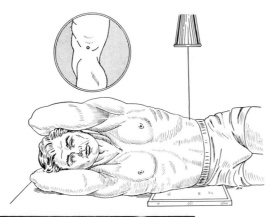

POINTS OF PRACTICAL INTEREST ABOUT FIGURE 9-10

1. In the right lateral recumbent position, the stomach tends to swing away from the spine. The points of fixation are the subdiaphragmatic portion of the esophagus (liver and diaphragm) and the postbulbar duodenum. Although the stomach is better depicted in this projection than in the left lateral erect (Fig. 9-13), the relation of the stomach to the retrogastric space and spine are not represented for detection of possible retrogastric space-occupying lesions. The left lateral erect view is better for the latter purpose.

2. The retroperitoneal part of the duodenum is, however, clearly represented in this view, and its relationship to the spine may be accurately studied.

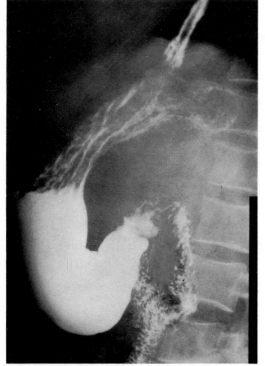

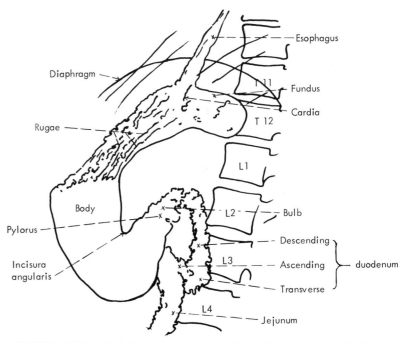

FIGURE 9-10. Right lateral recumbent view of stomach and duodenum.

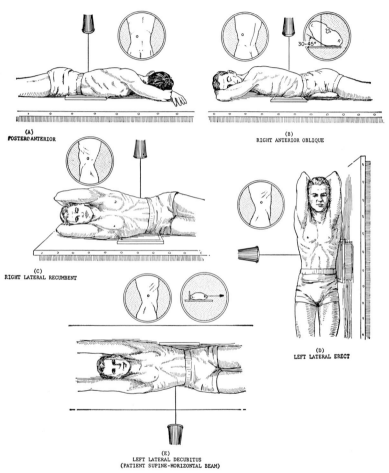

(A) POSTERO ANTERIOR

(B) RIGHT ANTERIOR OBLIQUE

(C) RIGHT LATERAL RECUMBENT

(D) LEFT LATERAL ERECT

(E) LEFT LATERAL DECUBITUS
(PATIENT SUPINE-HORIZONTAL BEAM)

FIGURE 9-11. Diagrams illustrating the routine positioning technique for radiographic examination of the stomach, apart from fluoroscopy.

RADIOGRAPHIC EXAMINATION OF THE
STOMACH *(Illustrations begin on page 278.)*

Anteroposterior View of Stomach in Slight Left Posterior Oblique
(Figure 9-12)

In this position, the air in the stomach rises and when mixed with the barium furnishes a double-contrast visualization of the body, antrum and bulb, and a completely barium-filled fundus. Filling defects and mucosal disturbances are thereby sometimes intensified in these areas.

Air Insufflation of the Stomach

As a special examination, air may be introduced into the stomach either by stomach tube or indirectly by Seidlitz powders or a carbonated drink. The stomach should be empty for this examination. Introducing air directly has the advantage of permitting the examination of the dry gastric mucosa, following which the addition of a small amount of barium mixture affords double contrast. The carbonated drink method has the disadvantage of diluting the barium, which interferes with its coating property.

In either case, the patient is first examined fluoroscopically in all projections, and films in any desired position are obtained.

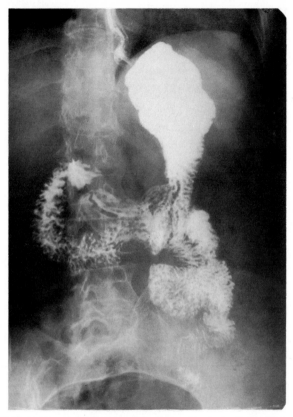

FIGURE 9-12. Anteroposterior view of stomach in slight posterior oblique. Note the excellent double contrast of the distal stomach while the fundus is completely filled with barium.

POINTS OF PRACTICAL INTEREST ABOUT FIGURE 9-13

1. The left lateral erect view is more accurate than the right lateral recumbent view (Fig. 9-10) for depicting the relationship of the stomach to retrogastric structures and the spine. Thus, it should be routine whenever a lesion is suspected in the lesser omental bursa or pancreas.

2. This view may be supplemented by a left lateral decubitus film obtained with the patient lying on his back, the film perpendicular to the table along his left side, and employing a horizontal x-ray beam.

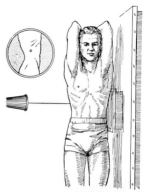

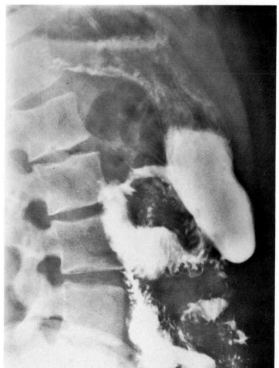

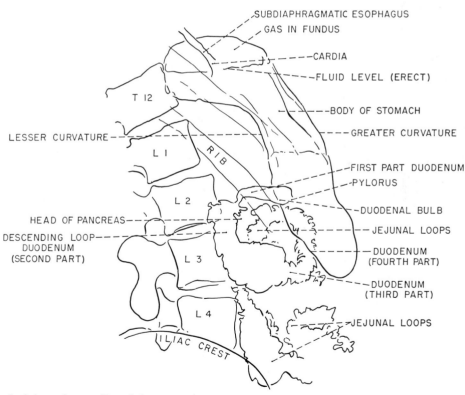

SUBDIAPHRAGMATIC ESOPHAGUS
GAS IN FUNDUS
CARDIA
FLUID LEVEL (ERECT)
T 12
BODY OF STOMACH
LESSER CURVATURE
GREATER CURVATURE
L 1
RIB
FIRST PART DUODENUM
PYLORUS
L 2
DUODENAL BULB
HEAD OF PANCREAS
JEJUNAL LOOPS
DESCENDING LOOP
DUODENUM
(SECOND PART)
L 3
DUODENUM
(FOURTH PART)
DUODENUM
(THIRD PART)
L 4
JEJUNAL LOOPS
ILIAC CREST

FIGURE 9-13. Left lateral erect film of the stomach.

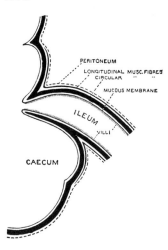

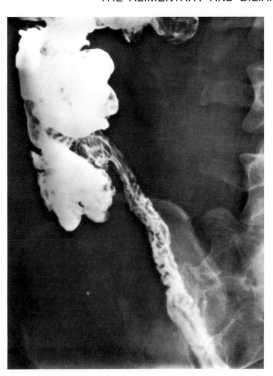

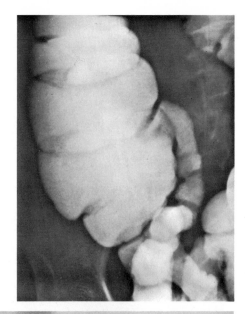

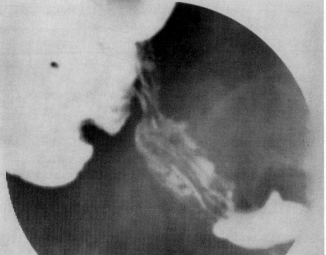

FIGURE 9-14. Ileocecal Junction: diagrammatic section (from Cunningham, D. J.: *Textbook of Anatomy,* edited by A. Robinson, Oxford University Press) and spot film studies.

RADIOGRAPHIC METHODS OF STUDY OF THE SMALL INTESTINE

Frequent-interval Film and Fluoroscopy Method (Figure 9-15)

Following a routine examination of the stomach and duodenum, the barium column is followed fluoroscopically until its movement in the jejunum is very slow. A large posteroanterior film of the abdomen is taken immediately, and at one-half to one hour intervals thereafter until the barium column has reached the ileocecal valve and cecum. The fluoroscopic examination is repeated whenever anything suspicious is seen on one of the interval films and again when the barium column has reached the ileocecal region, at which time spot film compression studies of this region are obtained.

An additional cup of barium sulfate suspension is desirable after fluoroscopy of the stomach and duodenum is completed.

Cold Isotonic Saline Method

Cold isotonic saline has been shown to increase motility in the small intestine, and to hasten gastric evacuation. Thus, after the administration of the barium sulfate and examination of the

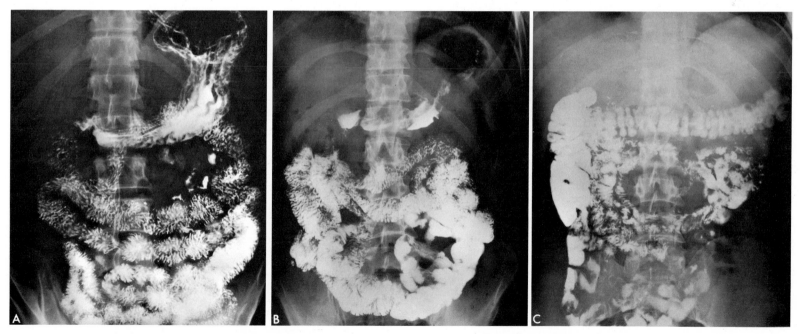

FIGURE 9-15. Illustrations to demonstrate frequent-interval film and fluoroscopy method for examination of small intestine: **A,** at one hour following administration of the barium; **B,** at two hours: **C,** at three hours.

stomach and duodenum, the patient is given a glassful of cold isotonic saline to drink. One-half hour later, he is given another glassful of the saline. Under these circumstances, the ileocecal region is reached in one-half to one hour instead of the usual longer intervals. The isotonic saline, however, tends to dilute the barium mixture slightly, and the contrast and detail are not quite so distinct as with the first method. This method has considerable value, since the continuity of the barium column can be more readily followed fluoroscopically, and hence the examination can be performed more efficiently.

Intubation Method

In this method, a Miller-Abbott or Cantor tube is passed into the small intestine as far as desired, and the segment of bowel in question is thereafter examined by the injection of barium mixture locally. The remainder of the small intestine can also be examined by gradually withdrawing the tube while, at the same time, continuing the gradual injection of barium mixture. This method has the advantage of permitting a more exact examination of a desired region of the small bowel without the interference of overlapping or contiguous loops of bowel. It has the disadvantage of requiring the passage of the tube, which is time-consuming and quite uncomfortable for the patient. However, it furnishes the most exact method of examining the small bowel.

Small Intestinal Enema Method

This method requires the passage of a tube into the duodenum. Thereafter, the barium is injected as rapidly as desired through the tube and thus forced on its way through the small intestine. As much as 1000 cc. of barium suspension can be injected in a very short time, and the entire small intestine examined fluoroscopically as well as by means of film studies at frequent intervals.

This method has the disadvantages of discomfort to the patient and overlapping of various segments of small intestine, but has the advantage that the examination requires less time.

In each of these examinations scattering of the barium in small clumps or flakes, distention of any segment of the small intestine, or gas in any part of the small intestine in the adult is abnormal. In the child, however, the normal feathery pattern of the small intestine does not appear in the first few weeks or months of life, and there is less tendency for the barium to move as a continous fine column. Gas in the small intestine of the infant is also normal (in contrast to the adult), and in the infant it is considerably more difficult to distinguish between the normal and the abnormal.

It is readily apparent that none of the methods of examining the small intestine is ideal, and all have their disadvantages, as well as advantages. There is still much to be desired in the proper study of the small intestine in the living subject, and our information regarding this examination is only just beginning to accumulate.

TECHNIQUE OF RADIOLOGIC EXAMINATION OF THE COLON

The methods of examination are: (1) the plain radiograph of the abdomen; (2) the barium enema, under fluoroscopic visualization, and accompanied by spot film compression radiography, in addition to certain routine film studies; (3) the barium meal, followed through until the colon is visualized, and thereafter at 6 hours, 24 hours, and further intervals if desired; and (4) the barium-air double-contrast enema.

POINTS OF PRACTICAL INTEREST ABOUT FIGURE 9-16

1. The exposure should be "high kilovoltage" to permit good penetration of the barium-filled colon. In this way, filling defects may be shown that otherwise could not be demonstrated readily.

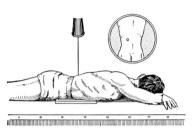
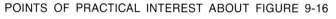

(A)
POSTEROANTERIOR

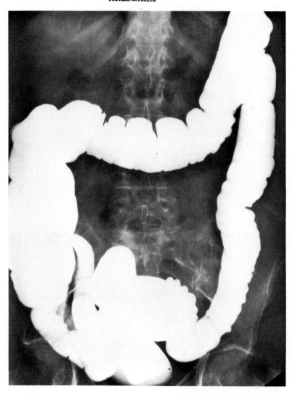

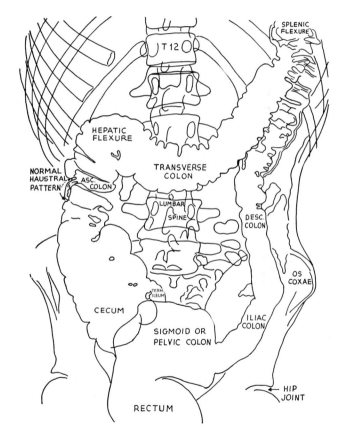

FIGURE 9-16.   Colon distended with barium: positioning of patient, radiograph and tracing.

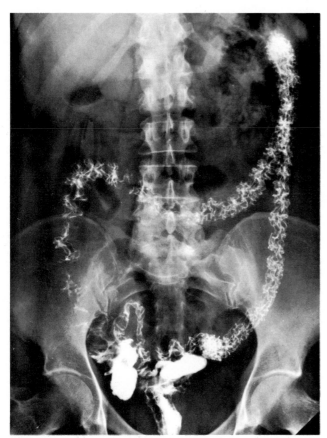

FIGURE 9-17. Radiograph of colon after evacuation of barium.

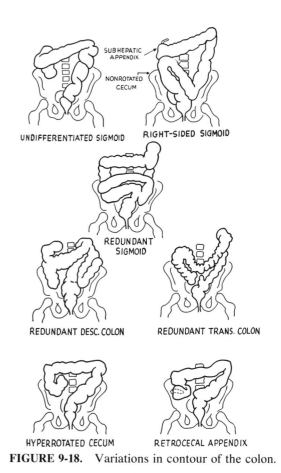

FIGURE 9-18. Variations in contour of the colon.

SCHEMATIC ILLUSTRATION OF DISTENDED BOWEL

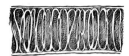

JEJUNUM
(NO INDENTED SEROSA;
COILED SPRING APPEARANCE)

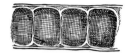

ILEUM
(NO INDENTED SEROSA)

COLON
(NOTE INDENTED SEROSA BY
HAUSTRA)

FIGURE 9-19. Differences in roentgen appearance of distended small and large intestine.

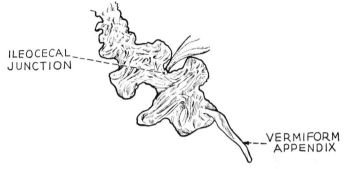

ILEOCECAL
JUNCTION

VERMIFORM
APPENDIX

FIGURE 9-20. Representative mucosal pattern of cecum.

The Barium Enema

Thorough cleansing of the colon prior to the barium enema is essential, since any retained fecal materal will obscure the normal anatomy and give rise to false filling defects and mucosal aberrations. This is usually best accomplished by means of 2 ounces of castor oil given on the night preceding the examination. This aperient has the advantage of not producing an irritation of the large intestine (since its physiologic effect is on small bowel primarily), and it ordinarily cleanses the large bowel quite thoroughly. If desired, other aperients are employed, but we have found them less satisfactory. Approximately two hours prior to the barium enema it is usually desirable to give the patient some cleansing enemas in addition; the two hour interval is efficacious in permitting adequate time for retained fluid to be reabsorbed in the colon. The cleansing enemas should be given until the returns are clear. Ordinarily the patient is examined without breakfast, since the breakfast meal will introduce gas in the stomach and, occasionally, in the colon.

The enema tip is introduced while the patient is on the fluoroscopic table. An ordinary tip may be employed, or special tips equipped with balloons that may be distended with gas or water to provide a rectal plug may be used to prevent involuntary evacuation. Care must be taken in the latter technique not to increase the pressure in the bowel excessively, since rupture of a weakened segment may occur. Ordinarily, if the head of the barium column is no more than 3 feet above the table, the pressure will not be excessive.

The barium suspension is made up of U.S.P. barium sulfate mixed with water in a 1:4 to 1:6 mixture depending upon preference. The barium is introduced slowly with the patient first lying on his left side (supine), and the rectum and pelvic colon are carefully studied fluoroscopically. It is usually advantageous to pause when the pelvic colon is filled to allow the colon to accommodate to the barium mixture, and also to obtain a spot film study of the pelvic colon in the right anterior oblique position (Fig. 9-21). Sufficient obliquity is employed to demonstrate the entire pelvic colon and the rectosigmoid junction.

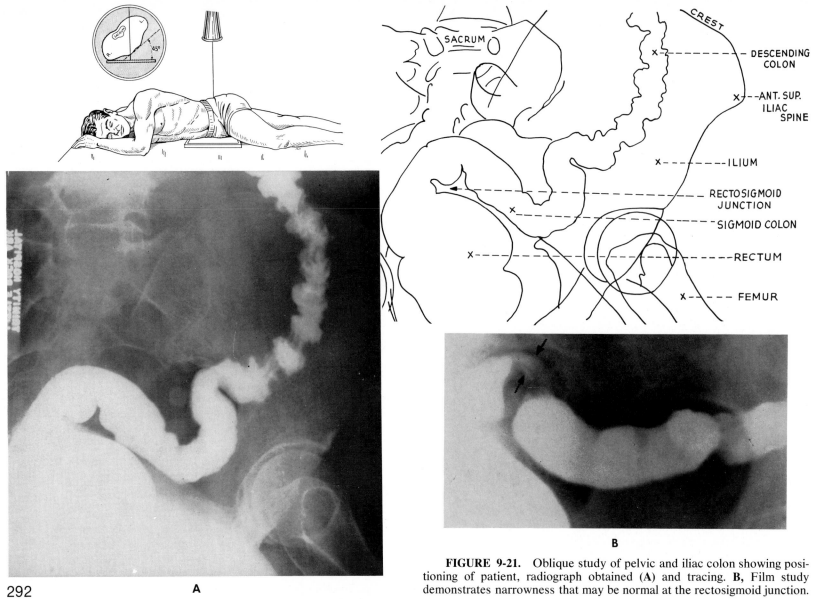

FIGURE 9-21. Oblique study of pelvic and iliac colon showing positioning of patient, radiograph obtained (**A**) and tracing. **B,** Film study demonstrates narrowness that may be normal at the rectosigmoid junction.

CREST

SACRUM

DESCENDING COLON

ANT. SUP. ILIAC SPINE

ILIUM

RECTOSIGMOID JUNCTION

SIGMOID COLON

RECTUM

FEMUR

A

B

POINTS OF PRACTICAL INTEREST ABOUT STUDY OF THE RECTOSIGMOID REGION

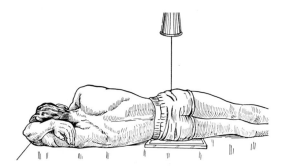

1. Figures 9-22 and 9-23 may be supplemented by a view obtained with the patient prone, and the central ray angled 15 to 30 degrees toward the head, centering over the anal canal. This position may be more tolerable for the uncomfortable patient than that illustrated in Figure 9-23, and a somewhat similar, distorted view of the rectosigmoid region will be obtained.

If the patient cannot be turned into the prone position, the central ray is angled similarly toward the feet, with the patient lying on his back.

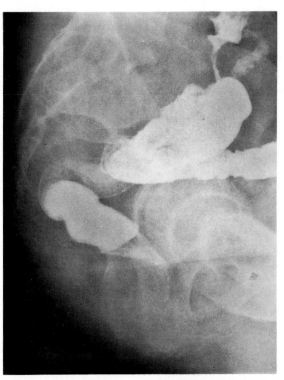

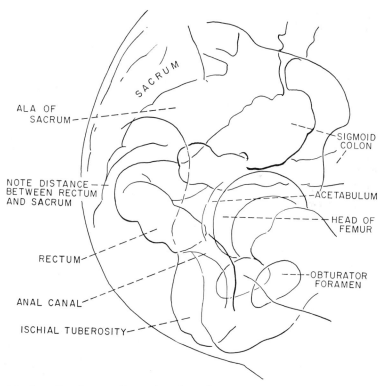

FIGURE 9-22.   Lateral view of the rectosigmoid: positioning of patient, radiograph and tracing.

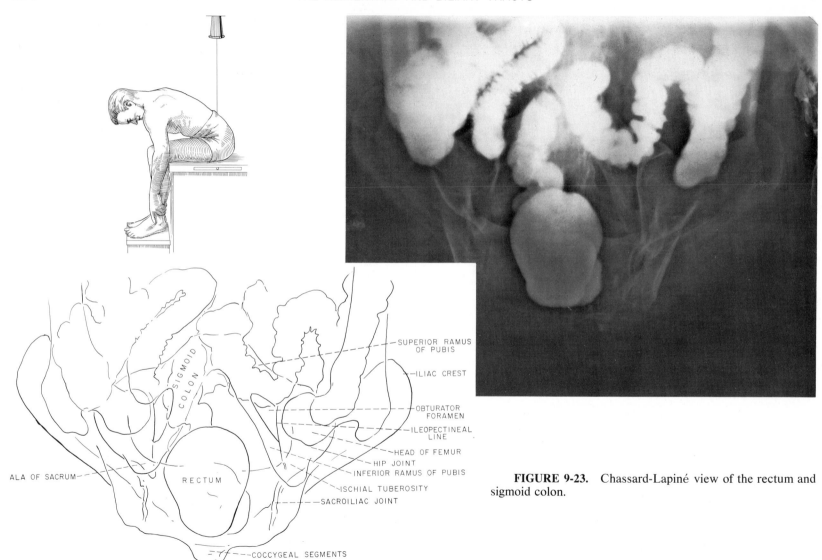

SIGMOID COLON

SUPERIOR RAMUS OF PUBIS

ILIAC CREST

OBTURATOR FORAMEN

ILEOPECTINEAL LINE

HEAD OF FEMUR

HIP JOINT

INFERIOR RAMUS OF PUBIS

ISCHIAL TUBEROSITY

SACROILIAC JOINT

ALA OF SACRUM

RECTUM

COCCYGEAL SEGMENTS

FIGURE 9-23. Chassard-Lapiné view of the rectum and sigmoid colon.

The Barium-Air Double-Contrast Enema

There are two types of double-contrast barium enemas: (1) a conventional technique performed after evacuation of a barium enema such as has been described and (2) a colloidal barium double-contrast enema. Following a complete evacuation of the barium enema, the large intestine may be insufflated with air. It may be necessary for the patient to evacuate more barium at this point to

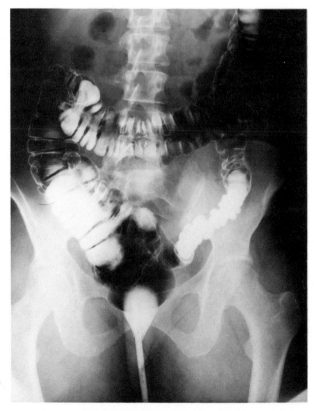

FIGURE 9-24. Colloidal barium and air double-contrast enema.

obtain a better mucosal relief pattern. However, after repeating this sequence until a fine coating of barium remains, air is once again insufflated, and plain or stereoscopic films of the colon are obtained in the posteroanterior, anteroposterior, decubitus and oblique projections (Fig. 19-24). These show the colonic walls as thin lines of barium, and these are widely separated by the gaseous distention. Any polypoid masses will be shown in a double relief pattern, being coated by barium. Unless the patient's colon has been thoroughly cleansed beforehand, the interpretation is hazardous since retained fecal matter would lead to a similar appearance.

The colloidal barium double-contrast enema may be performed in one of two ways: either the colon is partially filled with colloidal barium mixture to the splenic flexure or middle of the transverse colon, this is aspirated and then air is injected; or the colon is filled to the lower descending colon with colloidal barium mixture, followed immediately by the forceful injection of air, and the patient is rotated to assist in the proper dispersion of the heavy barium mixture (Fig. 9-24).

There are various colloidal barium sulfate preparations available, each with specific directions for mixture. Some of these are: Bariloid, which is easy to mix, Barotrast, Baridol and Stabarium. Since the colloidal barium mixture is viscous, pressure is required to force it through the enema tubing. This may be supplied by elevating the barium reservoir, by "milking" the tube, by "piston" type syringes or by pumping devices.

In both techniques, after introduction of the barium, the patient is turned under fluoroscopic guidance, even to the complete prone position, so that gravity will assist the air in distributing the barium throughout the colon.

Where suction and controlled drainage are required, various devices are available, i.e., the three-way valve box designed by Templeton and Addington that is attached to a sink and works on a Venturi siphon principle or simple Y-tube and clamp devices that permit drainage through one branch of the Y and injection through the other.

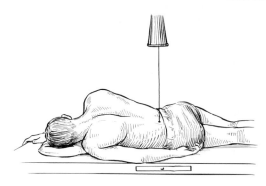

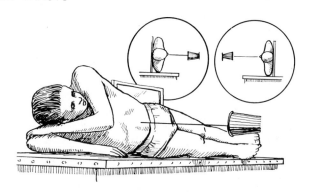

Indications for Single- and Double-Contrast Barium Enema

The single-contrast examination has wide usefulness in detecting most abnormalities of the colon including the right half of the colon, ulcerative disease, and terminal ileal disease in many cases. It is less efficient than the double-contrast enema in detecting small intraluminal tumors. It is unfortunate that both examinations cannot be done on the same day. They are best done one or two days apart as indicated by clinical history. It has been our practice to do the single-contrast study first. In patients with unexplained rectal bleeding (bright red or dark), with a history of polyps, or with polyps found at proctoscopy, the colloidal barium double-contrast enema is scheduled two days later, with a repetition of castor oil preparation the night before the second examination. Any dried barium or feces remaining from the previous study will interfere with the accuracy of the double-contrast enema.

We have also employed a low residue diet for three successive days, and X-Prep Liquid ® (2½ ounces) for three successive nights prior to the examination. This has given us successful preparation and is reasonably well tolerated.

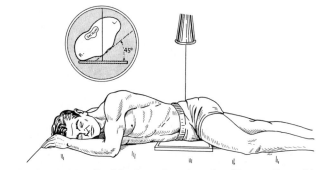

FIGURE 9-25. Positioning of patient for film studies with a double-contrast enema. In addition to the two oblique and the two horizontal beam views shown, straight posteroanterior and left lateral views are also obtained (Figs. 9-16 and 9-22).

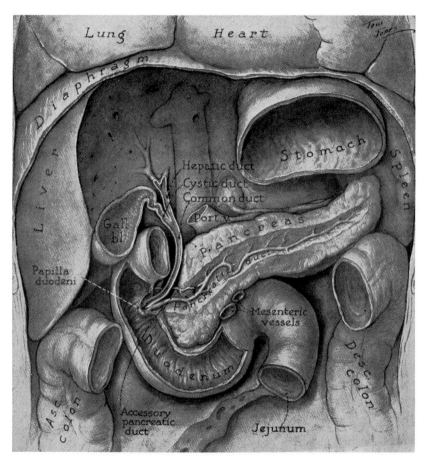

FIGURE 9-26. The gross anatomy of the biliary system. (From Jones, T.: *Anatomical Studies*. Jackson, Michigan, S. H. Camp and Co., 1943.)

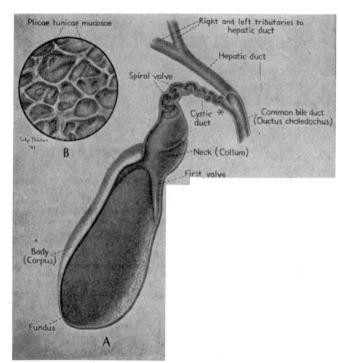

FIGURE 9-27. Gross anatomy of the biliary tract: **A,** interior of the gallbladder and cystic duct; **B,** surface of the mucosa of the gallbladder showing plicae. (After Boyden in Surgery. From Blount, R. F., and Lachman, E.: The digestive system, in *Morris' Human Anatomy,* 12th edition, edited by B. J. Anson. The Blakiston Div., McGraw-Hill Book Company, 1966.)

RADIOGRAPHIC EXAMINATION OF THE BILIARY TRACT

Prior to the gallbladder examination, it is well to remove as much gas and fecal material from the gastrointestinal tract as possible. Cascara sagrada or enemas given at least 24 hours before the examination may be of considerable assistance. Pitressin may be employed intravenously (0.5 to 1 cc.) in those patients in whom it would not be contraindicated on the basis of hypertension or arteriosclerosis.

It is also well to obtain a plain film of the entire right side of the abdomen, in the posteroanterior projection, prior to the administration of any dye. The gallbladder itself is not usually delineated with accuracy on such films, but if it should contain calcareous structure, this would immediately be evident from this preliminary study.

A visualization of the gallbladder requires that some form of contrast substance be introduced into it. Tetrachlorphenolphthalein had long been known to be secreted in the bile, and this substance had been used as a test for liver function. Graham and Cole (in 1924) introduced first the bromine radical, and thereafter the heavier iodine radical instead of the chlorine in this compound, and thus obtained a substance that was secreted by the liver in the bile, and concentrated with the bile in the gallbladder. This made it possible to render the bile radiopaque.

In recent years new compounds such as Priodax, Telepaque, Teridax, Monophen, and Cholografin (see Table 9-1) have been introduced which accomplish the same thing without many of the undesirable side effects attributed to the earlier contrast medium. Each of the newer compounds has certain contraindications and some adverse effects which are listed in Table 9-1.

The methods for cholecystography are as follows: (1) *intravenous dye*, such as Cholografin, (2) *oral dye*, such as those enumerated in Table 9-1, and (3) *cholangiograms*.

This latter may be an operative or postoperative procedure and involves the injection of a contrast medium into either the hepatic, cystic or common bile ducts, or percutaneously into any dilated hepatic biliary duct.

Details of Oral Procedure

On the day before the examination, a scout film of the abdomen is obtained. Thereafter, a fatty meal is given at noon to empty the gallbladder and a light fat-free meal is given at 6:00 P.M. Following this, 3 to 5 grams of the oral dye are administered. The drugs presently used are Telepaque, Teridax, Monophen and Priodax. All of the foregoing drugs depend upon their iodine content for visualization and depend upon concentration by the gallbladder. Occasionally they may produce nausea, diarrhea or dysuria (Table 9-1).

Nothing is allowed by mouth after the dye is administered until the patient appears for his examination the following morning, 14 to 16 hours after taking the dye.

Enemas are administered in the morning if advised by the radiologist. This is done particularly to cleanse the gastrointestinal tract of interfering shadows that may superimpose themselves upon the shadow of the gallbladder and thus obscure detail. On the other hand, some regard a visualization of the media in the colon as a check to note whether or not the dye was actually taken by the patient. When Telepaque is utilized the opaque material can be seen in the gastrointestinal tract. Priodax, on the other hand, is absorbed immediately and is excreted largely by the kidneys and hence is not detected in the gastrointestinal tract.

An exploratory film is taken 12 to 14 hours after the oral administration of the dye. Usually a sufficiently large film is employed to cover the entire area between the costal margin above and the iliac crest below the right lateral abdominal wall and the left lateral aspect of the spine. A scout film including this entire area should include a gallbladder anomalously placed either over the spine or in the iliac fossa (Fig. 9-28A).

Once the gallbladder is found, the patient is rotated in various positions to obtain a clear visualization of this organ on a second film. Every effort is made to obtain this visualization without super-

TABLE 9-1. Comparison of Some of the Major Compounds Employed for Gallbladder Visualization

	Pharmacology	*Contraindications*	*Accuracy and Adverse Effects*
Priodax	Phenylpropionic acid derivative Insoluble in water but soluble in alkali 51.38% iodine Excreted mostly by kidneys	Acute nephritis Uremia	35% less opacity than Telepaque 60% {nausea, diarrhea, dysuria} vs. 21.4% with Telepaque More patients require second dose (40%) than to visualize 12% of gallbladders visualized with Telepaque
Telepaque	Ethyl propanoic acid derivative Insoluble in water; soluble in alkali and 95% alcohol 66.68% iodine Excreted mostly via gastrointestinal tract	Acute nephritis Uremia Gastrointestinal diseases with disturbed absorption	Fails only in 3% of normal gallbladders or less with one dose Side reactions less than with Priodax Great opacity may obscure some gallstones
Teridax	Triiodoethionic acid (ethyl propionic acid derivative) Insoluble in water; soluble in alkali 66.5% iodine Excreted mostly by kidneys	Acute nephritis Uremia	Failure after one examination not always indicative of disease; but after second dose approaches 100% accuracy Not as well worked out as to side reactions as Priodax or Telepaque Said to produce density intermediate between Priodax and Telepaque
Monophen	Carboxylic acid derivative Insoluble in water 52.2% iodine Excreted mostly by kidneys	Acute nephritis Uremia	60% no adverse signs or symptoms 12% nausea 1% vomiting 9% diarrhea 9% cramps 3% dysuria Accuracy stated to be better (?) than Priodax

Cholografin	Iodipamide (triiodobenzoic acid derivative)
	For intravenous use (photosensitive)
	64% iodine
	With normal liver 90% excreted in feces, 10% in urine
	With poor liver function: mostly excreted by kidneys (hence pyelograms)
		Primary indication: Postcholecystectomy syndrome
		Contraindications:
		  Iodine sensitivity
		  Combined urinary and hepatic disease
			Sensitivity high
			Side effects minimal with slow injection
			77-85% successful biliary tree visualizations
			Visualization faint; usually gallbladder visualization too faint for significant accuracy
			Serious reactions: 2.5%
			Lesser reactions: 38.8%

Ipodate (Oragrafin) (Biloptin) (Solu-Biloptin)	Triiodohydrocinnamic acid derivatives (sodium or calcium salt) 61% iodine 42-48% excreted in bile in 24 hrs., equally in urine	Iodine sensitivity Combined renal-hepatic disease Severe kidney disorders Gastrointestinal disorders or liver disorders	Mild and transient nausea; vomiting; diarrhea

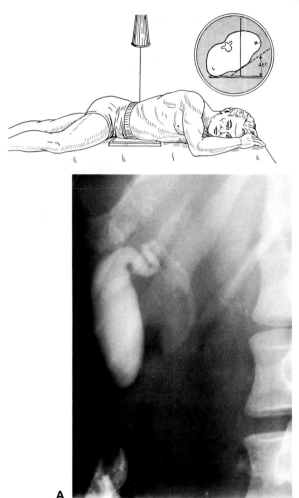

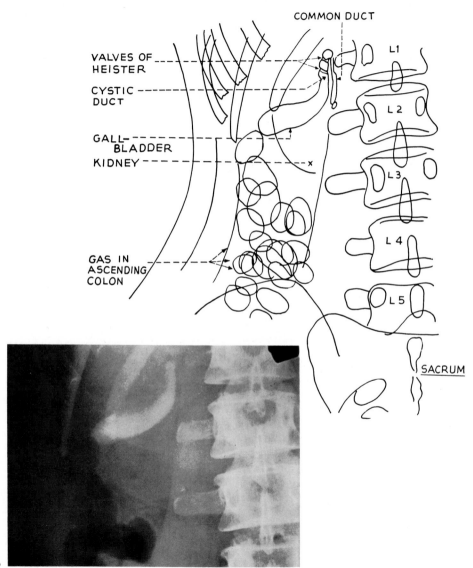

FIGURE 9-28. Radiographic study of the gallbladder: positioning of patient, radiographs obtained before (**A**) and after (**B**) fatty stimulation, and tracing of the latter.

position of rib shadows, calcified cartilages, gas shadows from the colon, or the other bony structures.

Occasionally it is necessary to place the patient on his right side so that the gallbladder drops by gravity and the gas shadows rise; thus, a clear visualization may be obtained employing a lateral decubitus horizontal x-ray beam (Fig. 9-29C).

An erect film of the gallbladder region should be routine since this may be an additional expedient for clearing the gallbladder of superimposed shadows (Fig. 9-29D). Moreover, if there are stones, very frequently they will either float or settle in the gallbladder and thus become more concentrated and more readily visualized. This should be a "coned-down" film.

After a satisfactory visualization of the gallbladder is obtained, a fatty meal or stimulant is given and films are taken at 15 minutes, 30 minutes, one hour, or two hours after the fatty meal until maximal emptying of the gallbladder is seen and until best visualization of the common duct is obtained (Fig. 9-28B).

The Intravenous Technique

Cholografin (Biligrafin in Europe) is an organic iodide administered intravenously in 20 to 40 cc. doses. It is secreted selectively by the liver in sufficient concentration, usually, to permit a faint concentration of the biliary radicles, common bile duct and gallbladder without dependence upon the concentration function of the gallbladder. Films are taken at 10 minute intervals for the first hour and at half hourly intervals thereafter until good visualization is obtained (up to four hours). This method is only moderately satisfactory (Fig. 9-30). It must be used when there is no fistula or tube in the common duct and when the patient continues to have serious symptoms postoperatively. The examination is contraindicated in the presence of fever (cholangitis or hepatitis) and is seldom successful in the presence of jaundice.

The primary indications for intravenous cholangiograms by this technique are:

1. The "postcholecystectomy syndrome": The patient continues to have right upper quadrant discomfort or pain after cholecystectomy.

2. When for any reason stones are suspected in the biliary tree above the level of the cystic duct.

3. When the gallbladder has not been visualized by oral techniques, and its visualization is still desired.

Testing of intravenous sensitivity to Cholografin should never be omitted prior to this study. Indeed, routine administration of antihistaminics prior to or with the media is advocated by some.

Intravenous cholangiography after cholecystectomy may at times reveal a saclike structure at the site of the amputated cystic duct. This may represent a "reformed gallbladder," and may account for the so-called postcholecystectomy syndrome in some patients. This may also represent a false sac created by persistent drainage into a walled-off saccular area at the site of the T-tube insertion in the common duct.

A scout film of the gallbladder area is first obtained. Once the hepatic ducts, the common bile duct, or the gallbladder are found, the patient is rotated in various positions so as to project these structures free from all interfering shadows such as overlying ribs, spine or gas. Ordinarily, the left anterior oblique recumbent projection will project the gallbladder upward toward the ribs, and the straight posteroanterior projection will project it closer to the spine. Every effort is made to obtain a clear visualization of the gallbladder and its adjoining structures.

The spiral valves of Heister must not be misinterpreted as small stones, since they may appear as small negative shadows alternating with positive shadows in the infundibulum and proximal portion of the cystic duct. A typical visualization of the gallbladder and biliary tree by this technique is illustrated in Figure 9-30.

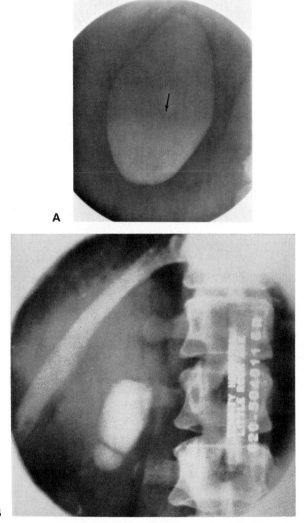

A

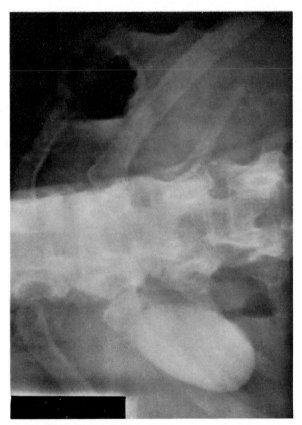

B

C

FIGURE 9-29.   Variations of gallbladder of radiographic significance. **A,** Sedimentation of Telepaque in erect position—a confusing normal variant; **B,** mucosal or serosal fold of gallbladder, known as a phrygian cap; **C,** horizontal beam study of the gallbladder with the patient lying on his right side.

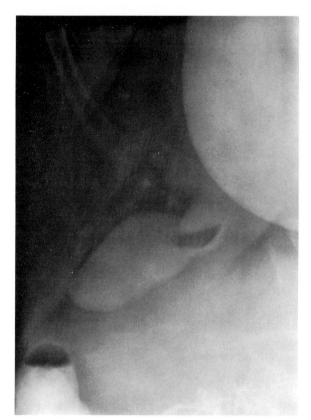

FIGURE 9-29. **D,** Horizontal beam study of the gallbladder with the patient standing erect.

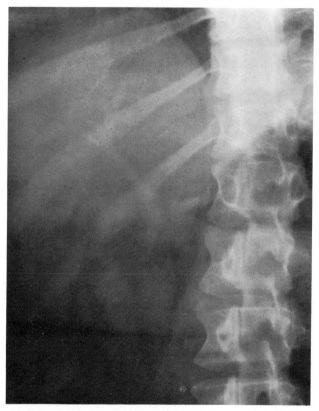

FIGURE 9-30. Faint visualization of the biliary tree by intravenous cholangiography with the aid of intravenous Cholografin. This is the order of density usually obtained. Sequential films are made at 10 or 15 minute intervals for 30 to 45 minutes; thereafter at 90 to 120 minutes; and occasionally at four hours. The first two films in this sequence are in the *right posterior oblique* position (patient supine), centering over the biliary tract; subsequent views are in the *left anterior oblique* position (patient prone). Later films, beyond 45 minutes, are obtained only if the gallbladder has not been removed surgically, since these are primarily for gallbladder (rather than biliary duct) visualization.

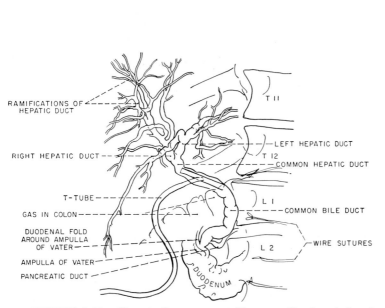

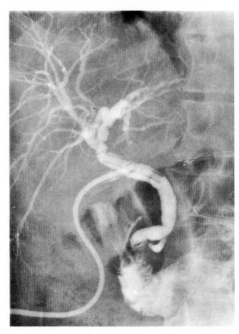

RAMIFICATIONS OF
HEPATIC DUCT

T II

LEFT HEPATIC DUCT

RIGHT HEPATIC DUCT

T 12

COMMON HEPATIC DUCT

T-TUBE

GAS IN COLON

L 1

COMMON BILE DUCT

DUODENAL FOLD
AROUND AMPULLA
OF VATER

L 2

WIRE SUTURES

AMPULLA OF VATER

PANCREATIC DUCT

DUODENUM

FIGURE 9-31. Twenty-five per cent Hypaque T-tube cholangiogram and its tracing. This contrast medium gives a more complete visualization of all hepatic radicles. This is extremely important since stones concealed in the hepatic radicles may descend later and cause a recurrence of symptoms.

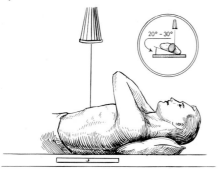

20° – 30°

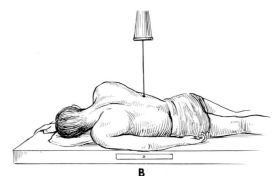

A

B

FIGURE 9-32. **A,** Right posterior oblique position of patient for first one or two films in intravenous cholangiographic series. **B,** Left anterior oblique position for later films in cholangiographic series, centering over gallbladder.

Chapter 10 — Specialized Angiologic Investigation, Including the Heart

INTRODUCTION

Apart from the previously described routine studies of the heart and major blood vessels, additional procedures are available to supplement the radiologic information obtained from the routine study. These include:

Orthodiagraphy: a method of outlining the cardiac contour accurately and a method which is very seldom used at this time.

Kymography: a method of estimating the presence of and recording abnormal pulsation.

Venous angiocardiography: the rapid injection of a radiopaque solution by an intravenous route and the subsequent serial filming of the heart chambers in sequence.

Selective angiography: the injection of the radiopaque solution through a catheter that has been previously introduced into the aorta or one of the major arteries or a cardiac chamber, and subsequent examination by films in rapid sequence. This may be combined with blood gas analyses and pressure studies.

Translumbar aortography: aortography by direct percutaneous puncture through the back of the aorta.

Venography: radiographic study of the inferior vena cava or other veins by catheterization methods.

Transosseous venography: venography in which the contrast medium is introduced by inserting an appropriate needle directly into a marrow-containing bone such as the rib.

Lymphangiography: the direct instillation in peripheral lymphatics of a suitable radiopaque substance, with films obtained in slow sequence thereafter to depict lymphatics as well as lymph nodes.

In general, these specialized procedures are outside the scope of the present text. Brief descriptions of the procedures and their

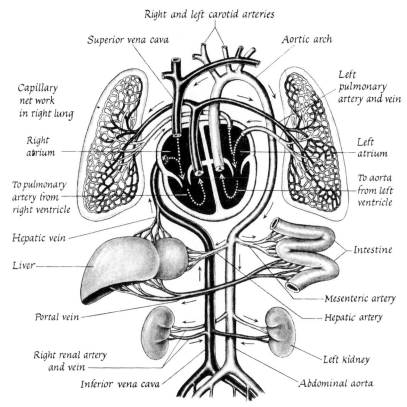

FIGURE 10-1. Diagram illustrating the *greater* circulation from heart to viscera, extremities and head; and the *lesser* circulation from heart to lungs. The head and extremities are not shown in the diagram. The coronary circulation is also not shown. (From Moment, G. B.: *General Zoology,* 2nd edition. Boston, Houghton Mifflin Co., 1958.)

related anatomy are undertaken because a general understanding is necessary for anyone embarking on a career related to diagnostic roentgenology.

ANGIOCARDIOGRAPHY

Angiocardiography refers to the visualization of the heart and great vessels by rapid sequence serial radiographs during the passage of contrast material through these structures (Kjellberg et al.).

In venous angiography the contrast material is rapidly injected into a systemic vein, with considerable pressure so that a large bolus of the contrast agent (approximately 35 to 40 cc. ordinarily) will pass through the cardiac chambers and the major blood vessels. The injection is made by special pressure injectors in one to one and one-half seconds.

In selective angiocardiography the contrast medium is injected under sufficient pressure through a catheter that has been previously passed directly into one of the chambers of the heart. The bolus of contrast agent in the latter instance is usually 8 to 10 cc., but here the pressure is ordinarily sufficient to permit the entire bolus to be injected in a matter of approximately one second.

Ordinarily, the catheter is introduced percutaneously as described by Seldinger, or by some modification of this basic technique. The catheter may be introduced into the femoral, the brachial or the axillary artery and passed to any desired level in the aorta.

The basic tray for catherization includes the standard equipment for sterile preparation of the skin and local anesthesia (Fig. 10-2). The scalpel is used to puncture the skin at the needle puncture site to facilitate the subsequent passage of the needle. The Cournand or Seldinger needle assembly is used (Fig. 10-2). When arterial flow is obtained, the needle is advanced through the opposite wall of the artery until flow is stopped. The obturator is then removed (Fig. 10-3), and the needle is withdrawn into the lumen of the artery until good flow is restored. Flexible tubing may then be connected to the needle. It should be of sufficient length to be attached later to a hand syringe, for hand injections, or to an automatic pressure controlled injector device, if the injections are to be made through this needle. A guide wire is passed through the needle in the classic Seldinger technique, and the needle is withdrawn over it while the wire is kept in position in the artery by pressure above the puncture site. A tapered (and appropriately curved) catheter is then passed over the wire into the artery. The open tip of the percutaneous catheter can be occluded with a small obturator, thereby converting the catheter to a side-hole type. Under image amplifier and fluoroscopic control, the catheter and guide wire are manipulated into the desired anatomic position. The guide wire is removed and the catheter flushed with heparinized saline. A small test injection of contrast agent is made to ascertain exact position. Films are taken as required during and following the injection. The catheter, ordinarily left in place until the films are viewed, is flushed intermittently with heparinized saline.

Direct left ventricular puncture for cardiography has also been employed, but the incidence of complications and even fatality is considerably higher by this technique (Bjork et al.).

Apart from the visualization of the cardiac chambers and major blood vessels, heart catheterization permits the measurement of pressures within the heart chambers and great vessels, estimation of the volume of blood flowing through the lungs and systemic circulation, and recognition of abnormal blood flows or shunts within the heart by measurement of carbon dioxide content and oxygen saturation.

The introduction of fluoroscopic image amplification has simplified and extended the usefulness of heart catheterization and selective angiocardiography. The amplified image may be studied directly by a number of observers through a closed circuit televison system; a television tape recording of the angiocardiogram or angiogram may be obtained and studied leisurely thereafter; or a movie film recording of the amplified image may be obtained at a rate as rapid as 64 frames per second, to be carefully studied thereafter. The movie frames may be viewed in slow motion or even individually by special projector devices.

Special film changers are available that are designed to obtain satisfactory sequential radiographs as rapidly as 12 per second in

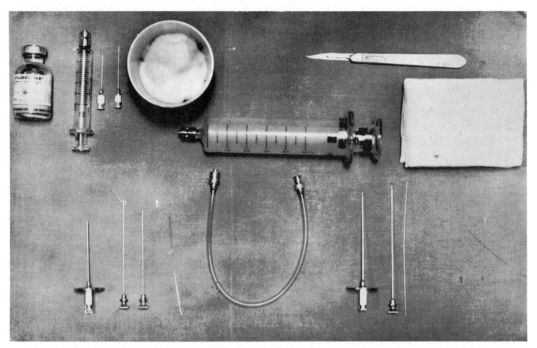

FIGURE 10-2. Assembly for peripheral arteriography by percutaneous puncture; Cournand needle assembly on the left and Seldinger assembly on the right. (From Keats, T. E.: Trends in peripheral arteriography. Radiol. Clin. N. A. *2*:484, 1964.)

two planes simultaneously and that have programming devices that allow one to obtain films for as many seconds as is deemed necessary in several different sequences.

In any of these techniques, one must be certain that the urinary tract of the patient functions adequately for excretion of the contrast medium injected.

With *venous angiocardiography,* the lesser circulation is quite well delineated, but by the time the contrast medium reaches the greater circulation, the left ventricle and the aorta, the contrast is relatively faint and detail may be far from ideal, particularly in heavy adults.

Angiocardiography is proving of great value in the investigation of both the congenital and the acquired heart diseases. It provides information needed by the internist and the surgeon to assess the operability of the case and the appropriate surgical technique to be employed, covering such matters as the site and extent of a stenotic lesion, the size and localization of a septal defect, the degree of overriding of the aorta and the appearance of the systemic arteries and pulmonary vessels. Usually selective angiocardiography affords the best opportunity to fulfill these many requirements.

Detailed descriptions of the technique of cardiac catheterization have been given by many writers (Cournand et al.; Dexter et al.; Mannheimer; Wood; Kjellberg et al.; Curry and Howland).

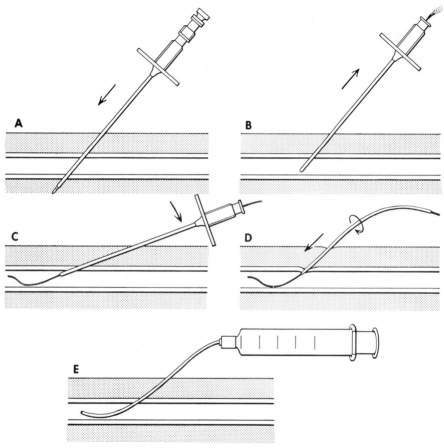

FIGURE 10-3. Application of Seldinger technique of arterial puncture. **A,** Puncture of both walls of the vessel. **B,** Retraction of tip of cannula into arterial lumen after withdrawal of needle insert. **C,** Passage of guide wire through cannula into artery. **D,** Passage of smoothly tapered catheter tip over guide wire into artery; gentle rotation of the catheter facilitates the entry. **E,** Catheter in lumen of artery after withdrawal of guide wire. (From Curry, J. L., and Howland, W. J.: *Arteriography.* W. B. Saunders, 1966.)

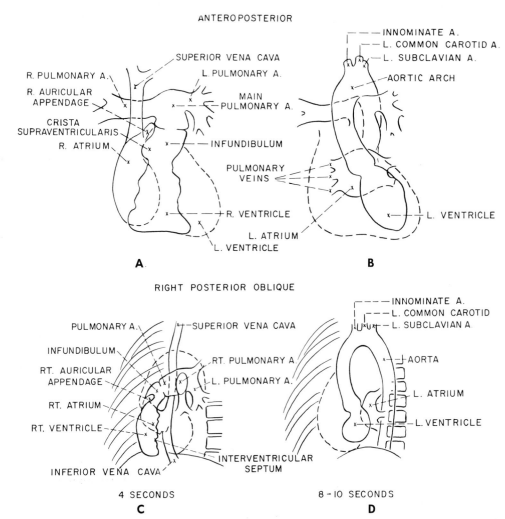

FIGURE 10-4. Major structures visualized in venous angiocardiograms: in the anterioposterior projection; **A,** lesser circulation phase and **B,** greater circulation phase: in the right posterior oblique projection, **C,** lesser circulation phase and **D,** greater circulation phase.

LEFT POSTERIOR OBLIQUE

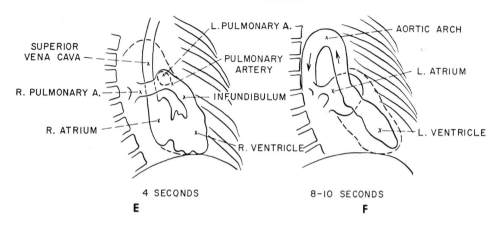

4 SECONDS

8-10 SECONDS

E

F

RIGHT LATERAL

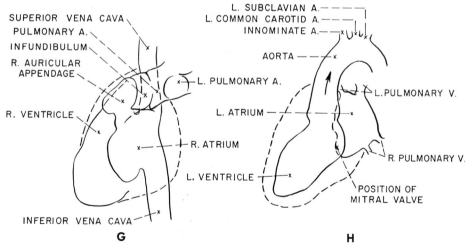

G

H

FIGURE 10-4. Major structures visualized in venous angiocardiograms: in the left posterior oblique projection; **E,** lesser circulation phase and **F,** greater circulation phase; in the right lateral projection; **G,** lesser circulation phase and **H,** greater circulation phase.

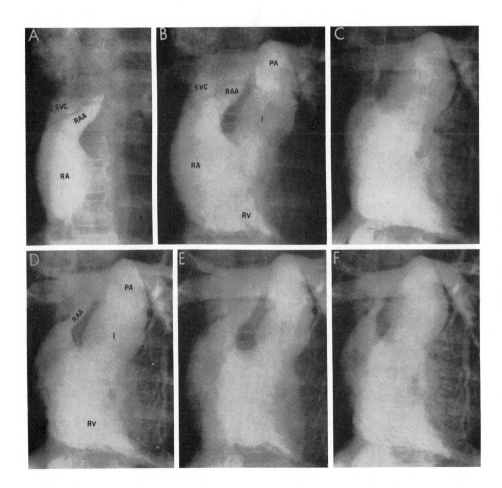

FIGURE 10-5.   A to F, Representative angiocardiograms, lesser circulation phase, frontal projection. Right auricular appendage lies directly to the right of the infundibulum and the right ventricle and lower part of the pulmonary artery, which consequently, in the lateral projection, are overlapped by the appendage. *I*, infundibulum; *PA*, pulmonary artery; *RA*, right atrium; *RAA*, right auricular appendage; *RV*, right ventricle; *SVC*, superior vena cava. (From Kjellberg, S. R., et al.: *Diagnosis of Congenital Heart Disease.* Year Book Medical Publishers, 1955.)

FIGURE 10-5. G and **H,** Normal frontal angiocardiograms of a four and one-half month old infant. At two seconds, most of the opaque material has traversed the superior vena cava and left innominate vein, which are still faintly seen. The right atrium, right ventricle, and pulmonary arteries are well filled. Just above the infundibulum of the right ventricle, localized lateral bulges in the pulmonary artery wall identify the sinuses of the pulmonary valve and clearly define the end of the pulmonary conus. Attention is directed to the arborization and tapering of the peripheral pulmonary arterial vessels. Their pattern contrasts sharply with that of the pulmonary veins, which are well seen at 3½ seconds (**I** and **J**). At this time, the left atrium is in full diastole, and the left ventricle has begun to opacify the aorta. *A,* aorta; *LA,* left atrium; *LAA,* left auricular appendage; *LPA,* left pulmonary artery; *LV,* left ventricle; *PA,* pulmonary artery; *PV,* pulmonary vein; *RA,* right atrium; *RPA,* right pulmonary artery; *RV,* right ventricle. (From Robinson, S. J., Abrams, H. L., and Kaplan, H. S.: *Congenital Heart Disease,* 2nd edition. The Blakiston Div., McGraw-Hill Book Company, 1965.)

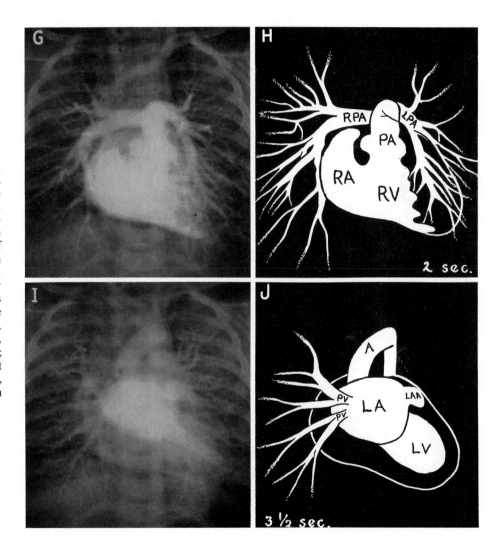

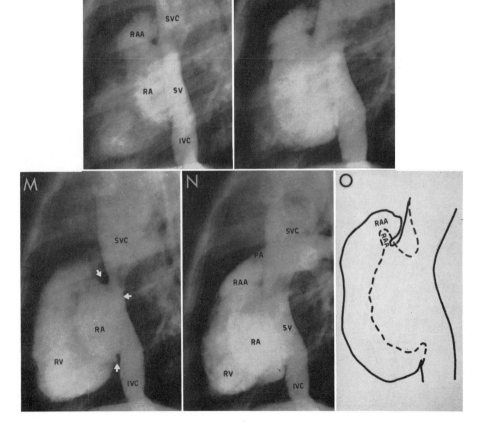

FIGURE 10-5. Representative venous angiocardiograms, lesser circulation phase, lateral projection. **K** to **N,** During atrial systole, the atrioventricular border is shifted dorsally while the dorsal wall of the atrium remains in the same position. The crista terminalis presses into the lumen like a membrane (**M,** lower arrow). Sphincter mechanism of the venae cavae is clearly visible. **O,** Collective picture of appearance of atrium in late diastole (solid line) and late systole (broken line). *IVC,* inferior vena cava; *PA,* pulmonary artery; *RA,* right atrium; *RAA,* right auricular appendage; *RV,* right ventricle; *SV,* sinus venosus; *SVC,* superior vena cava. (From Kjellberg, S. R., et al.: *Diagnosis of Congenital Heart Disease,* Year Book Medical Publishers, 1955.)

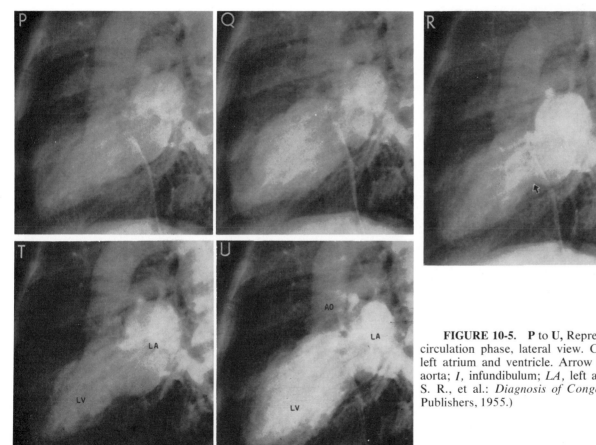

FIGURE 10-5.   **P** to **U,** Representative venous angiocardiograms, greater circulation phase, lateral view. Conditions during filling and contraction in left atrium and ventricle. Arrow in **R** points to atrioventricular plane. *AO,* aorta; *I,* infundibulum; *LA,* left atrium; *LV,* left ventricle. (From Kjellberg, S. R., et al.: *Diagnosis of Congenital Heart Disease.* Year Book Medical Publishers, 1955.)

Complications of Angiography and Angiocardiography

A well trained team and a well organized laboratory are essential for the successful application of these physiologic tools. The studies are carried out preferably under image amplification fluoroscopy, with every care taken to avoid excess radiation of the patients and members of the research team.

The entire team must be constantly conscious of various complications which may ensue. Some of the most important of these are:

Air Embolism. This is undoubtedly infrequent if appropriate precautions are taken in relation to all injections made.

Venous and Intracardiac Thrombosis. Venous thrombosis usually extends less than 5 cm. upward from the site of the catheter insertion. Hence in order to maintain free blood flow in the main brachial vein, it is important to choose as the site of the introduction of the catheter a branch of the basilic venous system which is distal to and at a distance of at least 5 cm. from the last confluence of veins of this system. When the saphenous vein is used it is best to tie it off as close to the femoral as possible at the close of the procedure if an open insertion has been employed. Intracardiac thrombosis has not been frequently reported.

Rhythm Disturbance. This is by far the most important complication to consider. Premature contractions are often observed during the manipulation of the catheter inside the heart. However, actual ventricular fibrillation as a fatal complication is indeed rare. Ordinarily, simultaneous electrocardiograms must be obtained which allow one to recognize ectopic beats or runs of ventricular tachycardia immediately and, if necessary, to withdraw the catheter in order to prevent further accidents. Moreover, an appropriate defibrillator should always be on hand in the event such an accident might occur.

Blood Loss. The volume of blood withdrawal during the procedure is ordinarily not less than 100 cc. This amount constitutes a fairly large proportion of the total circulating blood volume, particularly in young children and infants. Moreover it is likely to upset the circulation. In such cases it is important to estimate the volume of blood withdrawn during each step of the procedure and to replace it with an equivalent amount of donor blood whenever it is deemed necessary.

RETROGRADE AORTOGRAPHY AND SELECTIVE ARTERIOGRAPHY

This method involves the passage of a catheter through a peripheral artery to the aorta and subsequently to the blood vessel of maximum interest. The Seldinger percutaneous technique is most frequently employed. An appropriate amount of the contrast agent is injected rapidly, and serial films are obtained immediately as desired, usually at the rate of two per second for two to four seconds and one per second thereafter for a total of approximately eight seconds. This varies, however, from region to region. Good opacification is thereby achieved. Detail of this order cannot ordinarily be derived by conventional venous angiocardiography. The procedure is of great value in demonstrating any of the major branches of the aorta and many organs such as the brain, the lungs, the kidneys, the intestines, the urinary bladder and the extremities.

Catheterization of the coronary arteries has been found feasible and very helpful in the diagnosis of coronary artery disease as well as collateral circulation (Sones and Shirey).

TRANSLUMBAR AORTOGRAPHY

Prior to translumbar aortography, adequate hydration of the patient is important to avoid renal complications. The aortic puncture is accomplished with a 7 inch No. 17 thin-walled needle inserted through the left flank into the aorta opposite the twelfth thoracic or first lumbar vertebra. A flexible tube is attached to the needle to allow the operator to stand behind a specially constructed lead shield during the injection procedure. Twenty to 30 ml. of an appropriate contrast agent (80 per cent sodium iothalamate or 50 per cent Hypaque), previously warmed to body temperature, is injected by hand from a large bore syringe. During the latter part of the injection, radiographic exposure is made of the aorta and iliac ar-

teries. By means of a special film holder, sequential films may be obtained at desired intervals (Fig. 10-6). Rapid sequence films of the urinary tract may also be obtained thereafter, with those of the kidney area taken at two per second for the first four seconds, one per second for the next four seconds, and then at one minute intervals for approximately five or six minutes. With sodium acetrizoate a high incidence of neurologic and renal damage has been reported, but no such damage has been encountered with sodium iothalamate, sodium diatrizoate or methylglucamine diatrizoate.

(Text continues on page 327.)

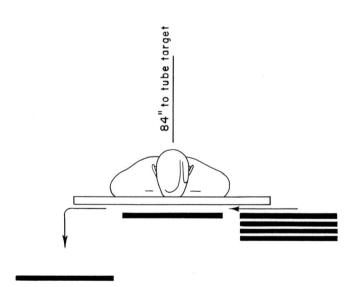

Schematic Design of "Long Film Cassette Changer"

FIGURE 10-6. The long cassette is drawn into position, the exposure is made, and the cassette then drops into a carrier device while the next one moves into position. (Modified from Clark, K. C.: *Positioning in Radiography.* London, Ilford Ltd. William Heinemann Medical Books, 1964.)

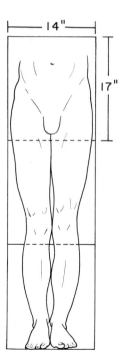

FIGURE 10-7. Diagram illustrating how a long cassette is loaded with three 14 by 17 inch films in tandem to cover indicated anatomic areas.

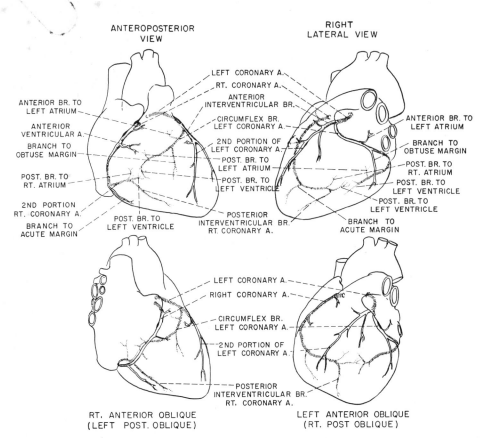

FIGURE 10-8. Diagram of coronary circulation as it might be seen in frontal, lateral and oblique projections. (Modified from Yuglielmo, L. D., and Yuttadauro, M.: Acta Radiol, Supp. 97, 1952.)

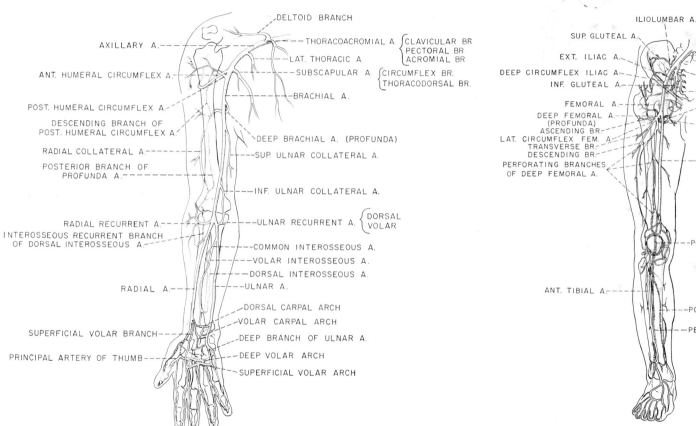

FIGURE 10-9. Diagram of arterial circulation of upper extremity.

FIGURE 10-10. Diagram of arterial circulation of lower extremity.

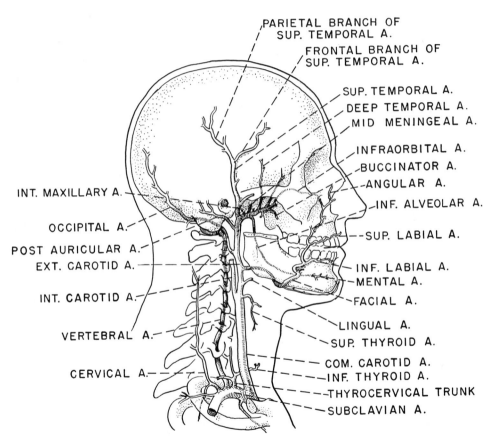

FIGURE 10-11. Major deep arteries of head and neck, lateral view (excluding brain).

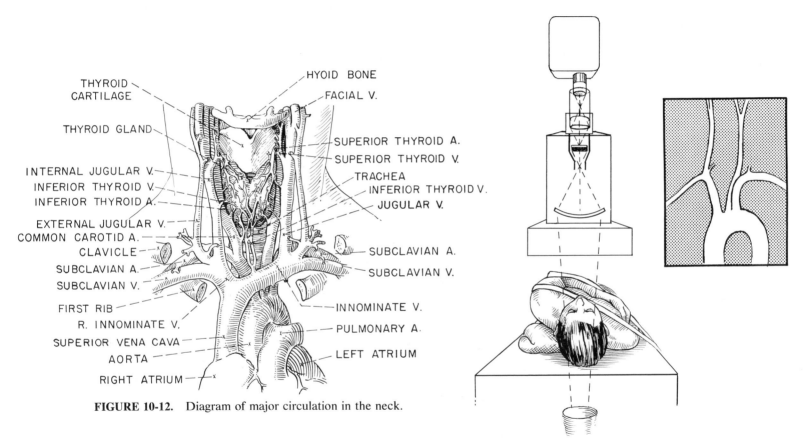

THYROID CARTILAGE
THYROID GLAND
INTERNAL JUGULAR V.
INFERIOR THYROID V.
INFERIOR THYROID A.
EXTERNAL JUGULAR V.
COMMON CAROTID A.
CLAVICLE
SUBCLAVIAN A.
SUBCLAVIAN V.
FIRST RIB
R. INNOMINATE V.
SUPERIOR VENA CAVA
AORTA
RIGHT ATRIUM

HYOID BONE
FACIAL V.
SUPERIOR THYROID A.
SUPERIOR THYROID V.
TRACHEA
INFERIOR THYROID V.
JUGULAR V.
SUBCLAVIAN A.
SUBCLAVIAN V.
INNOMINATE V.
PULMONARY A.
LEFT ATRIUM

FIGURE 10-12. Diagram of major circulation in the neck.

FIGURE 10-13. Diagrams illustrating position of patient for aortic arch angiographic studies.

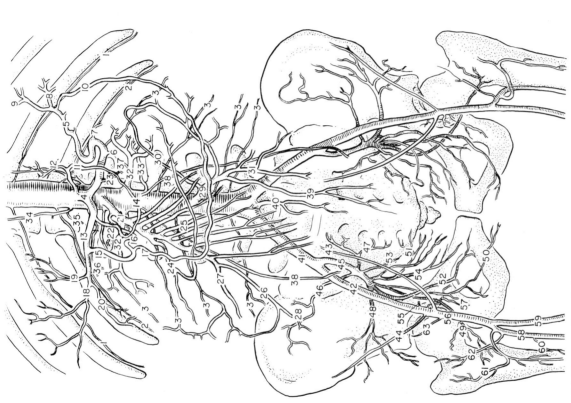

FIGURE 10-14. The arteries of abdomen, pelvis and thigh: 1, Intercostal; 2, subcostal; 3, lumbar; 4, celiac axis; 5, splenic; 6, dorsal pancreatic; 7, great pancreatic; 8, terminal branches to spleen; 9, short gastric branches; 10, left gastroepiploic; 11, left gastric; 12, esophageal branches; 13, common hepatic; 14, right gastric; 15, gastroduodenal; 16, anterior superior pancreaticoduodenal; 17, right gastroepiploic; 18, right hepatic; 19, left hepatic; 20, cystic; 21, superior mesenteric; 22, inferior pancreaticoduodenal; 23, inferior pancreatic; 24, middle colic; 25, intestinal branches; 26, ileocolic; 27, right colic; 28, appendiceal; 29, inferior mesenteric; 30, left colic; 31, sigmoid; 32, renal; 33, accessory renal; 34, inferior phrenic; 35, superior suprarenal; 36, middle suprarenal; 37, inferior suprarenal; 38, internal spermatic (or ovarian); 39, superior hemorrhoidal; 40, middle sacral; 41, common iliac; 42, external iliac; 43, inferior epigastric; 44, deep circumflex iliac; 45, hypogastric; 46, iliolumbar; 47, lateral sacral; 48, superior gluteal; 49, inferior gluteal; 50, internal pudendal; 51, middle hemorrhoidal; 52, obturator; 53, uterine; 54, vesical; 55, superficial epigastric; 56, common femoral; 57, superficial external pudendal; 58, deep femoral (profunda); 59, superficial femoral; 60, perforating muscular branches; 61, lateral femoral circumflex; 62, medial femoral circumflex; 63, superficial circumflex iliac. (Modified from Muller, R. F., and Figley, M. M., Am. J. Roentgenol. 77, 1957.)

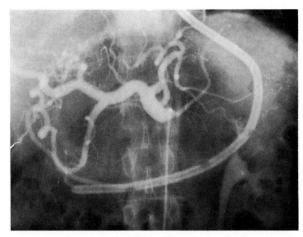

FIGURE 10-15.   Selective arteriogram of celiac artery.

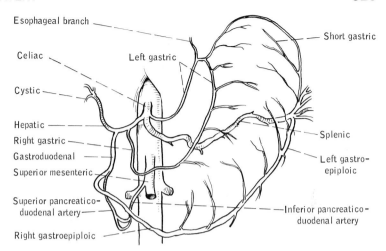

Esophageal branch

Short gastric

Celiac

Left gastric

Cystic

Hepatic

Right gastric

Gastroduodenal

Superior mesenteric

Splenic

Left gastro-
epiploic

Superior pancreatico-
duodenal artery

Inferior pancreatico-
duodenal artery

Right gastroepiploic

FIGURE 10-16.   Diagram illustrating arterial circulation around the stomach.

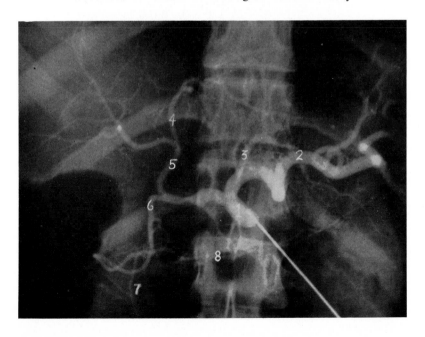

FIGURE 10-17.   Radiograph of the celiac artery and its major branches by the method of aortography. 1, Celiac artery; 2, splenic artery; 3, left gastric artery; 4, right gastric artery; 5, hepatic artery; 6, gastroduodenal artery; 7, superior pancreaticoduodenal artery; 8, right gastroepiploic artery. (Through the courtesy of Drs. Parke G. Smith, Arthur T. Evans, Benjamin Felson and Edward C. Elsey, Cincinnati General Hospital and Christ Hospital, Cincinnati, Ohio.)

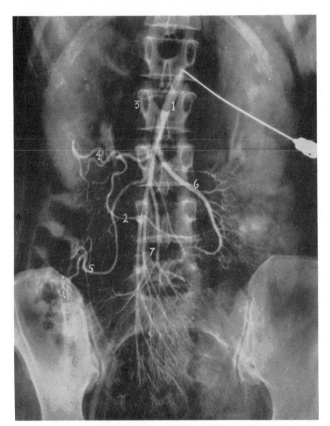 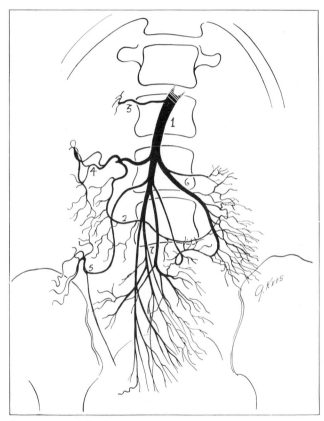

FIGURE 10-18. Radiograph and tracing of the superior mesenteric artery and its branches. 1, Superior mesenteric artery; 2, middle colic artery; 3, pancreaticoduodenal inferior artery; 4, right colic artery; 5, iliocolic artery; 6, jejunal artery; 7, ilial artery. (Through the courtsey of Drs. Parke G. Smith, Arthur T. Evans, Benjamin Felson and Edward C. Elsey, Cincinnati General Hospital and Christ Hospital, Cincinnati, Ohio.)

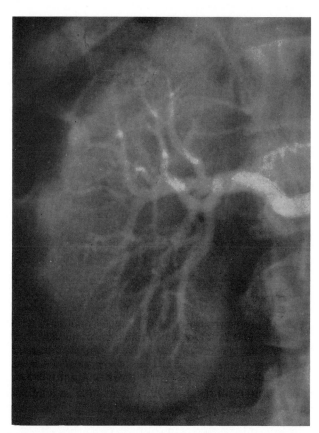

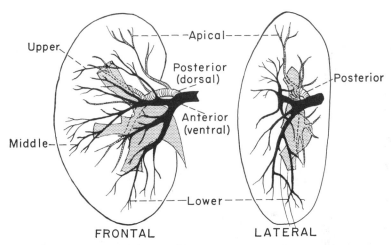

FIGURE 10-19B. Diagram illustrating the renal artery and its segmental branches in frontal and lateral perspectives, with the relationship to the pelvocalyceal system shown. (After Boijsen, E.: Acta Radiol., suppl. *183*:51, 1959.)

FIGURE 10-19A. Radiograph of the normal renal circulation as demonstrated by the method of aortography. (Through the courtesy of Drs. Parke G. Smith, Arthur T. Evans, Benjamin Felson and Edward C. Elsey, Cincinnati General Hospital and Christ Hospital, Cincinnati, Ohio.)

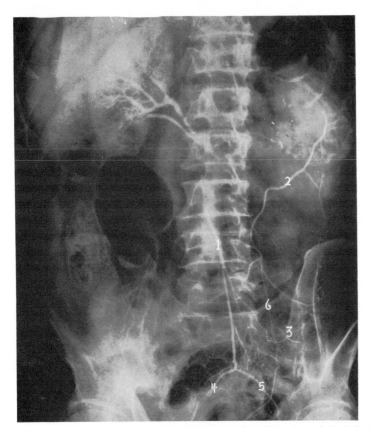

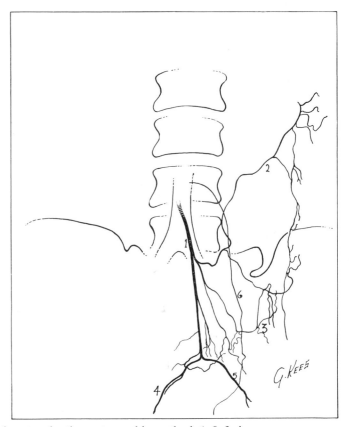

FIGURE 10-20. Radiograph and tracing of the inferior mesenteric artery by the aortographic method 1, Inferior mesenteric artery; 2, left colic artery; 3, sigmoidal artery; 4, right hemorrhoidal artery; 5, left hemorrhoidal artery. In addition 6 demonstrates the left spermatic artery. (Through the courtesy of Drs. Parke G. Smith, Arthur T. Evans, Benjamin Felson and Edward C. Elsey, Cincinnati General Hospital and Christ Hospital, Cincinnati, Ohio.)

VENOGRAPHY OF THE INFERIOR VENA CAVA

Venography of the inferior vena cava can be accomplished by catheterization of the femoral vein by the Seldinger technique, passing the catheter to the common iliac vein and injecting thereafter 50 to 90 per cent Hypaque in an appropriate volume (30 to 40 ml.). If a larger bolus of contrast agent is desired, bilateral percutaneous catheterization can be carried out with simultaneous bilateral injection of the contrast agent. Inferior vena cavography may reveal an enlargement chiefly of retroperitoneal nodes situated between the aorta and the vena cava and behind the latter structure. The vena cava is usually displaced forward and to the right in patients with retroperitoneal tumors at the level of the second lumbar vertebra. There is often a characteristic displacement of the right aspects of the vena cava with abnormalities which adjoin this vascular structure. Anteroposterior and lateral views must be employed for optimal utilization of this technique (Helander and Lindbom; Lockhart et al.; Lund et al.).

AZYGOGRAPHY

Intra- and extrathoracic disorders may modify the hemodynamics of the azygos venous system; thus a study of these veins has at times been valuable in the elucidation of certain clinical problems. The azygos vein on the right receives the right intercostal veins, except for the supreme intercostal vein which empties directly into the innominate vein. The left half of the azygos system consists of an inferior portion called the hemiazygos vein and a superior segment called the accessory hemiazygos vein. The hemiazygos vein receives blood mainly from the lower four to six left intercostal veins and several small branches directly from the mediastinum. The accessory azygos vein receives blood from the second to the fifth left thoracic segments. These veins and their various contributing channels are somewhat variable, but are worthy of par-

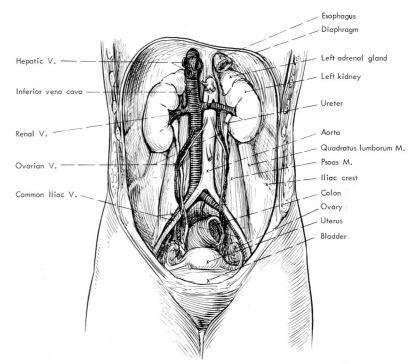

FIGURE 10-21. Diagram of the inferior vena cava and its main tributaries.

ticular consideration because of the structures that are in direct contact with or in close proximity to the azygos venous system: the lungs, posterior pleura, mediastinal lymph nodes, right bronchus, middle third of the esophagus, aorta, vertebral bodies, and thoracic duct. Expanding disease processes from these structures may impinge upon or displace these venous channels.

The technique recommended by Schobinger is as follows: 20 to 25 ml. of the organic iodide agent are injected in the tenth rib on the right in about 5 seconds or less. Anteroposterior, posteroanterior, or lateral films of the chest are taken during the introduc-

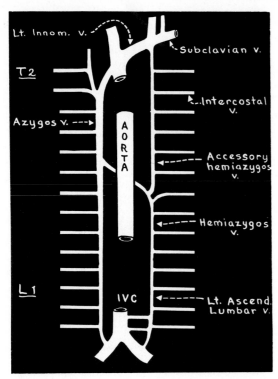

FIGURE 10-22. Diagrammatic representation of the azygos venous system. The segmental lumbar veins are joined to each other by a longitudinal vessel, the ascending lumbar vein. The right ascending lumbar vein, as it enters the thorax, becomes the azygos vein, and the left ascending lumbar vein is continuous with the hemiazygos vein. The hemiazygos vein crosses in front of the vertebral column at the level of T 8 or T 9 to join the azygos vein. The accessory hemiazygos vein is continuous with the hemiazygos, receives the upper thoracic veins on the left, and joins the left superior intercostal vein above. (From Abrams, H. L.: Radiology 69, 1957.)

tion of the last 2 or 3 ml. of the medium when the patient is apneic without straining. One film is usually adequate, although serial films may be employed.

Azygography may assist in the evaluation of middle third esophageal lesions, of pericardial abnormalities and of cardiac pathology. Obstructions of the portal vein may also affect the azygos venous system. Retrograde flow may, however, be produced by straining or by cardiac failure as well.

INTERNAL MAMMARY VENOGRAPHY

Bilateral internal mammary vein visualization may be obtained by the rapid injection (five to six seconds) of 15 to 30 ml. of 50 per cent Hypaque or its equivalent into the midline of the sternum opposite the fourth or fifth intercostal space.

Unilateral visualization may be obtained by injecting similarly into the fifth or sixth rib in the anterior axillary line.

This procedure is helpful in evaluating parasternal lymphadenopathy, particularly in patients with carcinoma of the breast. It may also be used for evaluation of other intra- and extrathoracic abnormalities.

PHLEBOGRAPHY OF THE LOWER EXTREMITY

Technique

Numerous slight variations in technique are described, but there is general agreement that the contrast medium should be injected into one of the superficial veins of the foot or ankle. The

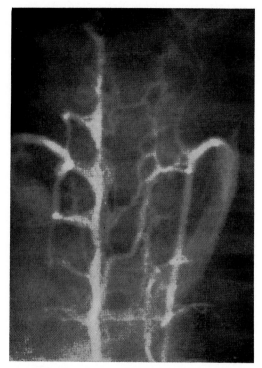

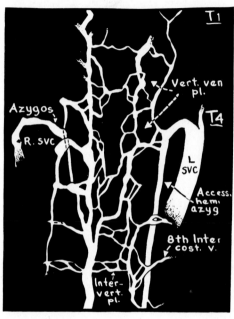

FIGURE 10-23. The vertebral veins at the upper thoracic level. The vertebral venous plexuses are opacified following the injection of the opaque medium into the left saphenous vein. The primitive paired arrangement of both the azygos and the superior vena cava is preserved, the accessory hemiazygos emptying into the left superior vena cava, and the azygos into the right superior vena cava. The medial portions of the intercostal veins are opacified. *R. SVC*, right superior vena cava; *L. SVC*, left superior vena cava. *Access. hemiazyg,* accessory hemiazygos vein. (From Abrams, H. L.: Radiology *69, 1957.*)

contrast media in common use in this country are 50 per cent solutions of either Hypaque or Renografin or an equivalent organic iodide.

In the method utilized by Epstein, Wasch and Loewe in their investigation of the normal phlebogram, 20 cc. of the medium was injected within 60 seconds into any available vein on the dorsum of the foot or over either malleolus with a hypodermic needle. Two and sometimes three exposures were made using the Potter-Bucky

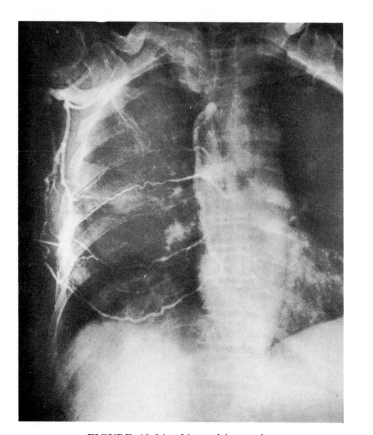
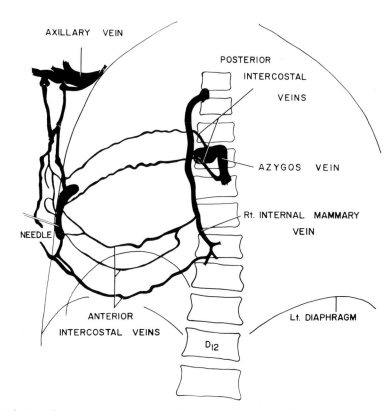

FIGURE 10-24. Normal internal mammary venogram. Injection performed into sixth rib in the right mid-axillary line. Anteroposterior projection. Contrast medium outlines two intercostal veins corresponding to the level of injection, the superior portion of azygos vein posteriorly, and the ipsilateral internal mammary vein. Note the opacification of extrathoracic veins (lateral thoracic, thoracoepigastric and axillary veins) through costoaxillary communications. (From Schobinger, R. A.: *Intra-osseous Venography.* Grune & Stratton, 1960)

diaphragm, each exposure being made as rapidly as possible as follows:

1. First exposure, leg slightly in inversion, made immediately upon completion of the injection, centering just below the knee.
2. Second exposure, centering just above the knee.
3. Third exposure, centering just below the groin.

They also studied some of the patients in the lateral projection as well.

The medium may also be injected in this manner while applying a 30 mm. of mercury pressure cuff around the calf in an effort to visualize the deep system of veins, since this pressure will occlude the superficial veins, but not the deep. We have found this method of considerable value particularly because the deep veins are of greater interest clinically.

An alternative technique for demonstration of competency of femoral vein valves is to catheterize the saphenous vein in the groin, pass the catheter to the femoral vein, and introduce 15 to 20 cc. of the dye rapidly *with the patient erect.* Films are obtained immediately of the thigh and leg, and thereafter at one minute intervals for four minutes. (Direct percutaneous puncture of the femoral vein in the groin may be employed in lieu of the catheterization method described.)

If the femoral valves are competent, the passage of the dye will be stopped almost entirely at the first set of valves approximately 8 to 10 cm. from the inguinal ligament. A very small amount of dye may escape down to the second set of valves, but no farther. This method may be referred to as the "gravity method" of phlebography. Another indication of abnormality is a visualization of an unusual number of the veins which communicate with the femoral vein in the thigh. Normally the dye should virtually disappear in less than one minute. Persistence for two minutes or longer is an indication of venous stasis and poor venous circulation.

Normal Anatomy (Figure 10-27)

The superficial veins form a continuous network around the leg and the thigh. The lesser saphenous vein (Fig. 10-29) begins behind the lateral malleolus, courses along the posterior surface of the Achilles tendon, and passes upward to enter the popliteal vein in the groove between the two heads of the gastrocnemius muscle. It anastomoses freely with the greater saphenous vein, which arises in front of the medial malleolus and courses upward on the medial aspect of the tibia, making a slight curve at the medial tibial and femoral condyles. It then extends upward on the medial and anterior aspect of the thigh to enter the femoral vein in the fossa ovalis. Numerous branches are received throughout its course and it communicates freely with the deeper veins (Fig. 10-25).

The popliteal vein is formed by the junction of the anterior and posterior tibial veins (Fig. 10-29), and this vein is very subject to slight variations.

The femoral vein (Fig. 10-28) and its tributaries constitute the deep veins of the thigh. It accompanies the femoral artery and terminates as it enters the pelvis as the external iliac vein. The femoral veins are said to contain two bicuspid valves, but usually it is possible to see three or four valves in the femoral vein radiographically.

The deep femoral vein has numerous tributaries, but since these are seldom seen radiographically in the usual examination, they need no further consideration in this text.

The great variability and the superposition of veins make the radiographic interpretation of venograms very difficult. Only those veins which happen to be patent at the time of examination will fill, and it is most unusual to obtain a complete filling of all the major veins in a single examination. Indeed, excessive filling of smaller tributaries is an indication of abnormality.

It is well to repeat these studies on several separate occasions

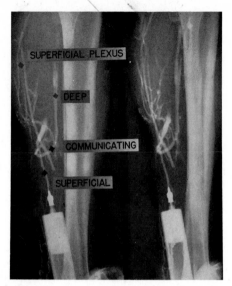

FIGURE 10-25. Venograms of leg demonstrating the communicating veins joining superficial and deep veins. (Courtesy of Dr. E. C. Baker, Youngstown, Ohio)

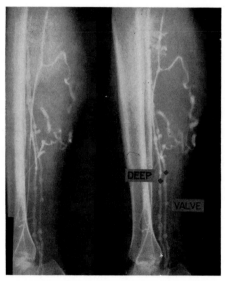

FIGURE 10-26. Venograms of deep veins of leg, showing their paired nature. (Courtesy of Dr. E. C. Baker, Youngstown, Ohio.)

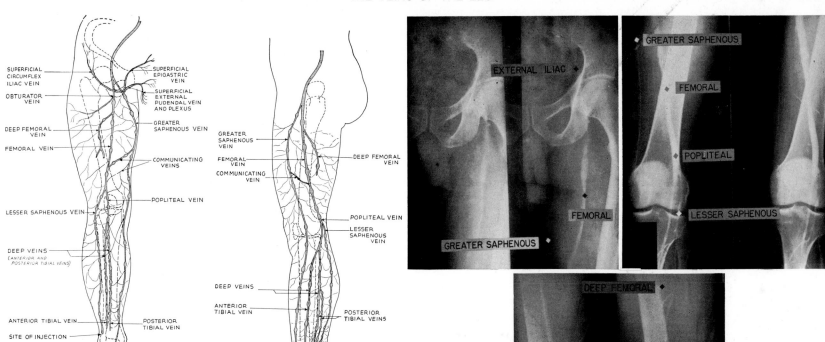

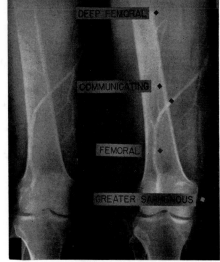

FIGURE 10-27. Diagram of the anatomy of conventional venograms of the leg: **A,** anteroposterior projection; **B,** lateral projection.

FIGURE 10-28. Venograms demonstrating the external iliac vein, the femoral vein, and its major tributaries. (Courtesy of Dr. E. C. Baker, Youngstown, Ohio)

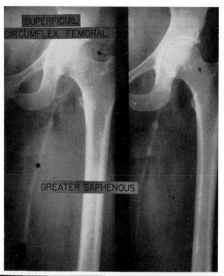

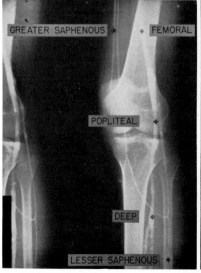

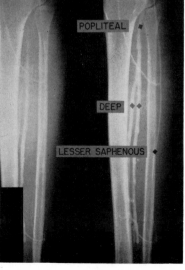

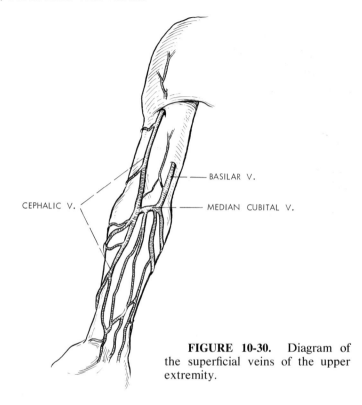

FIGURE 10-30. Diagram of the superficial veins of the upper extremity.

FIGURE 10-29. Representative conventional venograms of the lower extremity demonstrating primarily the lesser and greater saphenous veins and several deeper veins of leg and thigh. (Courtesy of Dr. E. C. Baker, Youngstown, Ohio.)

by the routine method of injection of a vein in the foot so that, when they are interpreted the constancy of a given finding will add weight to its reliability.

PERCUTANEOUS SPLENOPORTAL VENOGRAPHY

Three major methods are available for visualizing the portal circulation: (1) the direct approach through an abdominal incision; (2) the percutaneous approach by splenic puncture and (3) rapid serial film studies through the portal venous phase following mesenteric artery arteriography.

The percutaneous method requires general anesthesia and, preferably a rapid film changer. A 16 gauge needle is inserted in the midaxillary line of the ninth or tenth intercostal space. (This may be replaced by a suitable polyethylene catheter threaded through the needle into the splenic pulp.) The patient is maintained in apnea as the spleen is approached, to prevent laceration of the spleen. The needle is advanced about 2 or 3 cm. into the splenic pulp and, at this juncture, may be replaced by the polyethylene catheter threaded through the needle. Fifty ml. of 50 per cent Hypaque or similar contrast substance is forcefully injected in 5 or 6 seconds. Exposure rates of one per second for about 12 or 15 seconds are adequate. The patient is maintained in apnea during the injection and exposure.

It is apparently customary to find 50 to 100 cc. of blood in the peritoneal cavity when the abdomen is opened, although occasionally the blood loss may be greater. In occasional cases, splenectomy is necessitated. Under no circumstances should the procedure be done except prior to surgery for performance of a shunt. Its main purpose is to demonstrate patency of the various major vessels of the portal circulation, to save the surgeon hours of search for a nonexistent or thrombosed vein which he is hoping to utilize in the anastomosis.

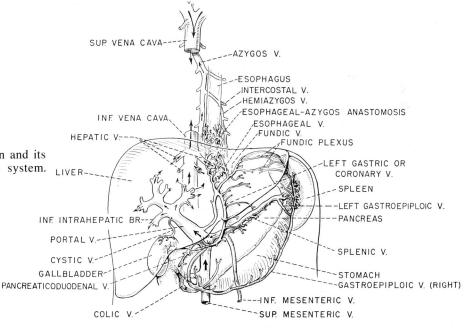

FIGURE 10-31. Anatomic diagram of the portal circulation and its relationship to the esophageal veins and the azygos venous system.

The basic anatomy of the area is illustrated in Figure 10-31. Typical splenoportograms are shown in Figure 10-32.

LYMPHANGIOGRAPHY

Various techniques for lymphangiography have been proposed. A vital dye is injected intradermally into the first interdigital webbed space on the dorsum of the hand or foot, permitting a visualization of the minute lymphatic channels in the webbed space or proximal to it. One lymphatic in each extremity is thereafter carefully can-

nulated and injected with Ethiodol, an ethyl ester of poppyseed oil containing 37 per cent iodine. The injection is carried out under low and constant pressure over a period of one to two hours. The patient remains supine throughout the entire procedure. This is apparently especially important for visualization of the thoracic duct.

The normal lymphatics parallel the veins throughout most of the body. In the lower extremity, they travel with the greater and lesser saphenous veins. Peripherally, there are usually one or two fine caliber channels that have a beaded appearance due to valves. The number of channels ordinarily increases to 8 or 12 near the in-

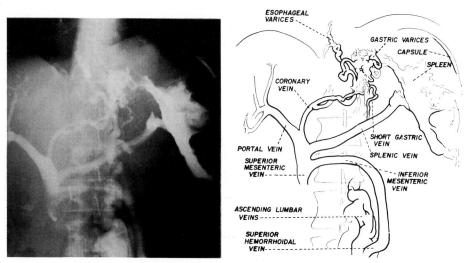

FIGURE 10-32. Roentgenogram at 12 seconds demonstrates coronary vein, gastric and esophageal varices. The anastomosis between the inferior mesenteric vein and superior hemorrhoid plexus is demonstrated. The latter is also seen to drain into the vertebral venous plexus. Tracing at right. (From Evans, J. A., and O'Sullivan, W. D.: Am. J. Roentgenol. *77*, 1957.)

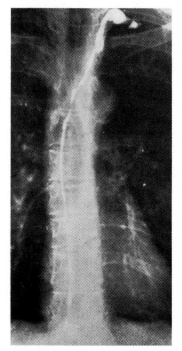

FIGURE 10-33. Normal thoracic duct (Busch and Sayegh, U.S. Naval Hospital, Philadelphia, Pa.)

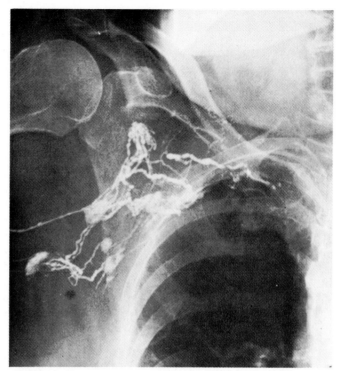

FIGURE 10-34. Normal axillary lymphatics and nodes; emptying into the subclavian vein is shown.

occurs abundantly. Injection of the lower extremity will ordinarily fill the inguinal, the external and common iliac nodes and the para-aortic nodes to the level of L 2, where the lymphatics empty into the cisterna chyli (Fig. 10-35). Thereafter the flow is through the thoracic duct until the supraclavicular nodes are seen (Fig. 10-33). The lymphatic channels will usually empty within a few hours, but normal lymph nodes will usually retain the contrast agent for four to six weeks or longer.

The thoracic duct empties into the subclavian vein, and a fine shower of opaque material may be seen in the lungs and occasionally in hilar lymph nodes.

The inguinal nodes actually fill within 5 or 10 minutes following the start of the injection; very often the thoracic duct may be seen as early as at 20 minutes, but it is best seen at 45 to 60 minutes.

In the arm, the lymphatics follow the basilic and cephalic veins, thereafter the axillary and supraclavicular lymph nodes, and finally reach the subclavian vein (Fig. 10-34). Roentgenograms are taken at the termination of the injection for visualization of the lymphatics, demonstrable for two to four hours. Re-examination is carried out in 24 hours for best demonstration of the lymph nodes. The lymph nodes may retain the contrast agent for approximately four weeks or even longer (as long as four to six months).

The lymphatics have been studied in this fashion in both normal and many abnormal states; the method is particularly valuable in assessing the extent of involvement by lymphosarcomas. On the 24 hour film studies, in addition to the anteroposterior projection, oblique and sometimes stereoscopic views are very helpful in assessing the extent of abnormality of the visualized lymph nodes. The total amount of oily contrast medium injected on each side should never exceed 10 ml. This procedure is ordinarily contraindicated in the presence of chronic or debilitating lung disease.

guinal nodes. The lymphatic channels are separate for the medial and lateral aspects of the extremity with only minor connecting linkages until the lymph node chains are reached. At the level of the sacrum, however, intercommunication between the two sides

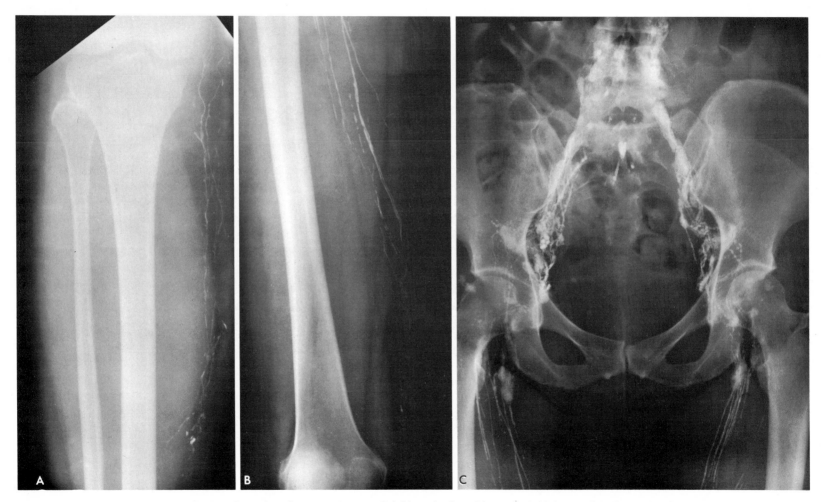

FIGURE 10-35   Lymphangiograms: **A,** superficial lymphatics of leg; **B,** of thigh; **C,** of groins and pelvis.

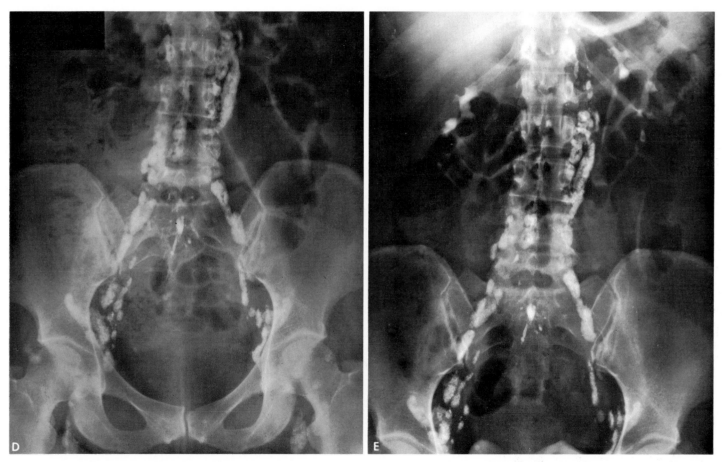

FIGURE 10-35 Lymphangiograms: **D,** 24 hour A-P study of pelvis and lower abdomen; **E,** 24 hour A-P study of abdomen showing cisterna chyli, upper left at L 2 level.

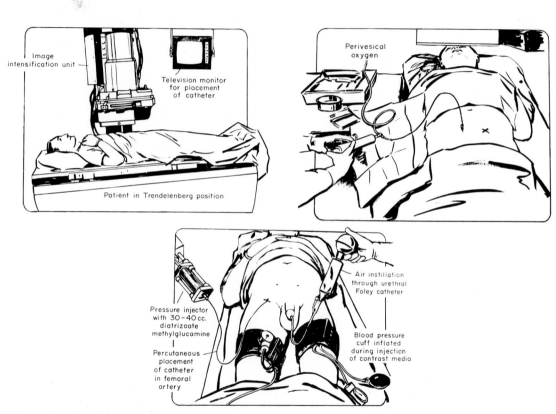

FIGURE 10-36. Pelvic pneumoperitoneum, air cystography and arterial angiography of the urinary bladder (triple contrast). (Courtesy Drs. S. C. Lacy, C. E. Cox, W. H. Boyce and J. E. Whitley, Depts. of Urology and Radiology, The Bowman Gray School of Medicine.)

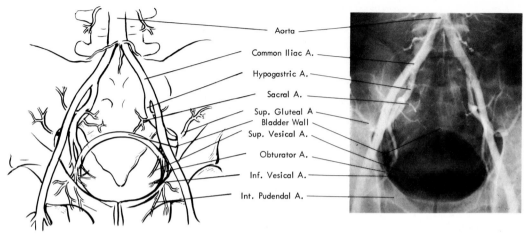

Aorta
Common Iliac A.
Hypogastric A.
Sacral A.
Sup. Gluteal A
Bladder Wall
Sup. Vesical A.
Obturator A.
Inf. Vesical A.
Int. Pudendal A.

FIGURE 10-36. *(Continued)*

"TRIPLE-CONTRAST" STUDY OF THE URINARY BLADDER

As a special study of the urinary bladder, the "triple-contrast technique" with the aid of perivesical oxygen, intravesical air and retrograde femoral arteriography may be used (Fig. 10-36). The patient is placed supine on the x-ray table in the Trendelenburg (head down) position. Image amplification and television viewing during the procedure are desirable. An 18 gauge needle is inserted in the extraperitoneal space just outside the urinary bladder (after appropriate skin sterilization and anesthesia), and approximately 300 cc. of air instilled, so that the urinary bladder wall is seen and its wall thickness is measureable when 300 to 500 cc. of air is injected into the bladder through a Foley catheter. The femoral artery is catheterized by the Seldinger technique and connected with a pressure injector.

Blood pressure cuffs are placed around each thich, peripheral to the femoral artery catheterization site. These are inflated above arterial pressure just prior to injection of the contrast agent into the femoral artery catheter, and the femoral arteries are thereby occluded during the injection. Thirty to 40 ml. of 50 per cent diatrizoate methylglucamine are used for the injection in about one second. Serial films of the pelvic region are obtained at three per second for three or four seconds, and one per second for an additional three or four seconds.

The films will show clearly the arterial distribution to the urinary bladder and to any tumor contained within its wall. Spread to or invasion of contiguous structures in the pelvis will thereby be demonstrated also. Tumor vessels and tumor staining are readily apparent. The triple-contrast technique is particularly helpful for assessment of total spread and degree of involvement.

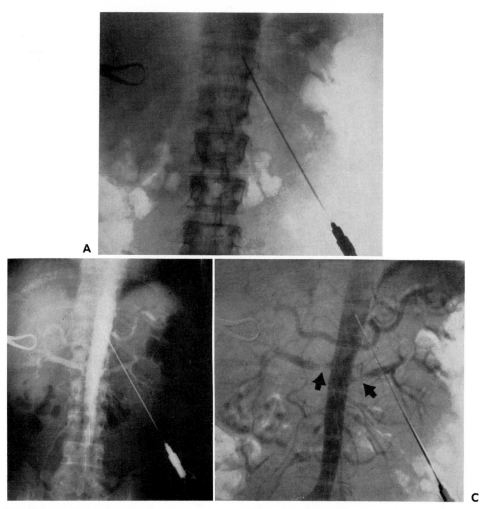

FIGURE 10-37.   Subtraction technique for more accurate delineation of vascular branches. A scout film is first obtained in a position identical to that to be used for delineation of the contrast-filled vascular region. This is reversed so that a negative film (**A**) is obtained In this film the bones appear black and the gas shadows appear white. Thereafter, the aortogram (**B**) is obtained in routine fashion. By superposition of film **A** over film **B,** the bone shadows are neutralized and "subtracted out " Film **C** is thereby obtained. The arrows point to bilateral renal artery stenosis noted more clearly on the postsubtraction film **C.**

SUBTRACTION TECHNIQUE

The principle of subtraction techniques has been carefully elucidated by Des Plantes. He demonstrated that if one obtains a radiograph prior to the introduction of a contrast agent, and thereafter a second radiograph with the contrast agent, one can intensify the appearance of the contrast agent more clearly by removing interfering bony shadows in the following manner (Fig. 10-37). A negative transparent "diapositive" is obtained from the control radiograph, and this negative is superimposed on the radiograph containing the contrast agent. Since in the negative diapositive of the control radiograph the bony structures appear black, this black-

ness will ordinarily neutralize out the bony structures as visualized on the second film when light is transmitted through the two films superimposed over one another. If a third film is then obtained, this neutralization process results in virtual obliteration of the bony shadows and a clearer demonstration of the contrast agent.

A further modification of this technique has recently been suggested by Oldendorf, and is illustrated in Figure 10-37. In this latter modification, a second-order diapositive is introduced to subtract more of the detail not subtracted by the first. The initial dye-free control film is contact-printed onto a Du Pont commercial S film or Eastman commercial film. These combined two diapositives are then superimposed over the succeeding films in an angiographic series, to obtain the final subtracted film.

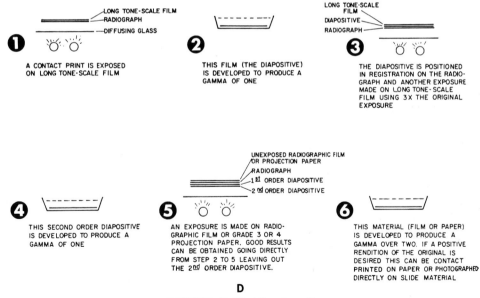

FIGURE 10-37. *(Continued)*

D, Steps in the modified subtraction method as recommended by Oldendorf. With complete subtraction by a good pair of diapositives, greater enhancement will result from using contrast paper in steps 5 or 6. (Part **D** from Oldendorf, W. H.: Neurology *15:*367, 1965)

In each instance, the control film prior to the introduction of the contrast agent must be obtained in exactly the same position as the later films with the contrast agent in order to get ideal subtraction.

ADVERSE REACTIONS TO RADIOPAQUE AGENTS

Physical and Chemical Aspects of Radiographic Contrast Agents

Contrast agents in radiology should have the following basic attributes: (1) They must contain a relatively heavy atom (such as barium or iodine) that will afford adequate radiopacity for diagnostic procedures. (2) For injection and ingestion purposes, such compounds should possess little or no toxicity. (3) When utilized as physiologic test agents, they must enter into the appropriate physiologic action without alteration of normal function.

In the gastrointestinal tract it will be noted that barium sulfate in its several forms has found wide usefulness because it is relatively inert, it is not absorbed from the gastrointestinal tract, and it does not alter normal physiologic responses. Also the barium atom is sufficiently heavy for good radiopacity.

For injection purposes in the vascular system, organic combinations with iodine have been particularly useful. Iodine is a relatively heavy atom that affords adequate radiopacity and also can readily be attached to organic molecules making compounds that have low toxicity and can enter into normal physiologic processes.

The generally accepted urographic contrast agents which also have many uses in vascular radiography are Hypaque-50, Renografin-60, Miokon-50 and Conray-60. The sodium salts (such as Hypaque) are as a rule less viscous than the methylglucamine salts (such as Renografin) in solutions of identical concentration. In high concentrations, the methylglucamine tends to give a syrupy solution, which is understandable in view of its close molecular resemblance to glucose. For low pressure injections into long catheters with small lumina, viscosity plays a very important role. It is probable also that some of the new high pressure, high speed injection devices produce flow rates with sufficient turbulence to introduce other important variables apart from viscosity. There is also some question whether under some circumstances these contrast agents when injected as solutions, are capable of forming peculiar complexes with some of the blood elements.

For gallbladder studies, substances are sought which are selectively excreted by the liver and concentrated in the bile. The compounds currently utilized for this purpose are: Priodax (iodoalphionic acid) and Telepaque and Teridax, (alpha-ethylpropionic acid benzene derivatives). An intravenously administered contrast agent, iodipamide (Cholografin), has been introduced for the visualization of the gallbladder and the common ducts. This compound contains a greater concentration of iodine per molecule than those previously mentioned, and hence a visualization of the biliary system can be obtained directly without dependence upon the concentration function of the gallbladder.

Contrast substances have also been devised in suspension for maintenance of local concentrations of these radiopaque materials. They are occasionally administered in an aqueous vehicle, thickened by such materials as methylcellulose. Applications of such compounds include bronchography, urethrography and myelography for visualization of the subarachnoid space already mentioned in prior chapters. Other applications include the visualization of sinus tracts, fistulas, abscesses, the uterus, fallopian tubes, the urinary bladder, biliary tract passages, paranasal sinuses, and salivary gland ducts.

Some iodinated organic compounds have been used as radiopaque substances for gastrointestinal examinations, particularly if they are not significantly absorbed from the alimentary tract. These substances have not gained wide acceptance because of the fact that barium sulfate is so innocuous, so inexpensive and yet so effective as a gastrointestinal radiopaque agent.

In view of the great importance of intravascular injections of contrast agents, it is important for us now to consider some of the adverse reactions induced by these compounds.

Adverse Reactions to the Intravascular Injection of Radiopaque Agents

Adverse reactions to radiopaque agents can involve the cardiovascular, respiratory, nervous, gastrointestinal, cutaneous and renal systems. Some of these reactions are nausea, vomiting, flushing, dizziness, mild stridor and local tissue pain. Less frequently one may see severe urticaria, various degrees of shock and severe tissue damage due to extravasation from the vessel injected. Occasionally albuminuria may also be found. A satisfactory explanation has not yet been developed for all the various reactions that have been observed. It would appear, however, that the injection of synthetic blood volume expanders such as Dextran can reduce the severity of some of them.

From extensive surveys it has been estimated that human mortality from intravenous injection of contrast agents for urography is about seven or eight for every million examinations. Anyone who uses these agents must be prepared for emergencies and have at hand appropriate medication and a plan of action for himself and his team of workers (Table 10-1).

Before injecting any contrast material, the physician should take a history of any sensitivity reactions in relation to previous injections, hives, asthma or other history of an allergic state. The physician, of course, should make doubly sure that the material he is injecting is exactly what is desired and that the dosage is accurate for the procedure in question. In anticipation of adverse reactions, a complete tray must be readily available to the physician and should contain certain medications within arm's reach and other medications within a syringe ready for utilization. For example, it is desirable to have Adrenalin ready within a syringe in the event of a reaction.

When the contrast material is injected, a small quantity such as 1 ml. is first instilled as a test dose; the physician should wait approximately one minute with the needle in position to see whether an adverse reaction is encountered. After completing the injection the physician should probably remain in attendance, or at least be readily available for several minutes in the immediate vicinity, so that he can be called for treatment if an adverse reaction occurs.

If an adverse reaction does occur, the patient's vital functions such as cardiac status and respiration must immediately be studied. Assuming cardiac resuscitation is necessary, the closed chest cardiac compression technique, in which the sternum is pressed inward and the heart is compressed against the spine, is recommended. This method is, of course, contraindicated in a patient with pneumothorax or an intrathoracic hemorrhage. The heel of one hand is placed just above the xyphoid process of the sternum with the other hand on top of it. The fingers themselves are kept off the chest wall since the point of application of force should be as small as possible. The compression is performed by a $1\frac{1}{2}$ to 2 inch thrust into the chest with a rapid release. In an infant or child the pressure must be correspondingly diminished. Such compression is ordinarily applied about 60 times per minute. If there is need for artificial respiration, it should be applied about every third or fourth cardiac compression or 15 or 20 times per minute. Preferably oxygen should also be available.

The presence of a palpable pulse is probably the earliest indicator of a satisfactory resuscitation response. When the blood pressure exceeds 70 mm. of mercury, cardiac compression can be stopped, and the introduction of a 1 per cent solution of Aramine or 0.2 per cent solution of Levophed is effective in maintaining the blood pressure or bringing it to the patient's customary blood pres-

TABLE 10-1.   Adverse Reactions to Radiopaque Agents

Clinical Reaction	Procedures*	Drug*	Dosage*
Cardiovascular collapse (faintness, sweating, rapid, weak pulse)	Oxygen through clear airway Extracorporeal cardiac massage if cardiac arrest occurs	Aramine I.V.	0.2-1.0 cc. (2-10 mg.) 5 cc. in 500 cc. saline (50 mg.) Solu-Cortef 100 mg. I.V.
Convulsions or jerky movements	Oxygen through clear airway Artificial respiration	Sodium pentobarbital (Nembutal)	25 mg. I.V. at two minute intervals until controlled
Bronchial asthma		Adrenalin S.C. Aminophylline I.V. Benadryl I.M. Solu-Cortef I.V. (in addition to above)	0.3 cc. 1/1000 aqueous 10 cc. (250 mg.) 2 cc. (20 mg.) 2 cc. (100 mg.)
Laryngeal edema (difficulty in breathing)	Tracheotomy may be necessary	Adrenalin I.V. Benadryl I.V.	0.05-0.1 cc. 1/1000 aqueous 1 cc. (10 mg.)
Pulmonary edema (shortness of breath with wet cough and sputum)	Phlebotomy 250-500 cc. or bloodless phlebotomy using tourniquets high on arms and legs, releasing one at a time for five minutes every half-hour	Adrenalin I.V. Demerol I.V. Solu-Cortef I.V.	0.1 cc. 1/1000 aqueous 1.0 cc. (50 mg.) 2 cc. (100 mg.)
Nausea, flushing, hyperventilation, urticaria, periorbital edema	Reassurance	Benadryl	10 mg. I.V.

*Physicians should advise and train their technicians for participation in this endeavor.

sure range. If a heartbeat is not obtained in approximately five or six minutes of cardiac compression, Adrenalin may have to be injected directly into the left ventricle while the compression is continued. This may be repeated in five minutes. Ventricular defibrillation by an externally applied defibrillator should be attempted.

If the patient is obviously apneic or demonstrates inadequate air exchange, the neck should be hyperextended with the chin brought forward and the head drawn to the side if drainage is desirable. Suction may be utilized and an endotracheal tube may be passed if one is skilled in its use; even a tracheostomy may have

to be performed by the physician in attendance. Once the airway is established, artificial respiration may be applied by mouth-to-mouth or mouth-to-nose techniques. A bag, mask, or the equivalent may also be used, and oxygen should always be available. Cardiac compression can be stopped after about one hour, particularly if the pupils are markedly dilated. Pulmonary resuscitation should be stopped only after many hours if the heart is beating, and the patient should then be turned over to a mechanical respirator if possible.

The physician should treat allergic reactions such as urticaria, angioneurotic edema, laryngeal edema, asthma, status asthmaticus, or anaphylactoid collapse by an injection of 0.3 to 0.5 cc. of Adrenalin (1/1000) subcutaneously or 25 to 50 mg. of Benadryl intravenously. Prednisolone phosphate, 100 mg. intravenously every four to six hours, may be utilized. For asthma, aminophylline, 25 mg./cc. in a 250 mg. intravenous drip given slowly, may be used at the rate of 1 cc. per minute.

In certain special radiographic procedures, topical anesthesia must be utilized, as in the case of urethrography or bronchography. All topical anesthetics carry some hazard. When adverse reactions occur to such patients, in about 98 per cent of the cases they are caused by toxic blood plasma levels having been attained; in about 2 per cent of the cases there is an allergic or psychogenic response. In using topical anesthetic agents, one must know the safe maximum topical dose and carefully check the concentration of the particular solution being employed. One should use as dilute a solution as is practical and ordinarily one should wait several minutes before adding more anesthetic to a previous application. Among the topical agents, it is noteworthy that Dyclonine is effective in 0.5 to 1 per cent solutions with a maximum tolerable dose of 500 mg. (100 cc. of the 0.5 per cent or 50 cc. of the 1 per cent solution). With any of these agents one may obtain either central nervous system stimulation or depression with apnea, coma, hypotension or cardiac arrest. When central nervous system stimulation is observed, the anesthetic drug should be immediately discontinued, oxygen applied by mask, and a short-acting barbiturate injected by the physician. When depression is observed, the airway should be established, oxygen applied, a vasopressor agent utilized and cardiac compression used if indicated.

A special emergency cart or tray should include all the drugs indicated for use in an adverse reaction, plus any of the equipment needed for the use of these various elements, including a cut-down

tray, tracheostomy tray, electrocardiographic equipment and defibrillator. An emergency cart designed by Dr. W. C. Talley and used at the University of Arkansas Department of Radiology is shown in Figure 10-38B.

Weigen and Thomas have designed an emergency kit in a single box with a drug and dosage chart prominently displayed on the cover. A photograph of the box is shown in Figure 10-38A. The emergency equipment recommended by them is as follows:

1. Oxygen tank and mask, pharyngeal airways.
2. Aramine, 1 cc. ampules (10 mg.) and 10 cc. ampules (100 mg.).
3. Adrenalin chloride, 1/1000 aqueous, 1 cc. ampules.
4. Aminophylline, 10 cc. ampules (25 mg./cc.).
5. Benadryl, 10 cc. ampules (10 mg./cc.).
6. Solu-Cortef, 100 mg. (2 cc. Mix-O-Vial).
7. Nembutal sodium, 5 cc. ampules (25 mg./cc.).
8. Aromatic ammonia, crushable vials.
9. Amyl nitrite, crushable vials.
10. Demerol, 2 cc. ampules (50 mg./cc.).
11. Syringes: 2, 5, and 20 cc.; 1 and 4 inch needles of various sizes.
12. Tubing adapters.
13. 30 cc. physiologic sterile saline.
14. 500 cc. physiologic saline and venocylsis set.
15. Sphygmomanometer and stethoscope.
16. Padded tongue depressor.
17. Instruction card, with type of reaction, drug to be used, and dosage recommended.
18. Suture kit, including scalpel.
19. Tourniquet.
20. Tracheotomy set.

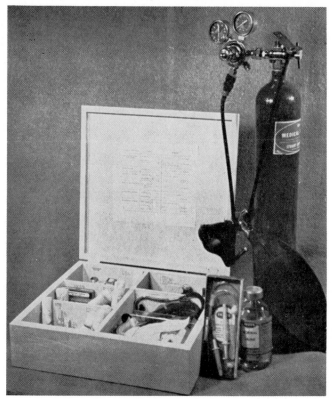

A

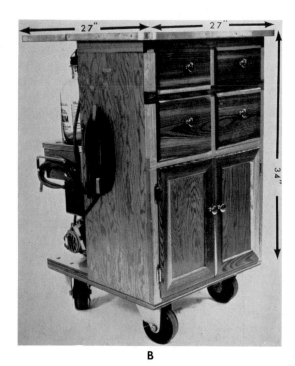

B

FIGURE 10-38. **A,** View of box containing drugs and accessories, with dosage chart on the cover, as well as emergency equipment for the treatment of reactions to intravenous medications. (From Weigen, J. F., and Thomas, S. F.: Radiology *71*:24, 1958.) **B,** Emergency cart designed by Dr. W. C. Talley and used at the University of Arkansas Department of Radiology. The drawers are compartmented as needed, and the contents of each drawer and door are labeled for quick reference. There is a suction motor on the back powered by 110 volts. The top of the cart is hinged to allow easy access to the suction and oxygen apparatus contained at the rear. The four drawers contain drugs; needles; airways and masks; and syringes, towels and sponges. Behind the doors are such items as a cut-down tray, a sphygmomanometer, a stethoscope and solutions. (From Barnhard, F., and Barnhard, H.: Radiol. Clin. N. A. *3*:61, 1965)

SUMMARY COMMENTS REGARDING SPECIALIZED CARDIOVASCULAR INVESTIGATIONS

There are a few fundamental principles which deserve emphasis:

1. As a general rule, it is important to obtain radiographs with as short an exposure as is consistent with dense opacification and highest possible detail. For best results, three-phase generator equipment with high output will give best results, along with selective catheterization of the blood vessel of primary concern.

2. There are a number of satisfactory film changers and automatic injectors available commercially. Whichever is chosen, it is extremely important that familiarity with design be achieved, since frequent and careful maintenance is necessary for good predictable results. Cineradiography and video-tape recording generally do not offer quite as good detail as direct filming, but with electronic improvements, it is conceivable that video tape recording may become the method of choice, particularly if a good kinescopic method of obtaining film records from the videoscreen are also developed.

3. It is essential that flow-rate curves be known for different sizes and lengths of catheters, and these curves should be attached to the pressure injector for ready reference if the pressure injector is of a type that can not be set to deliver a specific number of milliliters per second automatically. Ordinarily, the entire bolus necessary for an arterial region should be delivered within one to one and one-half seconds. It is probable, however, that even more important than the pressure setting are the position of the catheter tip and the proper choice of volume and type of contrast agent.

4. Needles used for arterial puncture must be kept meticulously sharp and clean, to avoid tearing the artery and other complications.

5. The catheter must be carefully prepared for use and cleaned after the examination is completed. Hydrogen peroxide, followed by flushing with distilled water, and the 0.1 per cent Detergicide solution may be used if the catheter is to be used again. The catheter should be flushed with isotonic, sterile saline before use. It is best also, before using it, to fit the catheter with a two-way stopcock, so that it can at all times be flushed with saline while in use.

6. Cardiac or aortic angiography should be undertaken only with a cardiac monitor in use during the examination and with a suitable defibrillator at hand.

7. Image amplification and video-monitor control for fluoroscopy is highly desirable. This will improve the accuracy of the examination, diminish exposure to the patient and enhance the team effort.

8. Every attention should be paid to diminishing exposure of all personnel during radiography. Monitoring devices should be worn at all times, and accurate records kept. If hand injection is used, this should be done only behind an appropriate lead screen. Lead protective aprons should be worn by personnel at all times, and exposure to the direct x-ray beam avoided completely.

9. To minimize the hazard of blood clots, 20 mg. of heparin should be added per liter of irrigating saline.

10. After the catheter or needle is withdrawn, one must continue to apply pressure over the puncture site for 5 to 10 minutes, then diminish the pressure slowly over the next 15 minutes, carefully observing the puncture site continually, and keeping the anatomic part at rest.

11. Immediately before withdrawal of a catheter or needle (or cannula), a small volume of 0.5 to 1 per cent procaine is injected, when the tip is proximal to the site of entry. This tends to minimize local spasm and is particularly important with extremity artery puncture.

12. The pulse should be carefully monitored after withdrawal of pressure over the needle puncture site. If the pulse does not

return in about 15 minutes, the possibility of thrombosis requiring surgical intervention should be considered.

13. Hospitalization for at least 24 hours after catheterization should be routine.

14. Direct major vessel arterial puncture should ordinarily be carried out only if pulsations are palpable to avoid trauma to an already diseased artery.

15. Intra-arterial injections are ordinarily made in a retrograde rather than antegrade manner, in order to avoid laminar flow and less satisfactory visualization.

16. Circulation in the upper extremity is somewhat more rapid than the lower, and serial film studies are more desirable than scan type exposures or single film studies. Films should be obtained at about two per second for two to four seconds, and then one per second for the next four to six seconds. This will allow demonstration of veins as well as arteries. The most appropriate timing for serial exposure of the lower extremity may be initially determined by isotopic records of circulation over the knee and foot, following injection in the upper femoral artery.

17. Where pulsations are palpable only in either the upper or lower artery, the palpable one is catheterized, and the catheter tip is manipulated *via* the aortic arch. When attempting axillary injection *via* the femoral artery route, it is best to inject the aortic arch to determine the status of major vessels arising from it.

18. If a good pulse is palpable in one femoral artery, but not in the other, the catheter or cannula may be introduced on the good side, and the antegrade flow of the contrast agent down the affected side studied by injection on the good side, or at the bifurcation of the aorta. A pressure cuff around the thigh of the good side below the level of the introduction of the catheter will materially assist the flow of the contrast agent toward the affected side.

19. The period of catheter examination should not, if possible, exceed approximately one hour, to avoid spasm and thrombosis. If significant spasm is encountered, the procedure should be abandoned after injection of 5 cc. of 1 per cent procaine into the affected artery.

20. Arch aortography is performed in the right posterior oblique projection of about 30 degrees, in order to obtain maximum visualization of the arch and its branches. The catheter tip is placed in position about midway between the aortic valves and the origin of the right innominate artery to avoid a large bolus (35 ml.) of contrast agent entering the brain in a short time (one to one and one half seconds).

21. In renal angiography, the three phases of the investigation include: aortography above the level of renal arteries, which will determine the presence of supernumerary arteries and renal artery stenosis at its aortic junction; selective renal arteriography circulation in all of its arterial, capillary and venous phases by rapid serial angiography; and pyelography, as indicated.

Because the origin of the renal arteries is at an angle (usually anteriorly) to the aorta, posterior oblique projections may be necessary to show the renal orifice clearly.

22. Phentolamine (Regitine) should be available for instant use when renal arteriograms are obtained in patients with hypertension—particularly paroxysmal hypertension—to avoid a hypertensive crisis in the presence of a pheochromocytoma. The inferior adrenal artery arising from the renal artery, when injected, may produce this.

GLOSSARY

Ab-: prefix meaning "away from."
Abdomen: that portion of the body which lies between the thorax and pelvis.
Abduct: to lift away from.
Abscess: a localized collection of pus.
Acetabulum: the cavity in which the head of the femur rests.
Achilles tendon: the thick tendon at the back of the heel.
Adnexae: adjacent parts (of an organ).
Aerated: air-containing.
Air embolism: the presence of an air bubble in a blood vessel.
Alar: pertaining to a process resembling a wing.
Albuminuria: the presence of albumin in the urine.
Alignment: arrangement in a straight line.
Allergic reaction: hypersensitivity reaction.
Alveolus: tooth socket; air sac of the lungs.
Amphiarthrodial joint: one that permits little movement, such as the intervertebral disc between two vertebral bodies (fibrocartilage between bones).
Anastomose: to communicate with (especially arteries and veins); to join together surgically.

Angiocardiography: the radiographic study of the heart and blood vessels.

Angiography: a radiographic study of the blood vessels after the injection of contrast media.

Angiology: a study of blood vessels.

Anode: the positive pole of a source of electricity.

Anomalous: irregular or unusual.

Anomaly: that which deviates from the normal.

Anteflexion: a bending forward.

Antegrade: in the direction of the natural flow; forward flow.

Antepartum: before birth.

Anterior: situated toward the front.

Antero-: prefix meaning "before" or "toward the front."

Anthropoid: having the form of man.

Antrum: a cavity within bone, especially in relation to the maxillary sinus.

Anus: the opening through which fecal material is expressed.

Aortography: investigation of the aorta by injection of a contrast medium and radiography.

Apical: toward the apex.

Apnea: temporary stopping of respiration.

Apophyseal joints: joints between the superior and inferior articulating processes of vertebrae. These are synovial joints.

Appendage: a part that is added.

Arachnoid: a delicate membrane applied closely to the brain.

Arborization: a branching (of bronchi or vessels).

Areola: a small space in tissues; the dark area surrounding the nipple.

Arteriogram: a radiograph of an artery after injection of contrast material.

Arthro-: pertaining to a joint.

Articulation: a joint between bones.

Ascites: excess fluid in the abdominal cavity.

Atresia: closure or absence of a normal opening.

Axial: directed from base to vertex or vice versa; also, pertaining to the spinal axis of the
body.

Axilla: the armpit.

Azygography: the radiographic study of the azygos vein after injection of contrast material.

Bacilluria: the presence of bacteria in the urine.

Balsa wood block: a wooden support used in radiology. This block readily permits the
penetration of x-rays, since it is so very light in weight and low in density.

Basal (basilar): the lowermost part (in radiology, especially, refers to the skull or lung).

Bi-: prefix indicating "two" or "twice."

Bifurcation: a division into two branches.

Bilateral: having two sides; referring to both sides.

Biopsy: removal of a portion of tissue for microscopic study.

Bolus: a term applied to the portion of material that is swallowed at one time.

Breech (birth): a birth in which the fetus presents with the buttocks instead of the head (normal presentation).

Bronchography: the radiographic study of the bronchi after instillation of opaque contrast media.

Bronchus: one of the two main branches of the trachea.

Bruit: a murmur that is heard by listening through the stethoscope.

Bursa: a cavity containing a thin layer of fluid placed so that friction is prevented and extending between muscles or arising from joints.

Buttocks: the prominent group of muscles at the base of the spine upon which one sits.

Cadaver: the nonliving body.

Calcaneus: the bone that forms the prominence of the heel.

Calcareous: containing calcium.

Calcification: the process by which calcium becomes deposited in a tissue.

Calcium: a silver-white metallic chemical element found in a chalk-like deposit opaque to x-rays, always in combination.

Calculus: a stone, as in the kidney.

Calvarium: the skull above its base.

Cannula: a tube for insertion into the body.

Canthus: the angle at either end of the slit between the eyelids.

Capitate (bone): a small bone of the wrist, lying between the trapezoid and hamate bones.

Capsule: a thick membrane that incloses joints; a portion of the brain or kidney.

Cardi-: pertaining to the heart (prefix).

Cardia: the upper portion of the stomach.

Cardiac: pertaining to the heart.

Cardiovascular: pertaining to the heart and blood vessels.

Cataract: an opacity of the lens of the eye.

Cathartic: medication that produces evacuation of bowel contents.

Catheter: a thin tube that drains fluid from a body cavity; also used for injection purposes.

Caudad: toward the feet.

Caudal: toward the "tail" end of the body.

Cephalad: toward the head.

Cephalic (presentation): head presentation of the fetus.

Chole-: prefix indicating relationship to bile or the biliary tract.

Cholecystectomy: removal of the gallbladder.

Chromosome: that portion of the cell nucleus which contains the genes.

Cineradiography: motion radiographs, rapidly obtained and projected.

Cirrhosis: a disease of the liver.

Cistern: a reservoir or open space.

Clavicle: the "collar bone" of the shoulder.

Coccyx: the small series of bones at the base of the spine.

Collateral circulation: a secondary or accessory circulation.

Collimate: to bring into a straight line; to make parallel.

Collimation: the making parallel of light or rays.

Colostomy: an operation that connects the large intestine with the exterior.

Coma: a state of loss of consciousness.

Commissure: that which joins adjacent parts together.

Concave: a curve directed inward.

Condyle: a rounded bony protrusion near a joint.

Confluent: flowing together to form one.

Congenital: descriptive term for a condition present at or before birth.

Conjunctiva: the outer membrane of the eye.

Contiguous: in close contact.

Contrast material: an opaque medium used to outline an anatomical part that is normally radiolucent.

Conventional: conforming to usual standards.

Convex: a curve directed outward.

Coronal: pertaining to the crown of the head; the plane of body from side to side in the direction of the coronal suture.

Costo-: prefix denoting relationship to a rib.

Costovertebral joint: the joint between the rib head and the vertebra.

Cranial: relating to the skull; toward the skull.

Cranio-: prefix indicating relationship to the skull.

Cuboid (bone): a small bone of the foot, lying between the calcaneus and the fourth and fifth metatarsal bones.

Cuneiform (bone): a small bone of the proximal segment of the foot.

Cusp: a portion of a heart valve; an elevation on the chewing surface of a tooth.

Cutaneous: pertaining to the skin.

Cyanosis: blue discoloration of the skin.

Cyst: a membranous sac that contains liquid, air, or semisolid material.

Cystitis: inflammation of the urinary bladder.

Cystogram: a radiographic study of the urinary bladder using contrast medium.

Cystourethrogram: a radiographic study of the urinary bladder and urethra using contrast material.

Decubitus: lying down. (The x-ray beam is always directed horizontally with "decubitus" studies.)

Defibrillation: to stop fibrillary motions of the heart and restore normal rhythm.

Delineate: to make an outline of or describe.

Demi-: prefix indicating half.

Dens epistrophei: a process of the second cervical vertebra; synonym of "odontoid process."

Dentin: the midportion of the tooth (between the pulp and the enamel or cementum).

Derma-: relating to the skin.

Diapositive: a positive image obtained from the regular x-ray film. The latter is actually a
    negative.
Diarthrodial: a term applied to a joint that moves freely in any direction and is lined by
    synovial membrane.
Diastole: the stage of dilatation of the heart.
Diploë: the layer of spongy bone lying between the two bony tables of the skull.
Distal: toward the far end.
Distortion: twisting out of a normal state or position.
Diuretic: a drug that promotes the flow of urine.
Diverticulitis: inflammation of a diverticulum or outpouching from the intestine.
Dorsal: pertaining to the back.
Duct: a passage with clearly defined walls, particularly for secretions or excretions.
Dynamic: pertaining to force; or to movement of elements or organs within the body.
Dyspnea: difficulty with breathing.
Dysuria: difficulty with passing of urine.

-ectomy: suffix meaning "removal of" (e.g., a cholecystectomy or removal of the gallbladder).
Ectopic: out of the normal place.
Ectopic beats: extra heart beats that occur out of sequence.
Edema: an abnormal accumulation of fluid in the cavities or tissues of the body.
Effusion: the escape of fluid into a space.
Electrocardiogram: a specialized study of the conduction mechanism of the heart.
Electron: an extremely small electrically charged particle that determines the physical and
    chemical properties of the atom; found in the orbits of the atom and sometimes in the
    nucleus.
Embolism: the blockage of an artery or vein by a clot brought by the bloodstream.
Embryo: the fetus in its earlier stages of development, prior to the third month.
Emissary (vein): leading out from inside the skull to the scalp.
Emphysema: the abnormal presence of air in tissues; increased air trapped in the lungs with
    ruptured interalveolar septae.
Enamel: the outer surface of the tooth.
Endo-: prefix meaning "inside of."
Enema: a liquid injected into the rectum and colon to cleanse, provide nourishment, or
    outline that organ with a contrast material.
Ependyma: the lining of the ventricles of the brain and innermost central canal of the spinal
    cord.
Epicondyle: a small bony protrusion near a joint, usually above a condyle.
Epilation: the removal of hair.
Epiphysis: portion of bone that, in early life, is separated by a thin layer of cartilage from the
    layer of adjacent bone, but later fuses with the main mass of the bone.
Erythema: redness (of the skin).

Erythroblastosis fetalis: a blood disorder of late fetal or neonatal life.
Esophagram: a radiograph of the esophagus using contrast material.
Eversion: a turning outward.
Ex-: prefix meaning "out of."
Exhalation: breathing out.
Extra-: prefix meaning "outside of."
Extravasation: escape from a blood vessel of its contents.
Exudate: material that has escaped from blood vessels as a response of body cells to irritation or inflammation.

Facet: a small flat surface, as on a bone. In vertebrae, these are the superior and inferior articulating surfaces on processes of the neural arch.
Falx: a thick layer of dura that divides the two hemispheres of the brain.
Fascia: a sheath of tissue surrounding individual muscles.
Feces: that which is discharged from the bowel.
Femur: the bone of the thigh.
Fetus: the child in the uterus, named thus after the third month.
Fibula: the smaller of the two bones of the lower leg.
Filament: a delicate wire-like structure.
Fimbria: a structure resembling a finger or fingers (applied especially to the end of the oviduct).
Fistula: a narrow abnormal canal between two organs or leading from the surface to the interior of the body.
Flexor hallucis longus: the long flexor muscle of the big toe.
Fluorescence: a luminescent property shown by some materials when irradiated.
Foramen: a perforation or hole, especially into or through a bone.
Foramen transversaria: a small foramen in the transverse process of the cervical vertebra through which the vertebral artery passes.
Fossa: a depression, especially in a bone.
Frontal poles: the two anterior poles of the brain deep to the frontal bone.
Fulcrum: the point of support around which a lever turns.

Ganglion: a group of nerve cells.
Gangrene: death of cells when blood supply is obstructed and the tissue undergoes decay.
Gastric: pertaining to the stomach.
Gastrocnemius: a muscle of the calf of the leg.
Gibbus: an acute posterior angulation of the spine.
Glomus: a small conglomeration of cavernous blood vessels.
Gluteal cleft: the line of cleavage between the buttocks.
Gluteal region: the area of the buttocks.

Gonads: the organs of reproduction; the ovaries and testes.

-graphy: suffix that when used with the name of a specific part of the body, may mean radio-graphic demonstration of that part (e.g., cystography, or demonstration of the bladder).

Gravitate: to move in accordance with the force of gravity.

Gyneco-: pertaining to women.

Gyrus: a fold (of the brain).

Hamate (bone): a small bone of the wrist, lying in the middle of the distal row of carpal bones.

Haustrum: a recess produced by one of the sacculations of the colon.

Hemodynamic: pertaining to the flow and forces of blood movement.

Heparin: a substance that prevents blood from clotting.

Herniation: the escape of an organ or part of an organ through an abnormal opening.

Hiatus: an opening.

Hilus: a depression or pit in an organ through which vessels and nerves enter and leave.

Hormone: a chemical compound produced by an organ, which produces its effects in another portion of the body after transmission via the bloodstream.

Humerus: the bone of the upper arm.

Hydration: the state of being combined with water.

Hyper-: a prefix meaning "overabundant" or "excessive."

Hyperemia: excess of blood in any part of the body.

Hypertension: elevated blood pressure.

Hypertonic: showing excessive tension, osmotic pressure, or activity.

Hypo-: a prefix meaning "under," or "low."

Hypoglycemic: having a deficiency of sugar in the blood.

Hypospadias: a defect on the under surface of the penis.

Hypotension: blood pressure lower than normal.

Hysterosalpingography: the roentgenographic study of the uterus and fallopian tubes after the injection of a contrast medium into the uterine cavity.

Ileus: obstruction of the intestine, either mechanical or reflex.

Iliac crest: the upper and outer margin of the bony pelvis.

Impacted: firmly lodged in position.

Increment: an increase.

Inert: without action.

Infarct: an area of necrosis of tissue due to blocking of the blood supply.

Inferior: lower than.

Infusion: the introduction of a fluid into a vein or tissues.

Inguinal ligament: a fibrous band extending from the ileum to the pubic spine.

Inguinal region: the region of the groin.

Inhalation: breathing in.

Innocuous: harmless.

Inorganic: having no living origin.

Instill: to put in drop by drop or gradually.

Insufflation: to blow a powder or air into a body cavity.

Intercostal: situated between the ribs.

Interosseous membrane: a membrane that connects the two major bones of forearm and leg.

Intra-: prefix meaning "inside of."

Intussusception: the invagination of one portion of the intestine inside another.

Inversion: the reversal of a normal relationship of a part.

Ion: an atom with a positive or negative electrical charge.

Ionization: the separation of a substance into its constituent ions.

Ischium: a portion of the bony pelvis.

Isotonic (solutions): solutions that are equal in osmotic pressure (usually designating a salt solution that, when injected into the blood, will not injure red blood cells).

-itis: suffix meaning "inflammation of" (e.g., mastoiditis, inflammation of the mastoid bone).

Jaundice: yellow discoloration of the skin due to the deposition of bile pigments.

Kinescope: an instrument that records photographically in motion pictures the images appearing on a television screen.

KUB: abbreviation for kidney, ureter, bladder.

KUB film: a film of kidney, ureter and urinary bladder.

Kymograph: an instrument for measuring the fine movements of an organ or part.

Kymography: a specialized radiographic procedure (see text).

Kyphosis: an acute curvature of the spine with the convexity directed backwards.

Laminectomy: removal of a spinal lamina.

Laryngogram: a radiograph of the larynx.

Lateral: pertaining to the side.

Lesion: any change in the appearance or function of an organ or tissue.

Leukemia: cancer of the white blood cells with uncontrolled production of white blood cells.

Ligament: a fibrous band that connects bones or organs.

Linear: pertaining to a line.

Lipoid: resembling fat.

Lipoma: a tumor of fatty tissue

Lordosis (lordotic): curvature of the spine in a forward direction.

-lucent: suffix referring to the ability of the x-rays to penetrate.

Lumen: the cavity within a tube or hollow organ.

Lymphadenopathy: pathology of the lymph nodes.

Lymphangiography: a radiographic study of lymphatics after the injection of contrast material.

Lymphatics: vessels that transport lymph.

Magnification: enlargement.

Malalignment: poor alignment.

Malleolus: the prominence on either side of the ankle, produced by the distal ends of the tibia and fibula.

Mammary gland: breast.

Mammography: radiography of the breast.

Matrix: the ground substance of an organ.

Meatus: an opening.

Medial: toward the midline of the body.

Medulla: bone marrow; the terminal portion of the brain; the inner portion of an organ.

Membrane: a thin layer of tissue.

Meninges: lining membranes around the brain or spinal cord.

Meningocele: protrusion of the meninges of brain or spinal cord through a defect in the skull or vertebral column.

Meniscus (of the knee): a cartilage within the knee.

Metacarpal bone: one of the small bones of the hand, lying between the wrist and the fingers.

Metastasis: the spread of disease from one organ to another without a direct connection.

Metatarsal (bone): one of the small bones of the foot, lying between the tarsus and the toes.

Modification: a slight change.

Molecule: the smallest particle of matter which retains the properties of that matter.

Monitor: to watch over.

Mucus: the secretion of the mucus glands.

Multangular bone: one of the small bones of wrist, in the distal row of carpal bones.

Mutation: a change in form or quality of an offspring from its parents.

Myelography: the radiographic examination of the spine and spinal cord after the injection of contrast material into the spinal canal (subarachnoid space).

Navicular (bone): a small bone of the wrist (in the proximal row of carpal bones) or ankle (between the talus and the three cuneiform bones).

Necrosis: death of a localized portion of tissue.

Neoplasm: an new or abnormal tissue formation, either benign or malignant.

Nephro-: relating to the kidney.

Neural: pertaining to a nerve.

Neurological: pertaining to the nervous system.

Nomogram: a chart on which annotations are made for statistical purposes; a chart to facilitate the representation of related values or numbers.

Nulliparous: an adjective describing a woman who has not borne a child.

Oblique (view): a slanted view, not directly frontal or lateral.

Obturator: a disc or plate that closes an opening; a foramen in the pelvis between the pubis and ischium.

Occipital poles: the two posterior poles of the brain deep to the occipital bone.

Occlude: to close, shut or block (of a passage).

Occlusal (film): film that is placed in the mouth between the teeth.

Occlusive disease: disease that follows the blockage of arteries or veins.

Odontoid: resembling a tooth. In the second cervical vertebra, this is a process that extends upward and acts as an axis for rotation of the first cervical vertebra.

-ography: suffix that, when used with the name of a specific part of the body, may mean radiographic demonstration of that part (e.g., cystography, or demonstration of the bladder).

-ology: (suffix) pertaining to a science or branch of knowledge.

Opacification: the act of making opaque.

Opacify: to make opaque by means of contrast material

Opaque: not permitting x-rays to pass through.

Operative cholangiogram: a radiograph after the injection of contrast material into the biliary tree at the time of operation.

Orbit: the bony socket containing the eyeball.

Organic: pertaining to living organisms, or any constituent part thereof; also pertaining to an organ or organ system.

Ortho-: prefix meaning "normal" or "straight."

Orthodiagraph: an apparatus for tracing the exact size of an organ, especially the heart.

Orthodiagraphy: a specialized radiographic procedure (see text).

Ossicle: a small bone.

Ossification: the formation of bone.

Ossify: to change to bone.

Osteo-: prefix indicating relationship to bone.

Palpable: perceptible to touch.

Para: prefix meaning "beside" or "adjoining."

Paraplegia: paralysis of the legs and lower part of the body.

Paraspinous: alongside the spine.

Parenchyma: the functioning portion of an organ.

Parietal: concerning the walls of a cavity; one of the bones of the cranium and lobes of the brain.

Pars interarticularis: portion of the neural arch of a vertebra which is situated between the superior and inferior articular processes.

Patella: "knee cap."

Patent: unobstructed; open.

Pathology: the study of disease.

Pedicle: one of two bases that connect the body of a vertebra with the lamina; the stalk of a protruding tumor.

Pelvimetry: the measurement of the size and capacity of the pelvis.

Pelvis: the bony framework of the lower trunk.

Penumbra: a secondary shadow.

Per-: prefix indicating "through."

Percutaneous: performed through the skin.

Peri-: prefix meaning "around."

Periosteum: the membrane that covers bone.

Peripheral: toward the outer side or edge.

Peristalsis: intrinsic movement of the gastrointestinal tract.

Peritoneum: the thin membrane lining the abdominal cavity.

Perivascular: around a blood vessel.

Peroneus longus: the long peroneal muscle of the leg and foot.

Phalanx: any bone of a finger or toe.

Pharynx: a space at the rear of the mouth common to both alimentary and respiratory tracts.

Phlebitis: inflammation of a vein.

Phlebo-: prefix meaning "pertaining to veins."

Phonation: the act of speaking.

Phosphor: a substance that luminesces when exposed to light or radiation.

Pineal gland: a small structure usually seen in the midline position of the brain in the posterior part of the third ventricle, frequently calcified in the adult.

Pinna: the cartilage of the ear.

Pisiform (bone): a small bone of the wrist, the medial bone of the proximal row of carpal bones.

Placenta praevia: a placenta situated close to the internal os of the uterus.

Placentography: radiography of the placenta.

Pleura: the lining membrane around the lung.

Pleural reflection: a change in the direction of the pleura.

Plexus: a network (usually of nerves or veins).

Pneumoarthrography: radiographic study of a joint after the injection of air into it for diagnostic purposes.

Pneumoencephalography: the radiographic study of the brain following the injection of air into the ventricles via the subarachnoid space surrounding the spinal cord.

Pneumo-: prefix indicating "air"; pertaining to the lung.

Pneumogram: a radiograph utilizing air as a contrast agent.

Pneumothorax: air within the thoracic cavity.

Poly-: prefix meaning "many."

Polyp: a pedunculated growth.

Portal (circulation): the passage of the venous blood from the spleen and alimentary canal through the liver and thence via the hepatic veins.

Posterior: situated toward the back.

Postero-: prefix meaning "behind" or "toward the back."

Pro-: prefix meaning "toward the front."
Process: a projecting point (of bone).
Projection: a view of a part of the body.
Pronate: to turn the palm of the hand down; to place in or assume a prone position.
Prone: lying with the face aspect down.
Psychogenic: originating in the mind.
Pulmonary: pertaining to the lung.
Pyelography: radiographic study of the renal pelvis and calyces.

Quadrant: one-quarter of a space or area, as of the abdomen.
Quantum: a unit whereby energy is measured.

Racemose: resembling a bunch of grapes.
Radicle: a small branch of a vessel or nerve.
Radiculitis: inflammation of the root of a spinal nerve.
Radioisotopes: two elements, chemically identical but physically different (isotopes), which
     have been made radioactive.
Radiopaque: x-rays are unable to penetrate; these substances appear white on ordinary x-ray
     films.
Radius: one of the bones of the forearm.
Ramification: a branching.
Ramify: to develop branches.
Ramus: a branch (of an artery); a portion of the pubic bone or mandible.
Rectum: the lower portion of the large intestine just proximal to the *anal canal,* which
     opens to the exterior.
Recumbent: lying down.
Redundant: more than necessary.
Resuscitation: the restoration to life or consciousness of one apparently dead.
Retro-: prefix indicating "behind," or "back of."
Retrograde: directed against the natural flow.
Retrograde aortography: a radiographic study of the aorta after injection of contrast material
     by catheter against the blood flow.
Retroperitoneal: behind the peritoneum.
Ruga: a ridge or fold.

Sacrum: the curved bone that forms the posterior boundary of the bony pelvis and the lower
     end of the spine.
Sagittal: from front to back (i.e., plane of the sagittal suture of the skull).
Sclerosis: an increase in the density of bone; eburnation.
Scoliosis: curvature of the spine.

Septum: a division.

Sequela(ae): that which follows.

Serial: in a series.

Sesamoid bone: a small bone of the hand or foot, found embedded in tendons or joint capsules.

Shunt: an abnormal communication, usually representing a shortened path.

Sialography: the radiographic examination of a salivary gland or duct after the injection of a contrast material.

Silhouette: an outline shadow.

Sinus: a hollow space; a dilated channel for venous blood; an air cavity within the bones of the skull; a tract that drains fluid from a part of the body.

Spasm: a sudden, severe, involuntary muscular contraction.

Sphincter: a ring of muscle that encircles a body orifice.

Sphygmomanometer: an instrument designed to measure blood pressure.

Spleno-: prefix indicating relationship to the spleen.

Spondylolisthesis: a slipping forward of one vertebral body over another, due to a defect in the neural arch of the slipped segment.

Sputum: the material from the throat and respiratory passages that is ejected from the mouth and that may be representative of disease of a portion of the respiratory tract.

Stasis: a cessation of flow, as of blood or other body fluid.

Static: at rest; standing.

Stereoscopic: combining several views to give a three dimensional appearance when viewed through a special instrument.

Sternum: the bone at the anterior aspect of the thorax; the "breast bone."

Stethoscope: an instrument designed to enable the physician to listen to sounds within the body.

Stridor: noisy respiration.

Sub-: prefix meaning "beneath."

Subarachnoid space: a space deep to the arachnoid membrane and continuous over the brain and spinal cord.

Subcutaneous: beneath the skin.

Subluxation: dislocation.

Sulcus: a groove, as of the brain.

Super-: prefix meaning "over," "above," "on top of."

Superimposition: the placing of one thing on top of another.

Superior: higher than.

Supernumerary: an excessive number of.

Supinate: to turn the palm of the hand upward; to place in or assume a supine position.

Supine: lying on the back.

Suture: the line of junction of two adjacent bones in the skull; also, a surgical tie or "stitch."

Symmetrical: equally distributed or arranged on two sides.

Symphysis: the line of fusion between two bones.

Synovial: a term applied to a joint lined by synovial membrane, which secretes fluid.

Synovial joint: a joint lined by synovial membrane, which secretes fluid (synovia).
Systemic: affecting the body as a whole.
Systole: the stage of contraction of the heart.

Tachycardia: excessively rapid heart action.
Talus: a bone of the ankle that articulates with the tibia and fibula.
Teleroentgenogram: a radiograph taken with a long distance between the x-ray tube and the
     film (usually 6 or more feet).
Temporal: pertaining to the temporal bone or lobe of the brain.
Tentorium: a layer of dura that separates the cerebellum from the hemispheres of the brain.
Thrombophlebitis: the development of a clot within the interior of an inflamed vein.
Thrombosis: the blockage of a blood vessel owing to clot formation.
Tibia: the larger of the two bones of the lower leg.
Tonsil: lymphatic tissue at the entrance of the pharynx; a small protuberance of an organ.
Topical: local.
Topical anesthetic: an anesthetic that is applied locally, rather than inhaled.
Tourniquet: an instrument designed to arrest the circulation (usually a piece of rubber tubing
     that is tied around a limb).
Toxicity: the quality or degree of being poisonous.
Tracheostomy: a surgical opening in the trachea connected with the exterior.
Transosseous venography: radiographic investigation of the veins after injecting the opaque
     medium into bones.
Transudate: a thin fluid that has passed through a membrane; sometimes a response of body
     cells to inflammation.
Trauma: injury by external force.
Tri-: prefix indicating "three."
Trigone: a triangular area, usually in relation to the urinary bladder, where the two ureters
     enter the bladder and the urethra exits from it.
Trimester: a three month period.
Trocar: an instrument with a sharp point used in conjunction with a cannula.
Tubercle: a protuberance of bone.
Tumor: an abnormal growth of tissue.
Turbulence: disturbance, agitation.

Ulcer: a break in the surface of an organ.
Ulna: a bone of the forearm.
Ulnar: pertaining to the ulna.
Unilateral: involving one side.
Urethra: the canal that connects the bladder to the surface.
Urethrography: the radiographic study of the urethra using a contrast material.

Urethroscope: an instrument to visualize the urethra.
Urography: radiography of any part of the urinary tract.
Urticaria: a skin eruption characterized by wheals.
Uvula: a small fleshy mass suspended from the soft palate.

Valve: a fold that prevents the flow of the contents of a channel from reversing.
Varices: enlarged and tortuous veins.
Varix: an enlarged, tortuous vein.
Vascular: pertaining to blood vessels; containing many blood vessels.
Venogram: a radiograph of a vein obtained after injection of contrast material.
Venography: investigation of the veins by injection and radiography.
Ventral: pertaining to the front aspects, as compared with the back (which is dorsal).
Ventricle: a cavity, referring especially to the brain or heart.
Ventricles (of brain): a series of intercommunicating cavities.
Ventriculography: radiographic study of the ventricles after the injection of contrast media.
Vertebra: one of the 33 bones of the spinal column.
Video-: prefix indicating relationship to television.
Viscous (fluid): sticky or slow to move.
Visualize: to make visible.
Volar: pertaining to the palm of the hand or the sole of the foot.

Ane, J. N.: Roentgen pelvimetry. New Orleans Med. Surg. J. *98*:497–502, 1946.

Ball, R. P., and Golden, R.: Roentgenographic obstetrical pelvicephalometry in the erect posture. Amer. J. Roentgenol. *49*:731–741, 1943.

Bauer, G.: Roentgenological and clinical study of sequels of thrombosis. Acta chir. scandinav. (Supp. 61) *86*:1, 1942.

Benson, R. C., Dotter, C. T., and Straube, K. R.: Percutaneous transfemoral aortography in gynecology and obstetrics. Amer. J. Obstet. Gynec. *85*:772–791, 1963.

Bjork, V. O., Cullhed, I., Hallen, A., Lodin, H., and Malers, E.: Sequelae of left ventricular puncture with angiocardiography. Circulation *24*:204–212, 1961.

Bowman, J. M., and Friesen, R. F.: Multiple intraperitoneal transfusions of the fetus for erythroblastosis fetalis. New Eng. J. Med. *271*:703–707, 1964.

Caldwell, W. E., and Moloy, H. C.: Anatomical variations in the female pelvis and their effect in labor with a suggested classification. Amer. J. Obstet. Gynec. *26*:479–503, 1933.

Camp, J. D., and Coventry, M. B.: Use of special views in roentgenography of the knee joint. U.S. Nav. Med. Bull. *42*:56–58, 1944.

Clark, K. C.: Positioning in Radiography. London, Ilford Ltd. William Heinemann Medical Books, 1964.

Chassard and Lapiné: Étude radiographique de l'arcade pubienne chez la femme enciente; une nuovele méthode d'appreciation du diamètre bi-ischiatique. J. Radiol. Electrol. *7*:113–124, 1923.

Chausse, C.: Suggestions for the radio-diagnosis of fractures of the labyrinth. Medico-legal importance. Brit. J. Radiol. *12*:536–546, 1939.

Chausse, C.: Trois incidences pour l'examen du rocher. Acta Radiol. *34*:274–287, 1950.

Colcher, A. E., and Sussman, W.: Changing concepts of x-ray pelvimetry. Amer. J. Obstet. Gynec. *57*:510, 1949.

Cournand, A., Baldwin, J. S., and Himmalstein, A.: Cardiac Catheterization in Congenital Heart Disease. New York, The Commonwealth Fund, 1949.

Curry, J. L., and Howland, W. J.: Arteriography, Principles and Techniques. Philadelphia, W. B. Saunders Company, 1966.

Des Plantes, B. G. Z.: Subtraktion Technique. Stuttgart, Georg Thieme Verlag, 1961.

Dexter, L., Haynes, F. W., Burwell, C. S., Eppinger, E. C., Seibel, R. E., and Evans, J. M.: Studies of congenital heart diseases: Technique of venous catheterization as a diagnostic procedure. J. Clin. Invest. *26*: 547–553, 1947.

Duggin, E. R., and Taylor, W. W.: Fetal transfusion in utero. Report of a case. Obstet. Gynec. *24*:12–14, 1964.

Epstein, B. S., Wasch, M. G., Lowe, L. L.: An evaluation of phlebography of the lower extremity. Amer. J. Roentgenol. *60*:650–657, 1948.

Etter, L. E.: Roentgenography and Roentgenology of the Middle Ear and Mastoid Process. Springfield, Charles C Thomas, 1965.

Etter, L. E., and Cross, L. C.: Projection angle variations required to demonstrate the middle ear, antrum, and mastoid process. Radiology *80*:255–257, 1963.

Feist, J. H., and Mankin, H. J.: The tarsus. 1. Basic relationships and motions in the adult and definition of optimal recumbent oblique projections. Radiology *79*:250–263, 1962.

Graham, E. A., and Cole, W. H.: Roentgenologic examination of the gallbladder. J.A.M.A. *82*:613–614, 1924.

Grashey, R.: Atlas Typischer Röntgenbilder von Normales Menschen *in* Lehmann's Medizinische Helanen, Vol. 5, 2nd edition, 1912.

Haas, L.: Verfahren zur Sagittalen Aufnahme der Sellagegend. Fortschr. Röntgenstrahlen *36*:1198–1204, 1927.

Haase: Charite Annalen, *2*:686, 1875, as cited in Williams, J. W.: Obstetrics, 8th edition by Henricus J. Slander. New York, Appleton-Century-Crofts, 1941, p. 155.

Helander, C. G., and Lindbom, A.: Venography of the inferior vena cava. Acta Radiol. *52*:257–268, 1959.

Kite, J. H.: Principles involved in the treatment of congenital club foot. J. Bone Joint Surg. *21*:595–606, 1939.

Kite, J. H.: The Clubfoot. New York, Grune and Stratton, Inc., 1964.

Kjellberg, S. R., Mannheimer, E., Rudhe, U., and Jonsson, B.: Diagnosis of Congenital Heart Disease. 2nd edition. Chicago, Year Book Medical Publishers, 1959, pp. 108–114.

Law, F. M.: Nasal accessory sinuses. Ann. Roentgen. *15*:32–51, and 53–76, 1933.

Lawrence, W. S.: A method of obtaining an accurate lateral roentgenogram of the shoulder joints. Amer. J. Roentgenol. *5*:193–194, 1918.

Liley, A. W.: Intrauterine transfusion of foetus in haemolytic disease. Brit. Med. J. *2*:1107–1109, 1963.

Lockhart, J., Gorlero, A. A., and Pollero, H. J.: Cavography in cases of testis tumors. J. Urol. *83*:438–444, 1960.

Lorenz: Die Rontgenographische Darstellung des Subskapularen Raumes und des Schenkelhalses im Querschnigt. Fortschr. Geb. Roentgenstrahlen *25*:342–343, 1917–1918.

Lund, R. R., Garcia, N. A., III, Le Blanc, G. A., Gartenlaub, C., and Richardson, J. F.: Inferior vena cavography in preoperative localization of pheochromocytoma. J. Urol. *83*:768–773, 1960.

Lusted, L. B., and Keats, T. E.: Atlas of Roentgenographic Measurement, 2nd edition. Chicago, Year Book Medical Publishers, 1967.

Mannheimer, E.: On the clinical diagnosis in congenital heart disease. Acta Paediat. *36*:671–679, 1947.

Mayer, E. G.: The technic of roentgenologic examination of the temporal bone. Radiology *7*:306–317, 1926. (Also see Owen, G. R.: A simplified method of producing the axial view of Mayer in chronic mastoiditis and antecholesteatoma. Amer. J. Roentgenol. *57*:260–263, 1947.

Meese, T.: Die Dorso-ventrale aufnahme der sacroiliacal-gelenke. Fortschr. Geb. Roentgenstrahlen *85*:601–603, 1956.

Merrill, V.: Atlas of Roentgenographic Positions, 3rd edition. St. Louis, C. V. Mosby Company, 1967.

Meschan, I., and Meschan, R.: Atlas of Normal Radiographic Anatomy. Philadelphia, W. B. Saunders Company, 1959.

Mokrohisky, J. F., Paul, R. E., Lin, P. M., and Stauffer, H. M.: The diagnostic importance of normal variants in deep cerebral phlebography, with special emphasis on the true and false "venous angles of the brain" and evaluation of venous angle measurements. Radiology, *67*:34–47, 1956.

Oldendorf, W. H.: A modified subtraction technique for extreme enhancement of angiographic detail. Neurology *15*:366–370, 1965.

Paulin, S., and Varnauskas, E.: Selective transseptal angiocardiography. Acta Radiol. *57*:3–10, 1962.

Pfeiffer, R. L.: Localization of intraocular foreign bodies with the contact lens. Amer. J. Roentgenol. *44*:558–563, 1940.

Pfeiffer, R. L.: Localization of intraocular foreign bodies by means of the contact lens. Arch. Ophthalmol. *32*:261–266, 1944.

Queenan, J. T.: Multiple intrauterine transfusion for erythroblastosis fetalis. J.A.M.A. *191*:943–945, 1965.

Roberts, D., Dotter, C., and Steinberg, I.: The superior vena cava and innominate veins. Amer. J. Roentgenol. *66*:341–352, 1951.

Ross, R. S.: Clinical applications of coronary arteriography. Circulation *27*:107–112, 1963.

Schobinger, R. A.: Intra-osseous Venography. New York, Grune and Stratton, 1960.

Schobinger, R. A., Cooper, P., Rousselot, L. M.: Observations on the systemic venous collateral circulation in portal hyperextension and other morbid states within the thorax. Ann. Surg. *150*:188, 1959.

Seldinger, S. I.: Catheter replacement of the needle in percutaneous arteriography. A new technique. Acta Radiol. *39*:368–376, 1953.

Selman, J.: Skull Radiography. Springfield, Charles C Thomas, 1966.

Shopfner, C. E.: Genitography in intersexual states. Radiology *82*:664–674, 1964.

Snow, W.: Roentgenology in Obstetrics and Gynecology. Springfield, Charles C Thomas, 1952.

Sones, F. M., Jr., and Shirey, E. K.: Cine coronary arteriography. Mod. Conc. Cardiov. Disease *31*:735–738, 1962.

Starkloff, G. B., Bricker, E. M., McDonald, J. J., and Litzow, L. T.: Proximal femoral venography. Ann. Surg. *131*:413–417, 1947.

Sweet, W. M.: Improved apparatus for localizing foreign bodies in the eyeball by the roentgen rays. Trans. Amer. Ophthal. Soc. *12*:320–329, 1909–1911.

Taveras, J. M., and Wood, E. H.: Diagnostic Neuroradiology. Baltimore, Williams & Wilkins, 1964.

Templeton, A. W., and Zim, I. D.: The carpal tunnel view. Missouri Med. *61*:443–444, 1964.

Templeton, F. E., and Addington, E. A.: Roentgenographic examination of the colon using drainage and negative pressure. J.A.M.A. *145*:702–704, 1951.

Ter-Pogossian, M. M.: The Physical Aspects of Diagnostic Radiology. New York, Harper and Row, 1967.

Thoms, H.: Pelvimetry. New York, Paul B. Hoeber, Inc., 1956.

Towne, E. B.: Erosion of the petrous bone by acoustic nerve tumor; demonstration by roentgen ray. Arch. Otolaryng. *4*:515–519, 1926.

Weigen, J. F., and Thomas, S. F.: Reactions to intravenous organic iodine compounds and their immediate treatment. Radiology *71*:24, 1958.

Wilson, M.: The Anatomical Foundation of Neuroradiology of the Brain. Boston, Little, Brown and Company, 1963.

Wood, E. H.: Special techniques of value in the cardiac catheterization laboratory. Proc. Mayo Clin. *28*:58–64, 1953.

INDEX

In this index, *italic* page numbers indicate illustrations;
roman page numbers refer to text.